T0275606

When considering influences on psychological ill health and mental illness, personal relationships are generally conceived to play an important role. It is therefore perhaps surprising that, despite much research in this area, there is so little evidence available from intervention studies to guide management practices. This second volume in a series looking at the social dimensions of mental illness, collates and critically examines the information currently available on social support as it affects mental health.

The international team of contributors, each actively involved in both clinical and research work in this field, collectively cover the whole range of perspectives from biological mechanisms through to psychological and social theory. An overview of the latest published evidence and a description of the nature and origins of social support is followed by evidence from observational studies and specific interventions and trials. The text concludes with a summary which will act as a valuable resource to practitioners in their evaluation of social and psychological treatments and should also serve to stimulate further research and intervention trials.

Practitioners and researchers in psychiatry, psychology and social work are certain to welcome this timely guide.

Social Support and Psychiatric Disorder

STUDIES IN SOCIAL AND COMMUNITY PSYCHIATRY

Volumes in this series examine the social dimensions of mental illness as they affect diagnosis and management, and address a range of fundamental issues in the development of community-based mental health services.

Series editor
PETER J. TYRER
Professor of Community Psychiatry, St Mary's Hospital Medical School, London

Already published:
IAN R. H. FALLOON AND GRÁINNE FADDEN: Integrated mental health care: A comprehensive community-based approach

Social Support and Psychiatric Disorder

Research findings and guidelines
for clinical practice

edited by
T. S. BRUGHA

Department of Psychiatry, University of Leicester

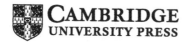

CAMBRIDGE
UNIVERSITY PRESS

CAMBRIDGE UNIVERSITY PRESS
Cambridge, New York, Melbourne, Madrid, Cape Town, Singapore, São Paulo

Cambridge University Press
The Edinburgh Building, Cambridge CB2 8RU, UK

Published in the United States of America by Cambridge University Press, New York

www.cambridge.org
Information on this title: www.cambridge.org/9780521442381

© Cambridge University Press 1995

This publication is in copyright. Subject to statutory exception
and to the provisions of relevant collective licensing agreements,
no reproduction of any part may take place without the written
permission of Cambridge University Press.

First published 1995
This digitally printed version 2007

A catalogue record for this publication is available from the British Library

Library of Congress Cataloguing in Publication data

Social support and psychiatric disorder: research findings and guidelines for
clinical practice / edited by T. S. Brugha.
    p.   cm. – (Studies in social and community psychiatry)
Includes index.
ISBN 0 521 44238 9 hardback
1. Social adjustment.   2. Mentally ill – Social networks.   3. Social networks –
Therapeutic use.   I. Brugha, T. S. (Traolach, S.)   II. Series.
[DNLM: 1. Social Support.   2. Mental Disorders – therapy.
WM 140 S678 1995]
RC455.4.S67S65   1995
616.89–dc20
DNLM/DLC
for Library of Congress   94–48028 CIP

ISBN 978-0-521-44238-1 hardback
ISBN 978-0-521-03805-8 paperback

Contents

Preface

The concept of social support is central to the thinking of many clinicians dealing with psychiatric patients. Patients, relatives and friends also attach great importance to the positive aspects and the problems of social relationships in relation to health maintenance. Therefore, it is surprising that there is very little evidence available from intervention studies upon which to base management decisions. But given this widespread feeling that personal relationships are of such importance, it seems timely to ask a group of workers who themselves have a background in clinical practice, particularly in psychiatry, psychology and the social sciences, and who have conducted empirical research in this area, to express their views about the implications for clinical practice of their own work and of related work.

It is hoped that these contributions can achieve two aims. First, that fellow practitioners who have read this book will approach the psychosocial aspects of the care of their clients or patients with a greater knowledge and understanding of what is known of the highly complex processes that are involved. At the very least it is hoped that this will result in a modest, cautious and questioning approach. Second, it is hoped that this collection will stimulate a much-needed expansion in formal clinical evaluation. Existing psychosocial intervention methods should be evaluated, whilst taking account of their effects on relationship variables. Also, it is hoped that well-designed clinical trials will be more forthcoming. Finally, it is hoped that in some way the necessary resources for such studies will be more readily available.

The book is laid out in four parts. Following an introductory overview of the latest published evidence on social support and psychiatric disorder, the first part of the book deals with the nature and origins of social support. Developmental and social psychology, evolutionary and biological mechanisms and structural, social network mechanisms are discussed. These contributions are largely original and will interest not only practitioners but also the academic and scientific community. The second part of the book deals with evidence from observational studies, this being the most substantial part of the scientific literature. All three chapters in this section give prominence to the fact that social relationships in themselves can have both positive and negative effects, depending on a variety of intervening factors including gender, age, individual attributes and the nature of network linkages. The third part of the book deals with a number of contributions on specific interventions and clinical trials and the lessons that can be gained from these. It is hoped that these contributions will help stimulate others to do further work of that kind. The book ends with two chapters designed to draw together what lessons can be learnt and how best to make use of them in day-to-day clinical practice. Included is a discussion of some well-evaluated psychosocial methods of intervention – family, marital and interpersonal – which may be highly relevant to the topic of social support. The busy practitioner may wish to begin with this section of the book and then choose which other aspects of the volume he or she is most likely to gain from studying in detail.

The aims of this book are intended to be modest. We hope to have dispelled some myths without erecting too many new ones to replace them. We hope to stimulate a fundamentally important field of enquiry at a time when, perhaps, it has become less fashionable but, we believe, in some ways more objective in its approaches. We do not in any way wish to challenge or question the value of biological approaches to the understanding of mental disorders and their treatment. Rather, we wish to emphasise instead the importance of interactions between individuals and their environments, in a way that good biology, psychology and social science always has. We have not set out to eschew the use of any particular fashion or form of terminology or language, in the belief that interdisciplinary communication will be best fostered by the wider acceptance of a more precise use of existing terminology, rather than by factional attempts at its replacement, which rarely gain universal acceptance. Thus we hope that this interdisciplinary approach will result in more patients *and* clients benefiting from more varied combinations of carefully chosen social, psychological and physical interventions, which are more critically evaluated and more effectively delivered in what it is hoped will be a more therapeutic relationship.

Traolach S. Brugha

Contributors

TRINE ANSTORP
Department of Psychiatry, Ullevål Hospital, Avd.A, Kirkeveien 166,
N-0407 Oslo 4, Norway

BRYANNE BARNETT
Paediatric Mental Health Service, 13 Elizabeth Street, Liverpool
NSW 2170, Australia

KIRSTEN BENUM
Department of Psychiatry, Ullevål Hospital, Avd.A, Kirkeveien 166,
N-0407, Oslo 4, Norway

WILLIAM R. BREAKEY
Department of Psychiatry and Behavioral Sciences, Johns Hopkins
Medical Institutions, Baltimore, MD 21287, USA

CHRIS R. BREWIN
MRC Social and Community Psychiatry Unit, Institute of Psychiatry,
De Crespigny Park, London SE5 8AF, UK

TRAOLACH S. BRUGHA
Department of Psychiatry, Clinical Sciences Building, Leicester Royal
Infirmary, PO Box 65, Leicester LE2 7LX, UK

LORNA CHAMPION
Department of Clinical Psychology, Philips House, University College
London, Gower Street, London WC1E 6BT, UK

ODD STEFFEN DALGARD
Department of Psychiatry, Ullevål Hospital, Avd.A, Kirkeveien 166,
N-0407 Oslo 4, Norway

PAUL GILBERT
Mental Health Unit, Masson House Pastures Hospital, Mickleover,
Derby, DE3 5SQ, UK

DEIRDRE KIRKE
Department of Sociology, St Patrick's College, Maynooth, Co. Kildare, Ireland

LIZ KUIPERS
Institute of Psychiatry, De Crespigny Park, London SE5 8AF, UK

CAMILLE LLOYD
Student Counselling Service, University of Texas Health Sciences Center, 7000 Fanin Suite 1600, Houston, Texas, USA

PATRICK McC. MILLER
Alcohol Research Group, University of Edinburgh, Royal Endinburgh Hospital, Morningside Terrace, Edinburgh EH10 5HF, UK

GORDON PARKER
Paediatric Mental Health Service, 13 Elizabeth Street, Liverpool NSW 2170, Australia

GLENYS PARRY
Sheffield Health Authority, Argyll House, 9 Williamson Road, Sheffield S1 9AR, UK

ANNELLE B. PRIMM
Community Psychiatry Program, Johns Hopkin's Medical Institutions, Baltimore, MD 21287, USA

TOM SØRENSEN
Department of Psychiatry, Ullevål Hospital, Avd.A, Kirkeveien 166, N-0407 Oslo 4, Norway

GRAHAM THORNICROFT
Institute of Psychiatry, De Crespigny Park, London SE5 8AF, UK

HANS O. F. VEIEL
Forensic Psychiatric Institute, Port Coquitlam, British Columbia, Canada V3C 5X9

1

Social support and psychiatric disorder: overview of evidence

TRAOLACH S. BRUGHA

Background

There is growing evidence that social support is important for physical and psychological health as well as for survival (House *et al.*, 1988). Unfortunately there have been few experimental studies and hardly any randomised controlled clinical trials to evaluate the effects on illness or survival of enhancing personal social support networks, or of enhancing the ability of such individuals to recruit support more effectively. Therefore, the need for a critical, experimental and evaluative approach to the topic and for a deeper understanding of the technical difficulties involved in doing so needs to be emphasised at this time.

A considerable diversity of research measures and designs have been used to study support–illness associations, making the use of more formal methods for evaluating the current published evidence largely impractical. The reviewer must also be aware of the possibility of biases introduced by the publishing process, which may tend to favour positive findings over 'non-significant' ones. Nonetheless, in this introductory chapter, emphasis will be given also to negative studies, many of which may reveal useful lessons for future researchers, and which may be of interest also to practitioners working with clients and patients.

The chapter begins by tracing the origins of the idea of social support within medicine and public health or social medicine. The theoretical background to the subject will then be explored in relation to the psychology and social sciences literature and then in relation to biological models that may also explain underlying mechanisms linking social behaviour and emotional and other states of arousal. Recent behavioural genetics studies that may add significant weight to evidence for the importance of both environmental and genetic components will be discussed. The nature of psychiatric disorder will be discussed briefly, particularly for the benefit of readers who are relatively new to the subject. A discussion of methodological issues will precede a consideration of a selection of the empirical literature, with particular emphasis on more recent prospective and experimental studies of the relationship between support and psychiatric disorder. A final discussion will focus on issues relevant to clinical practice and will point to the last chapter in this book, which deals in depth with that topic (Brugha, 1995).

A brief history of support

It could be argued that the concept of social support has no identifiable beginning in the sense that, rather like parenthood, it has always been there and its importance has always been taken for granted. Recent empirical work confirms the intuitive importance of social relationships to people's life goals (Lam & Power, 1991). The fifteenth-century Oxford vicar, Robert Burton, in his lengthy treatise *Melancholia* (Burton, 1621), quoted from a number of classical writers. On the value of the attention of friends, Plutarch was said to have written: 'if it be wisely administered it easeth grief and pain'; and Tully: 'I am much eased when I read thy letters'; and the physician Galen: 'many have been cured by good counsel and persuasion alone'.

In our own century, the concept of social support has developed within a number of different disciplines and different theoretical frameworks. Within psychiatry, early ideas on attachment theory, as exemplified in the writings of Bowlby (1969, 1977), also referred to in the chapters by Brewin and by Champion in this volume, emphasised the importance of early social relationships, particularly with one parent, in a developmental perspective. Similarly, in the biological field, secure attachment behaviour was shown to be damaged experimentally by extreme separation experiences in the early weeks of life (Harlow, 1960), which had long-term effects into adulthood. Ethological studies in the wild suggested a similar paradigm for what appeared to be an animal model of clinical depression due to separation in non-human primates, as illustrated in the work of Goodall (1973).

The *public health* concept of support was centred upon a network of community-based sources of medical, social and welfare assistance, which were to be organised around community mental health centres (CMHCs). The President's Commission on Mental Health (1978) in the United States promoted a policy to foster natural support systems in the wider community. However, empirical research on social support has focused almost exclusively on the emotional and perhaps more subtle, qualitative aspects of personal social support, particularly in relation to depressive disorders (Brugha, 1988a). Two pioneering review papers by Cobb (1976) and by Cassel (1976) emphasised the importance of the nature of information received from others about ourselves. Two other aspects of support have also dominated much writing. These have been termed instrumental (or tangible or material) and emotional (or esteem enhancing) support (Tolsdorf, 1976; Schaefer *et al.*, 1982; Lin & Dean, 1984).

Plutarch's view (quoted above) that the attention of friends 'easeth pain' has found its place in modern thinking also. The so-called *stress buffering* model of social support seems to derive some of its modern inspiration from Cassel's (1976) review of animal and human studies. He developed the hypothesis that the social environment affects host resistance both to biological noxious stimuli, such as infectious agents, and to psychological stressors. Dohrenwend & Dohrenwend (1974), similarly to Brown & Harris (1978), came to the field of social support from their pre-eminent positions in research on the relationship between adversity (stressful life events) and psychiatric disorder. Both groups were interested in finding a variable that explained why only some people exposed to adversity developed a subsequent illness. The topic has been extensively reviewed by Alloway & Bebbington (1987). Elsewhere in this volume, parallels between the development of the dual concepts of adversity and social support are historically traced in an illuminating and original way by Lloyd.

Interpersonal relationships

What kinds of social relationships provide emotional support? The importance of a single dyadic social relationship has been particularly emphasised in the earlier work of Brown & Harris (1978). This social relationship would normally be with a sexual partner and would involve closeness and confiding, in which there is trust and a free expression of feelings. This conceptualisation of support has been reconsidered in more recent work from the same group (Brown *et al.*, 1986). Other workers have emphasised the potentially considerable importance of a much wider network of close social relationships with others (Henderson, 1977; Schaefer *et al.*, 1982; Brugha, 1988*a*). This view is also closer to a sociological view of the way in which wider social structures may impinge on the important social relationships around an individual (Wellman, 1981). Thus, Mitchell (1969) defined the *social network* as a 'specific set of linkages among a defined set of persons, with the property that the characteristics of these linkages as a whole may be used to interpret the social behaviour of the persons involved'. The term 'social network' derives from the work of sociologists and social anthropologists, who chose as their unit of observation the collective links between people with *high* levels of social interaction (Mitchell, 1969). Within medicine and psychiatry the term came to be used in the fields of public health and community psychiatry (Caplan, 1974), medical sociology (Brown & Harris, 1978), psychiatric epidemiology and psychotherapy (Henderson, 1977). In this volume Kirke discusses the influence of peer support on drug-taking behaviour of teenage peer social networks, studied in a suburban community.

Social support, health outcomes and survival

In addition to mental health, general life course development (Olds *et al.*, 1988), physical health (Orth-Gomér *et al.*, 1993) and survival (House *et al.*, 1988), have been considered to be outcomes that may be predicted by levels of social support. The well-replicated finding in general population cohort studies that poor social support predicts early mortality, discussed by House and her colleagues (1988), not only adds weight to the validity of the concept of social support but gives practitioners an additional reason for devoting time and effort to helping their patients achieve a more supportive social environment. However, note should be taken of the fact that most survival studies have been conducted on male cohorts and that in certain age groups women with high social support may be at increased risk of early mortality (Shumaker & Hill, 1991). Elsewhere in this volume, Veiel explores in detail the role of gender in modifying the relationship between support and health.

Social support theory

A rich and varied theoretical literature is now available on the subject of social support (Barrera, 1986; Coyne & Downey, 1991; Brugha, 1991*a*; Henderson, 1991). A particularly accessible overview by Lloyd can be found elsewhere in this volume. In this section, psychosocial and biological aspects, emphasising some more recent contributions, will be discussed selectively on the basis of their possible value in relation to guidance on clinical and psychosocial intervention.

Social support concepts

There is general agreement amongst writers that the concept of social support is ill-defined and requires careful specification (Barrera, 1986; Thoits, 1986; Brugha, 1988*a*). Recent empirical work has tended to confirm the existence of distinct dimensions of social support that would appear to accord with the ideas of many writers. Newcomb & Chon (1989) employed data gathered from 793 individuals and derived three latent traits that satisfactorily accounted for their answers to questions about support. The first was *support type*, referring to the amount received and satisfaction with it. This dimension is probably common to all measures and, indeed, simple, self-completion questionnaires may be very satisfactory in tapping this common dimension (Sarason *et al.*, 1985), although in a therapeutic situation more detail would be required in order to identify sources of dissatisfaction. The second latent trait was accounted for by *sources* of support, such as family, friends and organisations. Social support network measures would appear appropriate for tapping this (Brugha *et al.*, 1987*a*). The third trait was that of support *functions*, which subsumed both affectively important functions such as intimate relationships and psychological and emotional distress (i.e. emotional support), and more instrumental functions (i.e. tangible support) such as finances, health, work and, perhaps of more ambivalent status, drug use (discussed in this volume by Kirke).

Thoits (1986) has conceived of support as a form of *coping assistance* in response to environmental demands on the individual (Lloyd, this volume). An interesting suggestion, perhaps of clinical usefulness (see also Gilbert, this volume), is that support is most likely to come from socially similar others, relevant to social comparison theory (Thoits, 1986) and to rank theory (Gilbert, 1992 and this volume).

Defining personal relationships

Hinde (1979) has made two important general points about personal relationships. First, it is necessary to consider not just their *behavioural* (directly observable), but also their *cognitive* and *affective* aspects [my italics]. Second, in order to understand and adequately describe human relationships it is necessary to take account of the way individuals relate over time. At a general behavioural level, relationships consist of episodes of *social interaction* over time, and the quality, content and diversity of these interactions should be taken into account. Important *cognitive factors* specific to human relationships include the nature of exchanges and rewards and how these are perceived by the participants (Hinde, 1979); the latter emphasis is particularly relevant to the theme of this volume. Recent advances in the assessment of dyadic or marital interaction using behavioural observation and sequential analysis have been considered by Hahlweg *et al.* (1984).

Psychosocial theory

Psychosocial theories relevant to our topic include cognitive aspects (Brewin, this volume), interpersonal aspects, social skills including assertion, attachment theory (Brewin, Champion, Barnett & Parker and Gilbert, this volume), social comparison, exchange and rank theory (Gilbert, this volume), social learning theory, coping and self-esteem (Lloyd, this volume) and social development (Champion, this volume). *Individual*, or personality factors, are repeatedly mentioned throughout each of these contributions and are discussed later in relation to the empirical evidence linking support to illness.

The importance of low self-esteem, which can be a trait or a temporary state interacting, with, for example, a depressive state, may be particularly relevant to our topic. This is because *rank theory* predicts that sources of affiliation and support will tend to be confined to others of similar rank (Gilbert, this volume). This may restrict the already depressed individual to engaging in interpersonal transactions with a very limited range of others of low self-esteem and low rank, who themselves may have very little scope for providing assistance.

Interpersonal theory is also of relevance to understanding how individuals who are already depressed may be less able to obtain or benefit from potentially available support because their behaviour alienates others (Coyne, 1976). Lane & Hobfoll (1992) were able to show in a correlational study carried out on 89 adults with severe chronic breathing difficulties that angry behaviour also resulted in increased anger from supporters. In a more complex study, using self and observer ratings of telephone conversations (Belsher & Costello, 1991), there was a significant tendency for *depressotypic speech* to be echoed by the other member of a dyad. Most notably it was found that depressed subjects were alone in avoiding changing the tendency of the confidant to use a particular style of speech; arguably, this would tend to promote the tendency of a partner to continue to use depressotypic speech. The relevance of this to marital and family interventions will be discussed in the final chapter of this volume. An important question to ask is whether this tendency continues when the depressive state has remitted. Work by Birtchnell and colleagues (1992) seems to indicate that the negative relating of depressed patients is very much a part of the depressive state.

Social skills and particularly *assertive behaviour* (Rakos, 1991) might be expected to be important topics because the support that an individual receives might be largely a function of the interpersonal skills he or she employs. This aspect of theory may therefore deserve more attention. Hogg & Heller (1990) found that relational competence was related to initial friendship formation in elderly community subjects. Observer and peer ratings of social skills deficits were found during an episode of depression but social skills had returned to normal again following remission from depression (Zeiss & Lewinsohn, 1988).

However, inconsistent results have emerged from research on assertiveness skills in relation to social support. In a study of individuals with spinal cord injuries (Elliott et al., 1991), it was shown that although non-assertive persons were less depressed, assertiveness and support were not highly correlated. Correlations were both positive and inverse, implying a more complex interrelationship between the two variables. Complex interactions were also found, although, apparently, these have yet to be replicated: non-assertive persons were less depressed if support levels were high, whereas persons who reported a greater willingness to be assertive in tense situations were more depressed if they reported higher levels of guidance (support from professionals). The same research group also conducted two studies among college students (Elliott & Gramling, 1990). Once again, their results were complex. For example, the expected results occurred in relation to *social integration*, with the more assertive persons who had higher levels of social integration becoming less distressed. In contrast, the rather more unusual support variable, *opportunity for nurturance*, originally proposed by Weiss (1974; see also Brugha, 1991*a*), was associated with increased levels of depression in those who were more assertive. The authors suggested that those who felt responsible for another person, which is what opportunity for nurturance taps, might also feel more *responsible* for the effects of stressors on those others.

In a study conducted in a work setting, an investigation was carried out to study whether others would respond supportively to assertive behaviour, whilst taking gender into account (Geller & Hobfoll, 1993). These investigators were concerned to examine the possibility that assertiveness may be counterproductive, leading others to provide less support. Males and females tended to respond preferentially towards others of their own gender, with ratings of similarity (i.e. similarity to one self) being somewhat more significant than ratings of a wish to be supportive towards and to evaluate more highly the other person. The authors emphasised, quite correctly, that it would be unwise to generalise these findings beyond the workplace.

An important monograph on correlational studies of assertiveness in various populations (Arrindell *et al.*, 1990) furnished very little evidence for a relationship between this and social support; in one study, it was found that in a non-clinical sample of females on a social skills training course there was an association between several support items and assertiveness. This group of researchers also reported the interesting finding that assertiveness is a subcomponent of a larger, more (statistically) coherent dimension of social *shyness*, which in turn is independent of neuroticism.

Clearly it is much too early at this stage to judge what role, if any, assertiveness skills will play, whether positive or negative, in explaining the relationship between support and disorders such as depression. Work that examines whether patients with depression and low self-esteem, and possibly also deteriorated social and occupational functioning, might show a benefit from assertion training mediated via improvements in the support they obtain from others. Until clearer evidence is forthcoming, these concepts may also aid clinical understanding.

In order to understand psychological aspects of personal relationships, considerable importance has also been attached by Hinde (1979) to *exchange theory* and interdependence theory, and to conflict and power. The latter will be covered below in the discussion of biological contributions to theory. Social comparison and exchange theory and the contribution they could make to the topic of social support have recently been the focus of particular consideration (Buunk & Hoorens, 1992). Like many others, these workers feel that a large part of the social support literature lacks a firm basis in theory. For example, social comparison theory may be used to explain the paradoxical finding that access to social support produces a deleterious effect in some individuals exposed to major stressors. When a stress implies strong emotions and embarrassing experiences or experiences that may evoke social disapproval, affiliation may aggravate the emotional impact on such individuals.

This selective discussion of psychosocial theory in relation to social support would be incomplete without at least a brief reference to *behavioural theories* and the work of Lewinsohn and his colleagues on social relationships as a fundamental source of reward and reinforcement, which others have discussed in greater detail than space permits here (however, see also: Gotlib & Hammen, 1992; Gilbert, 1992). According to this theory, a failure to obtain 'response contingent positive reinforcement' may be due to social skills deficits on the part of the subject, an environment that lacks social stimulation or a reduction in the person's capacity to enjoy positive experiences, as might occur in an episode of clinical depression. The importance of rewarding behaviours will be discussed further in relation to treatment, in the final chapter of this volume.

Measurement of support

Having considered some theoretical contributions to our knowledge of the nature of support, its assessment needs to be considered. A measure of supportive social networks should be capable of providing reliable information about some if not all of the theoretical dimensions already discussed. It should state from whom support has been obtained and therefore should gather reliable data about the social relationships that are important to the subject and in which there is some acknowledgement of closeness. Tangible and emotional support should be covered. It is also important that actual behaviour (i.e. who did or said what, when support was last needed) is distinguished from hypothetical or perceived support (i.e. who you feel you could call on when the need arises) (Brugha, 1988*b*). Negative as well as positive aspects of interpersonal transactions should be described; the former may be a more powerful predictor of symptoms in some populations (Schuster *et al.*, 1990), as well as being of particular relevance to certain kinds of effective interventions such as interpersonal psychotherapy (IPT: Klerman *et al.*, 1984).

These information-gathering requirements may only be possible to achieve reliably by setting a time limit on the social behaviour to be enquired about and by using an interview-based rather than a questionnaire-based approach (Brugha, 1988*b*). The Interview Measure of Social Relationships (IMSR), developed by this author and colleagues, was designed to achieve these aims and its reliability and validity have been tested in a number of studies (Brugha *et al.*, 1987*a*, 1990*a*, 1993). It is flexible enough to be used in a more informal or 'clinical' way.

A disadvantage of questionnaire or self-completion measures is that the items covered must be clearly understood by the respondent. Investigator-based measures allow the researcher to develop and assess his or her own conceptual models of social interaction either from data gathered at interview or from records of directly observed behaviour, which are rated by the investigator, often masked to other information about the respondent such as health status. Clearly these more costly measures cannot be employed in large-scale studies, where self-completion methods are more practical. A notable example of the investigator-based approach to measurement has been used, however, in a small general population survey focusing on a specialised group: inner city working class mothers (O'Connor & Brown, 1984). This will be discussed in the next section. A subset of the IMSR, covering self-completion items only, is being employed in large-scale national surveys in Great Britain administered by professional survey interviewers (Meltzer *et al.*, 1994).

The more specialised investigator-based assessment of attachment behaviour (West *et al.*, 1987), family emotional atmosphere (Kuipers, this volume) and marital or dyadic relationships (Hahlweg *et al.*, 1984) may also be worth considering in clinical settings. Work on interpersonal measures that does not ordinarily appear under the 'social support rubric' may be especially relevant to our topic and should not be overlooked by workers in the field. The Camberwell Family Interview (CFI: Brown & Rutter, 1966) is a clear example of this. In a study of recent-onset schizophrenia (Hahlweg *et al.*, 1989), in which the CFI was used together with other social interaction measures, ratings were also made of observed behaviours by means of a measure of positive and negative dyadic interactions (Hahlweg *et al.*, 1984), referred to above. It was found that relatives with low expressed emotion (i.e. whose behaviours and comments were rated from an audiotape interview as less critical and less emotionally overinvolved with the patient) were also actively supportive towards the patient, and provided a 'positive non-verbal climate, show[ing] concern for the patient and [trying] to find solutions to problems'. The basis of the CFI measure is discussed briefly later in this volume by Kuipers.

Measurement validity

The validity or *accuracy* of a measure, may be difficult to assess. Reporting of the supportive behaviour of close others could be distorted by attributes of the individual such as a tendency to denial, or plaintive set (a tendency to seize any opportunity to describe life in its blackest terms) (Henderson *et al.*, 1981; also discussed by Lloyd, this volume). Clearly, independent, direct observations of behaviour that incorporate rule-based ratings by the investigator of verbal content and interactional style are to be preferred (Hahlweg *et al.*, 1984; Kuipers, this volume). Goering *et al.* (1992), in an interesting study showing that married, depressed women had a poorer 6 months outcome than was predicted by their ratings of spouse support, came to the conclusion that these reports were accurate. Individual or personality variables may play an important role in this area – a subject reviewed by Monroe & Steiner (1986). A more detailed review and discussion of social support measurement issues, and a description of measures that have been tested for their reliability and validity, may be consulted by those needing further information (Brugha, 1988*b*). Further information on specific instruments is included in later sections of this chapter.

Determinants of social support

If deficits in social support influence the onset or course of psychiatric disorder, correcting such deficits requires a knowledge and understanding of their possible determinants or causes. In the discussion of psychosocial theory it was apparent that the nature of support may be mediated by a variety of, as yet, poorly understood psychological mechanisms. In this section the discussion is widened to include both antecedent factors and external factors that may influence the provision of support.

The term 'social' would seem to suggest that social networks and social support are influenced exclusively by factors in the social environment. With the possible exception of the public health and epidemiological concept of support, no other theoretical model would appear to have favoured this exclusively 'environmental supposition'. Concurrent socio-cultural factors have surprisingly little effect on levels of social support measured at a personal level (Brugha, 1991*a*), although they may have a developmental importance (see Champion, this volume).

Developmental influences

The effects of early developmental experiences on social support in adulthood are likely to be of importance. Institutional care in childhood has been shown to be related to small adult networks (Brugha *et al.*, 1990*b*) and a greater tendency to choose a sexual partner who already has significant social problems (Rutter & Quinton, 1984). Social networks appear to have considerable temporal stability (Brugha, 1984; Brugha *et al.*, 1987*a*, 1990*b*; Steinglass *et al.*, 1988) although the correlations achieved leave it to other factors to explain at least half of the variation in their size. This evidence suggests that concurrent environmental influences are no greater in their importance than are other constitutional or long-term developmental factors. However, perceived satisfaction with social support shows relatively little temporal stability and may therefore be more strongly environmentally influenced (although, as pointed out later, perceived support may be less environmental and more heritable than is available support).

Individual and social influences

Monroe & Steiner (1986) and Brewin *et al.* (1989) have reviewed studies showing effects on social support of a variety of individual or *personality factors*, such as self-esteem, sociability and locus of control. Lloyd (this volume) expands on this topic in relation to the life events literature. Effective social functioning, not surprisingly, may be another significant influence (Sarason *et al.*, 1985) but not a major one (Brugha *et al.*, 1993). Champion (1990) has recently provided some evidence of significant overlap between the *life events* and the widely used intimacy measures of Brown & Harris (1978). Two studies by the present author have shown that recent adversity explains very little variation in levels of social support (Brugha *et al.*, 1990*b*). Brugha and his colleagues (1990*b*) found no evidence for contamination of their own IMSR (Brugha *et al.*, 1987*b*), by the Brown & Harris Life Events and Difficulties Scales (LEDS: Brown & Harris, 1978), following a careful prospective investigation in a large series of hospital-treated depressives. The IMSR gathers data about the interactional characteristics of named close others in the social network, covering support, negative interaction and adequacy of interaction. The IMSR has also been shown to be largely independent of detailed measures of *social functioning* (community living skills) in a sample of long-term psychiatric patients (Brugha *et al.*, 1993). However, rare but severe forms of behavioural disturbance did seem to be significantly, although not very strongly, associated with the availability of close relationships. As mentioned above, relational competence and the mood of a confidant are important modulators. The effect of violence, including *sexual abuse*, has received surprisingly little study in relation to social support provision. However, it has been pointed out that sexually abused women expend considerable effort to prevent angering their spouses and that such efforts often compromise potentially supportive relationships with other network members (Coyne & Downey, 1991).

Influences on social support have also been experimentally tested. In an early study of 29 non-psychotic, female psychiatric inpatients (Kiecolt-Glaser & Greenberg, 1984) it was noted in a high-stress-load condition that task performance could be enhanced using the experimental provision of social support in which the active 'treatment' included the presence of a 'warm interviewer'. However, there is little evidence available from outside the rather artificial setting of the social psychology laboratory attempting to manipulate levels of social support in order to achieve health gains. Two contributors to this volume, who have conducted randomised controlled trials, had notably little success in modifying levels of social support (Barnett & Parker and Dalgard *et al.*, this volume). Randomly allocated couples (dyads) who received behavioural marital therapy, when contrasted with a waiting list condition, were found to show changes in the expected direction in their interactional patterns to the extent that they became indistinguishable from non-distressed (i.e. 'normal') couples (Hahlweg *et al.*, 1984). A number of open, non-experimental studies have provided somewhat encouraging, if less convincing, evidence that change can be achieved in the wider social network of patients. The COSTAR community outreach programme, described in this volume by Thornicroft *et al.*, produced some changes in the social networks of longer-term attenders. In a similar population, consisting mainly of long-term patients with a diagnosis of schizophrenia, Segal & Holschuh (1991) found that supportive rather than transitional, high-expectation environments contributed to the development of emotionally and instrumentally supportive social networks. Similar findings emerged in a small follow-up study of a group of day hospital service users with neurotic disorders (Sims *et al.*, 1993). At this stage it is perhaps safer to presume that producing change in social support networks may take a long time and that we do not yet appear to have a clear idea of the most effective ways of achieving this. However, a growing understanding of the possible internal and external determinants of social support, discussed here and later in the volume, should help us to achieve more effective intervention strategies.

However, some of the newest evidence for environmental influences on support provision has been provided recently by workers using behavioural genetic methods. This important topic is dealt with in the next section. According to Dunn & Plomin (1991) aspects of the environment that siblings do not share may be a very powerful source of influence, suggesting a promising line for future researchers. Personality characteristics, such as *extroversion*, which are partly inherited are also thought to be involved.

Heritability, environmentality and the determinants of social support

Bridging the apparent distance between the social and molecular poles of biology may seem improbable. But the most recent evidence for the influence of the environment on social functioning and social support has come from the field of behavioural genetics. This new line of work is likely to be viewed as controversial by at least some social scientists. But space is given to the topic as there has been little discussion of it elsewhere and readers with a broad background in medicine and biology may find this to be worthy of attention.

Behavioural genetics was founded by Francis Galton, who first introduced the use of twins in 1876, in order to assess the roles of nature (inheritance) and nurture (environment) (Plomin *et al.*, 1990). Plomin and his colleagues have recently made use of a large series of twins to study the effects of inheritance, and of the shared and non-shared environment, on certain aspects of social support (Bergeman *et al.*, 1990, 1991). The design and interpretation of studies in this area is complex and readers who are interested but unfamiliar with the underlying scientific methodology are recommended to read the major primer on this subject (Plomin *et al.*, 1990). Amongst the complicating factors is that inheritance affects not just a single individual but also genetically related individuals, who, as in the case of family members, may also be a key support source to one another. Dunn & Plomin (1991) have produced a helpful discussion of the significance of differences in sibling experience within the family, which it is to be hoped will stimulate research on developmental influences on social support.

Evidence for both environmental and significant inherited influences on social support has come from an analysis of the Swedish Adoption/Twin Study of Ageing (Bergeman *et al.*, 1990). A short version of the Interview Schedule for Social Interaction (ISSI: Henderson *et al.*, 1981; and see below), covering quantity of social relationships and perceived adequacy, was administered as part of a battery of questionnaires sent to 25 000 pairs of same-gender twins born in Sweden between 1886 and 1958. A subsample of twins aged 50 years and above consisted of reared-together and reared-apart monozygotic and dizygotic pairs (MZT, MZA, DZT and DZA, respectively). Statistical model fitting analyses took account of heredity, shared and non-shared environment and correlated environment (due to twins being reunited in later life). The results showed that 30% of the variance in perceived support and none of the variance in quantity of relationships was due to additive genetic effects (inherited). All of the remaining variance in perceived support was due to non-shared environment (physical or social experiences that differed between twin pairs). However, 27% of the variance in quantity of relationships was due to correlated environment, either due to the twin pair sharing the same environment or due to each contributing to the other's environment. Ten per cent of the variance in quantity of relationships was due to shared rearing environment and 63% was due to non-shared environment.

In further analyses of these data (Bergeman *et al.*, 1991) the association between perceived support and psychological dysfunction has been studied and is included here for convenience. A subset of 424 twin pairs, 50 years and older, was used. Bergeman and colleagues concluded that associations between adequacy of support and depression and life satisfaction involve genetic and non-shared environmental components in about equal amounts. They plan to gather follow-up data in order to extend these cross-sectional findings to prospective analyses of support and psychological outcome. Somewhat similar findings were obtained by Kessler and colleagues (1992) using a measure of perceived ('hypothetical') and received support in a study conducted on 821 sets of female (non-adopted) twins, also studied cross-sectionally and more recently prospectively. In a further report, perceived support was directly related to the onset of major depression but the genetic determinants of perceived support were not related to vulnerability to major depression (Kessler *et al.*, 1994). Numerous difficulties with the analysis and interpretation of these data make fascinating reading (Kessler *et al.*, 1992, 1994); these workers also acknowledge the advantage of the adoption twin design and data available to Bergeman and colleagues, referred to above. Future analyses are planned using data gathered by direct interview from their female twins and their parents, in order to study *intergenerational transmission* more carefully.

Further confirmation of the importance of environmental influences comes from a third twin study (Simonoff & Heath, 1989). Using questionnaire data from 2077 pairs of twins, data on spouse support was obtained, and in a small test–retest analysis was found to be reasonably stable over a 3–6 month period. No evidence for heritability could be found, when model fitting was carried out, and this surprising finding appeared to be specific for social relationships with individuals that the twins chose themselves. Kessler *et al.* (1992) found this to be true for marriage but not close friendship, where genetic influences were also important, and suggested that marriage, in contrast to close friendship, is kept 'intact' by socio-cultural constraints and laws, which would of course be exclusively environmental.

Two important caveats are required here. First, these studies were conducted using questionnaires (self-completion) measures of social support; their limitations are discussed in this chapter. Second, behavioural genetic research of this kind is still at an early, rapidly developing stage; interested readers may wish to evaluate further up-to-date reports before making any firm conclusions.

Elsewhere in the volume Gilbert provides a synthesis of biological and psychological evidence discussed in relation to attachment and rank theory. A number of thought-provoking contributions to the literature from a biological perspective have also been discussed by the author of this chapter (Brugha, 1991*b*; Brugha & Britto, 1992). Included are references to areas of general and growing interest, such as the relationship between aggression and affective disorders (van Praag, 1986), dominance acquisition, aggression and brain serotonergic functioning (Raleigh *et al.*, 1991), and the effects of anti-depressive drugs on loss induced 'depression' in non-human mammalian brains (Suomi *et al.*, 1978; Delini-Stula & Vassout, 1981). Although, at first sight, the evidence for interrelationships between group social functioning and neurobiological regulatory systems which these studies appear to reveal seem potentially exciting areas for further investigation, finding ways of studying these factors in normal and clinically depressed human beings has raised enormous technical difficulties, which cannot be considered here. However, such work does provide an important reminder of the possible underlying biological and physiological components of some of the major themes running through this volume; as will be argued in the final chapter on intervention, they also help provide a theoretical basis to the importance of emphasising to some patients that *both* physical and psychosocial treatments may be needed in order to achieve and maintain health.

Influence of symptoms

Symptoms, particularly if severe and long-standing, may also produce more lasting deficits on the provision of support by others, such as family members. Of course certain symptoms of, for example, depression, phobic anxiety or paranoid psychosis may represent specific examples of withdrawal from social contact with others. Our own attempts to study this have, however, shown that such connections, where confirmed, are not substantial in quantity (Brugha *et al.*, 1993).

To summarise, heritable and individual influences, environmental and developmental influences have all been shown to play some part, at least, in determining levels of social support assessed by means of self-completion questionnaires. Interactional and interpersonal theory, learning theory, cognitive theory and social comparison theory may all contribute to our eventual knowledge and to our understanding of the factors that determine support levels and perhaps the nature of support itself. As will be argued again in the final chapter, in the individual clinical example, the most valuable information about determinants or causes may come from a careful and systematic exploration of the person's field of close and important social relationships, of patterns of interaction, with particular emphasis on examples of negative and conflictual interaction, and on the person's appraisal of their relationships with others including causal attributions (Brewin, this volume). All of these matters may be of particular value in deciding on the use of therapies discussed in the final chapter, including, for example, cognitive behaviour therapy (Beck *et al.*, 1979), interpersonal psychotherapy (Klerman *et al.*, 1984), behavioural marital therapy (O'Leary & Beach, 1990) and family work (Kuipers & Westall, 1992; Kuipers, this volume).

The nature of psychiatric disorder

A brief note on language, terminology and 'names' may help at this point. Because of the stigma that has invariably been attached to the victims of psychiatric disorder, and in spite of the illuminating contributions of labelling theory, the naming of psychiatric disorders continues to attract some opposition. The medical historian Charles Rosenberg (1992) has succinctly seen off those who would criticise the fundamental legitimacy of attempts by psychiatrists (and nowadays their fellow colleagues) to give names to the different conditions or forms of suffering that their patients describe, with the following words: 'Criticism of the theoretical frameworks used most frequently in the past half century to explain such conditions cannot obviate the implacable reality of the conditions themselves. And such explanatory frameworks have a certain legitimacy of their own, even if they are arbitrary and perhaps ultimately inadequate'. For the researcher, such issues must be arbitrated upon if progress in quantification and the making of comparisons is to take place in a way that is reproducible. In practice, it has been possible to proceed in this way without in any way taking for granted the underlying difficulties involved. Much research on social support has been conducted using self-report checklist or questionnaire measures of the commoner *psychiatric symptoms* including anxiety, depressive and otherwise unexplained physical (psychosomatic) symptoms. Ease of use and low cost has encouraged their adoption rather than any real faith in their power to capture adequately the true nature of people's personal experiences (Coyne & Downey, 1991). The use of trained raters, applying clearly defined concepts of abnormal feelings, emotions, perceptions and forms of thinking and experience, as embodied in the Present State Examination (Wing *et al.*, 1974) is generally accepted as a major but more costly advance. A more complete overview of the instruments and measurement tools now used in psychiatric research can be found in a recent edited volume by Thompson (1988).

Social support and psychiatric disorder: the evidence

This extensive literature has been the subject of a number of detailed review and comment articles by the editor of this volume (Brugha, 1988 to 1992). In this chapter a selection of key studies, and some notable recent studies, will be covered, paying particular attention to their relevance to the topic of intervention and treatment. The final section of this chapter will provide a more general overview of current knowledge. Whilst the articles may well have been selected in a biased way, it is hoped that the balance of both 'positive' and 'negative' studies will be reassuring to the more sceptical reader. As far as possible, only reports of empirical findings that have been subject to peer referee are included. The Parts II and III of this volume should also be consulted by the interested reader.

Methodological issues

A number of methodological considerations should be taken into account by those new to this kind of evidence. Samples studied should be randomly chosen and *representative* of clearly defined populations. In practice this is often difficult to achieve; in these instances, the findings reported can only be generalised within the limitations of the sample chosen. A greater difficulty arises if the sample is not obtained randomly, because sampling bias may make generalisability impossible. For example, an otherwise very impressive, large-scale, prospective cohort study reported recently (Lewinsohn *et al.*, 1988) was conducted on 1213 adults out of 20 000 postal invitations to participate in the survey (a response rate of 6%). Studies in which initial recruitment is by personal contact interviewing by experienced and professionally trained survey interviewers can achieve 80–90% response rates – a much more satisfactory and reliable basis for such work.

A second methodological issue, mentioned earlier, centres on the use of either *self-completion measures* or *investigator-rated measures*. Similar principles apply in the area of social investigation as in clinical measurement, although the case for investigator measures may be said to be even greater in the latter example (see above for further discussion). Relatively few studies have been carried out on clinically ill psychiatric patients. Thus, the bulk of evidence on social support derives from studies of the commoner forms of psychiatric disorder (depression and non-specific non-psychotic disorders) identified in community surveys, and from studies carried out in more homogeneous groups, such as university students, using questionnaire measures of psychological dysfunction and (sometimes) depressed mood. Although of lesser relevance to a book on social support and psychiatric disorder, a selection of these general population studies must be included for completeness.

Examples of research designs include case–control (Brugha *et al.*, 1982), cross-sectional survey (Brown & Harris, 1978), prospective cohort (Brugha *et al.*, 1990*a*) and randomised controlled trials (Dalgard *et al.*, and Barnett & Parker, this volume). However, it is at the level of interpretation and inference that the most important questions of *causal logic* arise. Given the existence (in non-experimental studies) of statistical associations between psychiatric disorder and deficits in social support networks, are these due to:

1 Deficits in support leading to the initiation or poor later course of psychiatric disorder?
2 Psychiatric disorder leading to deficits in social support?
3 A combination of (1) and (2) acting over time? (A clinically useful model favoured by psychological and developmental theorists.)
4 A third variable that is associated with both giving rise to a *spurious association* between them (sometime termed a confound) and probably impossible to rule out completely without conducting a randomised controlled experiment?

In a review of the literature on social support networks in the schizophrenias, Henderson (1980) concluded that it has 'proved very difficult to know the direction of causality; whether the social variable was altered by the psychosis or its prodromata, including premorbid personality; or whether the social variable contributed appreciably to the onset, if not the course of the disease and other people's response to it'. However, as we shall see later, this 'either/or' view, though common in public health medicine and epidemiology, does not appropriately address the issues raised by more psychosocial, reciprocal and systems-based views of 'causality'. In general, psychosocial theories favour a systems model in which environmental and individual dispositions interact over time. However, as Parry (1988) has pointed out, a systems model may be extremely difficult to test except within an experimental design. Thus, it may be best to ask to what extent illness results from *and* gives rise to deficits in social support. Taking all of these difficulties and objections together, in selecting evidence to discuss here, we shall be confining ourselves almost exclusively to longitudinal and experimental studies. We begin with an important question for clinicians: Is the form or type of psychiatric disorder an important consideration?

The form or type of psychiatric disorder

The 'understandability' of symptoms or complaints greatly preoccupies researchers. Workers have attempted to examine whether it is important to make a distinction between mild, common or neurotic types of depression and the more severe or endogenous-psychotic types of depression. Billings & Moos (1984) compared newly referred cases of depression, attending psychiatric services for 1 year, diagnosed according to the Research Diagnostic Criteria of Minor and Major Depression (RDC: Spitzer *et al.*, 1978), which was a forerunner of DSM-III (American Psychiatric Association, 1980). They found no differences between these two diagnostic groups in relation to such social support variables such as number of friends, number of network contacts and quality of significant social relationships. In a replication of a pioneering study entitled 'The patient's primary group' of Henderson *et al.*, (1978), Brugha and his colleagues (1982), using the PSE (Wing *et al.*, 1974), found very similar deficiencies in the social networks of patients with neurotic depression (CATEGO N), but were unable to show as many such deficits in the patients with retarded depression (CATEGO R).

In a more recent attempt to confirm the value of such a diagnostic distinction, a larger series of depressed patients, falling into these two subtypes, was examined and *both groups* were found to be very significantly deficient in their social support networks, described by means of the IMSR (Brugha *et al.*, 1987a, b). However, when these patients were followed up approximately 4 months after first contacting the psychiatric hospital, there appeared to be a clearer association between social support and subsequent recovery in the 'neurotic' than in the 'endogenous' patients (Brugha *et al.*, 1987b). More recently, Romans & McPherson (1992) found that the social networks of bipolar patients were more impoverished the longer the illness continued, particularly if manic episodes occurred. Brugha and colleagues (1993) found the social networks of long-term psychiatric patients to be smaller than those of acute cases. However, the social networks of those with a diagnosis of schizophrenia (confirmed by the PSE) were no smaller than those of other long-term patients such as those with recurrent affective disorders. The topic of schizophrenia will be revisited in the next section. Rarer neuro-psychiatric and neuro-developmental syndromes, sometimes recognised in psychiatric practice, have largely gone unstudied; however, the important topic of Asperger syndrome (Frith, 1991) will receive some mention in the final chapter.

Further information on the relationship to rarer psychiatric symptoms, such as obsessional symptoms and acute psychotic symptoms (treated and possibly untreated), in all age, gender and socio-economic groups are hoped for from the use of a series of measures of social contacts, close relationships and perceived support that have been incorporated into linked national surveys of psychiatric morbidity in England, Wales and Scotland, mentioned earlier. Initial results of these surveys (including data on 10 108 household members in Great Britain) became available late in 1994 (Meltzer *et al.*, 1994).

Cross-sectional studies with paradoxical results

Although most cross-sectional (e.g. case–control) studies have confirmed the existence of deficiencies in support in those with psychiatric disorder (Brugha, 1991*a*) a number of somewhat unexpected findings have come from some recent studies. A not entirely surprising finding by Barrera & Garrison-Jones (1992) in a study of 94 adolescent psychiatric inpatients, was that the level of depression was lower if family and particularly father support was high; however, depression was greater when adolescents reported a greater number of support functions obtained from their peers outside the family. The authors suggested that distressed adolescents might turn to their peers as a reaction to their problems – a possible example of reverse causality. The findings reported by Kirke elsewhere in this volume, showing the transmission of drug use between the peer group members of housing estate social networks, are interesting in the light of the findings of Barrera & Garrison-Jones (1992): could it be that exposure to hazardous behaviours among such young adults is more likely to occur in the presence of pre-existing psychological distress? Also discussed in this volume, by Veiel, is an association between larger family networks and a worse clinical outcome in women only who were followed up longitudinally after discharge from psychiatric inpatient care. Prospective studies are less open than cross-sectional studies to bias due to contamination between sources of data.

Longitudinal observational studies of onset

Although evidence from studies of course and outcome in psychiatric patient services are of more direct relevance to this volume, some aetiological prospective studies should be considered. A notable study, in this regard, has been reported by Andreasson and colleagues (1987). They found that when they carried out a 15 year follow-up of 45 570 Swedish conscripts, there was little increase in the relative risk of developing *schizophrenia* in those who had reported a smaller number of friends in personal contact with them. This study would seem to suggest that the social network deficits of people with schizophrenia are entirely a result of their illness and not a primary aetiological factor. This conclusion does not allow for a shorter causal lag between social disruption and the subsequent onset of disorder. The subject of schizophrenia is taken up again below and in two other contributions to this volume by Kuipers and by Thornicroft *et al.*, concerning the course and outcome of that form of disorder.

A particularly influential, longitudinal study of the effects of social support on psychological health and *common psychiatric disorder* was carried out in the general population in Canberra, Australia, by Henderson and his colleagues (1981). Trained lay interviewers carried out initial and three follow-up interviews, over a 1 year period. The measure of psychological ill health was the self-completion General Health Questionnaire (GHQ: Goldberg, 1972) and the measure of social support, the Interview Schedule of Social Support (ISSI: Henderson *et al.*, 1981) mentioned in the earlier discussion of behavioural genetic studies. The ISSI is based on Weiss's six 'provisions of social relationships' (Weiss, 1974): attachment, social integration, opportunity for nurturance, reassurance of self-worth, reliable alliance, and obtaining guidance. A subset of the survey respondents were also administered the clinically rated Present State Examination (PSE: Wing *et al.*, 1974), but sufficient PSE data were not available for the planned risk factor analyses. The Eysenck Personality Questionnaire (EPQ: Eysenck & Eysenck, 1975) was administered, though not at the initial interview. Perceived (adequacy of) social support and adversity both accounted for significant amounts of the subsequent variance in the GHQ score. But when neuroticism was included as an additional variable in their model, the predictive effect of social support disappeared. There has been considerable debate, some of it controversial, about the use of a measure of neuroticism in predictive studies of this kind: a particularly well described study of the issues involved in differentiating stable and unstable measures of psychiatric symptoms has since emerged in re-analyses of the Canberra and other not dissimilar general population data sets (Duncan-Jones *et al.*, 1990).

Evidence that independent ratings of environmental social support, obtained from others, are related to concurrent psychological dysfunction (Repetti, 1987) and subsequent depression (Cutrona, 1989) has also emerged more recently. Cutrona found that informants' ratings of the social support available to pregnant teenagers significantly predicted later, postnatal depression symptoms. Repetti found that when all of the staff in a variety of different branch offices of a bank provided information on the supportiveness of the office social environment, symptoms were explained by the ratings of those who were still healthy and not just by those who were ill.

Brown and his colleagues (1986, and numerous other reports since) investigated social support and adversity in normal subjects who were followed up subsequently, to compare those who went on to develop an episode of *depression* with those who remained well. This study was carried out as part of a survey of inner city working class mothers, a high risk group for clinical depression. A new measure of support, the Self

Evaluation and Social Support schedule (SESS: O'Connor & Brown, 1984), was developed from their already well tried and widely adopted investigator-rated Life Events and Difficulties Scales (LEDS: Brown & Harris, 1978). The PSE was also used in this study. Only 2 of the 32 onset cases had not had a provoking agent (severe life event or difficulty arising during the intervening year) retrospectively assessed at the follow-up interview (1 year after the initial interview). The authors presented their results on social support and self-esteem for women who had experienced adversity only. Thus they did not consider in their report the question of whether lack of support itself predicts subsequent depression in its own right in women who have not experienced a major life event or difficulty. The study showed that lack of emotional support and 'being let down' in the presence of adversity were indeed related to fresh onsets of illness. The presence, at the first interview, of a close confiding social relationship bore no relationship to the subsequent development of depression a year later in women experiencing adversity. However, a particularly interesting finding was that, among the married women, confiding at first interview was significantly related to the husband later providing crisis support (measured at the second interview), which in turn was related to remaining well. Thus different but logically related kinds of social support were consistent over time.

Risk factor studies such as these should incorporate, in addition to simple (crude) analyses, further analyses involving *adjustments* that control for and examine possible confounding effects. Such a study, carried out on women only, has been reported in a series of papers from Edinburgh (Miller *et al.*, 1987, 1989). A group of 333 women in the general population were interviewed at three points over a 1 year period. This work showed that impaired social relationships predicted the onset of disorder, when self-esteem and life event stress were controlled. At the time of writing, preliminary GHQ and PSE data from a prospective cohort survey of over 500 women, during and following their first pregnancy, has showed that network size (IMSR) was not predictive of later onset of psychiatric disorder (Brugha *et al.*, 1993). However, the support given to these women at the time they became pregnant predicted a better symptomatic outcome (GHQ depression items), particularly if the pregnancy was unplanned or unwanted (a significant conditional effect: see further examples later). In future reports adjustments for neuroticism, individual and family psychiatric history are planned.

Longitudinal studies of course and outcome

The PSE has also been used in prospective research on adults (including men) who were already *clinically depressed*. A longitudinal study of 130 male and female psychiatric patients, of whom 120 were successfully followed up typically 4 months later, also appeared to show that the type of social relationships and support assessed at interview by the IMSR, which predict subsequent recovery from depression, differ according to gender and are not just limited to perceived support (Brugha *et al.*, 1990*a*). For example, living as married was related to recovery in men only, and having a larger number of close relatives and good friends was related to subsequent recovery in women only. All of these findings held when significant clinical predictors of recovery (the initial severity and duration of the episode) were controlled, using mathematical modelling techniques. In this study the correlation between neuroticism and severity at outcome did not alter the predictive power of the previously obtained social support measure. Further analyses from this study suggest that social support is related to a better outcome in those who are in a relapse as distinct from an initial, first-onset episode of depression (Brugha, 1991*c*). Both negative and positive aspects of support predicted outcome (Brugha *et al.*, 1990*a*), a finding reported in a similar-sized series of married men and women, with major depression diagnosed by means of a structured lay interview, identified in an urban community survey (McLeod *et al.*, 1992).

In a study by George *et al.* (1989), 155 middle-aged and *elderly* adults in the north-eastern United States, with a diagnosis of major depression, were followed up 6–32 months after a period of inpatient treatment. Subjective social support was significantly related to subsequent outcome and there was some evidence that this effect was greater in men than in women. Further analyses showed this association to decrease with increasing age (Blazer *et al.*, 1992).

A recent report from the World Health Organization multinational, 10-country study of the determinants of outcome of schizophrenia (Jablensky *et al.*, 1992), in which 1371 patients were followed up over a 2 year period, showed that there were fewer relapse episodes in those with greater contact with close as well as casual friends and in those who were married. But some social relationship variables were unrelated to outcome, including avoidance of the patient by their close or casual friends and the affective quality of the relationship with a spouse. Those who had no contact with close friends had the least favourable outcome, using a wide range of outcome indices of psychopathology and treatment required.

Conditional associations and independent replication of study findings

A number of the studies mentioned so far report finding conditional associations (also termed interactions) between support and outcome

(Brugha *et al.*, 1990*a*; Blazer *et al.*, 1992) – a topic which forms the basis of the contributions to this volume by Veiel and Miller. An important methodological caveat is required at this stage. The finding described above that certain support variables are related to outcome in men and that different ones are related to outcome in women (Brugha *et al.*, 1990*a*) must be *replicated* by other workers before it can be accepted. The general principle that study findings must be replicated needs to be emphasised even more firmly in relation to the reporting of such interactions. Such findings can occur due to chance; and are often difficult to replicate without very large samples and greater statistical power. Further evidence for the gender social support interactions discussed here has also been covered in a separate article that expands further on the topic (Brugha & Britto, 1992).

Negative or contradictory prospective observational studies

The possibility, not strongly favoured by its authors (Kessler *et al.*, 1992), that genetic factors may better explain the stress buffering effects of support on depression have already been discussed earlier; other potentially negative findings in prospective non-experimental studies are considered here.

A *4 year* follow-up of 352 men and women with RDC depression has been reported by Swindle and colleagues (1989). Family conflict, which had relatively high stability over the period, significantly explained the outcome variance in depression symptoms, whereas social resources, which was a less stable variable, failed to explain depression outcome. The authors concluded that the lack of association between positive aspects of personal relationships (i.e. social resources) and outcome may have been due to the changes in social resources over time, perhaps because of depression-related conflict.

Elsewhere in this volume Miller reports further data on a study conducted on medical students in Texas and Edinburgh, focusing on the effect of social relationships after taking account of levels of certain *personality characteristics*: suspiciousness, reserve and aloofness (see also Miller & Lloyd, 1991). For students with high levels of suspiciousness, reserve and aloofness, a close personal relationship actually carried a high cost, whether the relationship was gained or lost. In the same study, many effects were specific to one of the two training centres. It was noted that first-year medical students in Texas are several years older and therefore more mature than their UK counterparts. The authors discussed a number of personality characteristics that may determine the costs or benefits of close relationships in particular populations. In a further study in this volume by Veiel, possible detrimental effects of close family relationships on the outcome of an episode of major depression are discussed. If confirmed, these somewhat paradoxical findings could have important implications for social interventions in clinical practice, a topic returned to in the final chapter.

Husaini & Von Frank (1983) followed up 235 subjects from an original mixed-race, general population sample of 676, over a 6–18 month period. They found that the level of self-reported symptoms of depression at follow-up was unrelated to life events (a 52 item list) and only weakly associated with social support, as assessed at the initial interview. A general population study that was criticised above for its sampling difficulties (Lewinsohn *et al.*, 1988) also produced negative findings prospectively gathered. The same depression symptom measure was employed as in the study by Husaini & Von Frank, and the mean time lapse was 8.3 months. As commented upon earlier in relation to the longitudinal study of Brown and colleagues (1986), it may be that levels of support alter over longer periods of time and are likely to predict symptomatology significantly unless intervening factors are taken into account.

A recent report by Holahan & Moos (1991) accords with this last prediction. A general-population random sample of adults contacted by a combination of telephone and mail produced a final response rate of 84%, although the response rate in Caucasians was higher. Ninety-one per cent of these completed the full 4 year follow-up phase. Respondents returned postal check list questionnaires (but were not personally interviewed). Data gathered included stressors, depressed mood, social and personal resources (family support, self-confidence and an easy-going disposition as a single latent trait, of which family support accounted for the largest component) and coping. These data were analysed by means of a form of path analysis, based on structural equation modelling. This allowed intervening factors to be taken into account over longer periods of time. In simple (crude) correlational analyses family support (cohesion, expressiveness and conflict) was correlated with later depression. The structural equation and path modelling findings for social and personal resources, combined as a single latent trait (although not particularly strongly interrelated with each other), were that under high levels of stress, personal and social resources predict better future health (less depression) *indirectly*, through more adaptive coping strategies. Under low levels of stress, resources predict later depression more directly. The findings were essentially the same in each gender. Although these adjusted findings do not give a specific answer for family support on its own (after taking account of other variables) they do point towards an approach to intervention that emphasises the need for change in the individual *and* in others – a point taken up in the final chapter and by many other contributors to this volume.

Before concluding this first chapter, we shall now consider evidence based on experimental studies using randomised designs. Although such studies also have methodological drawbacks (Brewin & Bradley, 1989), randomisation does eliminate known and unknown sources of systematic error and bias of the kind that can interfere with the interpretation of the results of observational studies.

Experimental studies based on randomised designs

Laboratory experimental studies on normal volunteers have shown reduced anxiety (Bowers & Gesten, 1986) and enhanced performance at a problem-solving task (Sarason & Sarason, 1986) following a series of supportive statements, and reduced perceived stressfulness of a laboratory task (Lakey & Heller, 1988) when completed in the presence of a friend. However, it is difficult to evaluate the clinical significance of these laboratory studies, together with the extensive literature on non-clinical forms of psychological dysfunction, which have not been discussed here.

Experimental studies in the field have focused almost exclusively on *non-clinical* populations (those not referred to or attending services for people with recognised psychological problems). Although clinical/ treated populations are of prime interest in this volume, much has now been learnt from the work about to be described, and in the final chapter some lessons from the same literature will be suggested for consideration for use in clinical populations.

Studies have been conducted by epidemiological and social psychiatrists and by community psychologists, and the work of the former group will be described first. Elsewhere in the volume, Barnett & Parker discuss the background and some additional analyses and comments on a controlled experimental intervention study on highly anxious primiparous mothers identified during a survey and previously reported in the psychiatric literature (Parker & Barnett, 1987). The experimental treatment consisted of either lay or professional assistance, in the expectation that improvement in the treated mothers would be attributable to the therapeutic ingredient of social support. Social support was assessed by means of the ISSI, mentioned earlier. State and trait anxiety were measured using established scales (Spielberger et al., 1970). The intervention cases did show a significant improvement, in contrast to the controls. But there was no evidence that this was due to a change in the reported levels of social support. Similarly, in this volume Dalgard and his colleagues in Oslo used a population screen to identify a group of socially isolated middle-aged women at high risk of minor psychiatric morbidity, and commenced a long-term intervention experiment based on 'network stimulation' on this subgroup (see also Dalgard et al., 1986; Benum et al., 1987). Members of the randomly allocated experimental treatment group ($n = 50$) were invited to take part in various community-based group activities. This work showed that the women's social participation and perceived quality of life improved, but that the effects on their mental health were not so clear or significant. Two subgroups could be differentiated in retrospect: one much more socially active and the other more passive, with the positive effects of increased participation in social activity having been apparent only in the first subgroup. The more participant women were observed to be better at 'communicating, listening and empathising', but they could not be distinguished from the less participant women with regard to the severity of their prior psychiatric symptoms. Further, longer-term outcome data are reported by Dalgard *et al.* elsewhere in this volume.

Social support orientated experimental work of *community psychologists*, working almost exclusively in North America, has received little attention outside the field of community psychology. An issue of the *American Journal of Community Psychology* (1991) has been devoted to the topic of support interventions. Most extensively reported has been a randomised controlled experiment conducted on 928 unemployed respondents in Michigan, who agreed to be randomised either to receive a job-finding information pack (control group) or to participate in eight, 3 hour group training sessions over a 2 week period, designed to prevent the development of depression and to increase re-employment levels (Price *et al.*, 1992). Analyses were based on 'intention to treat'. Although many respondents declined to participate in the interventions there was a significant beneficial effect on self-reported depression at 1, 4 and 28 months post-intervention. Explicit social support aspects of the training package were described as follows: supportive behaviours by trainers, such as expressions of empathy, validation of participants' concerns and feelings, encouragement of coping; and group exercises designed to 'provide opportunities and reinforcement of participants' supportive behaviours toward each other' (Price *et al.*, 1992). However, as debated elsewhere in this chapter and particularly in the final chapter of the volume, the intervention contained other components, rendering less certain a final inference about the treatment *specificity* of a social support effect; the other ingredients being a job search skill training component, and an emphasis within the group on the anticipation of possible setbacks or barriers to job seeking, termed 'inoculation against setbacks'. A second, but far smaller randomised study of an advocacy intervention programme for women with abusive partners produced beneficial treatment interaction effects favouring the intervention group in relation to higher levels of social support and overall quality of life, but not in relation to post-shelter abuse (Sullivan *et al.*, 1992).

Considerable attention has been devoted to an experiment that failed to produce the intended treatment effect (Heller *et al.*, 1991). Following a detailed interview at home, socially isolated elderly women were randomised and those in the treatment group received supportive, friendly telephone calls for 10 weeks. Because of its potentially useful implications for the design of 'treatments', the possible reasons for the apparent failure of this low-cost intervention to produce a treatment interaction will be discussed in the final chapter.

Two other recent experimentally evaluated intervention programmes have also focused on the support needs of carers of the elderly, a group consisting almost entirely of female relatives who have to bear a considerable part of the burden of care in the community. Professionally led support groups produced beneficial effects in psychological functioning (Toseland *et al.*, 1989); and respite care, a form of instrumental support, produced a significant reduction in subjective burden (Montgomery & Borgatta, 1989).

Overview and conclusions

Social support is a heterogeneous concept, (Cobb, 1976; Cassel, 1976). Therefore specific definitions of support must be used in research and in clinical practice to facilitate measurement reliability (Brugha *et al.*, 1987*a*). Although at first theoretical discussions of the subject were lacking, there has been a growth in useful contributions more recently (see also Part I of this volume). Psychosocial theory has been particularly fruitful, given the growing acceptance that both *individual and environmental* factors should be taken into consideration. Social network theory has not been as successful. Developmental approaches clearly deserve far greater prominence (Champion, this volume).

Amongst the psychologically or psychiatrically unwell, measurement may well be contaminated by symptoms (Brugha, 1988*b*), although to a relatively small degree. Prior levels of symptoms should be controlled (adjusted) for in prospective cohort studies, both for this reason and because of their more general predictive importance. Psychosocial and systems theory suggest, and there is some evidence for this in practice, that the relationship between support and, for example, depressive symptoms, is reciprocal. The external validation of measures of support has received little attention (Brugha, 1990) and may well be a complex issue because of the difficulties involved in interpreting the meaning of disagreement between informants. But there is now evidence from two studies adding to the predictive validity of the concept (Repetti, 1987; Cutrona, 1989).

Social networks and social support appear to be influenced by a variety of environmental and constitutional factors including inherited characteristics (Bergeman *et al.*, 1990), temperamental characteristics such as sociability (Monroe & Steiner, 1986), and ongoing developmental factors such as extreme and early social disruption and deprivation (Rutter & Quinton, 1984), as well as by such later environmental factors as 'where you work' (Repetti, 1987) and who you end up with as your 'life partner', family and friends (Rutter & Quinton, 1984; Cutrona, 1989). Compared with these factors, cultural differences appear to be of relatively minor importance (Brugha, 1988a), although their importance in relation to early development deserves to be considered (Champion, this volume).

In general, evidence for the association between social support and later clinical or psychological state (i.e. outcome) is much more firmly based in studies on those who already suffer from psychiatric disorder (McLeod *et al.*, 1992) than it is in relation to initial illness onset, particularly if one is specifying the onset of clinically significant 'diagnosable' psychiatric disorder. Further, *onset* factors may differ from factors that influence *recovery* (Goldberg *et al.*, 1990; Brugha *et al.*, 1993). Deficits in social support are associated with an increased risk of developing symptoms that can be described as psychological dysfunction or 'neurotic' (Henderson *et al.*, 1981). The stress buffering literature has been somewhat inconclusive (Alloway & Bebbington, 1987), although the importance of adversity as an initiating factor is less often disputed now. Personality factors (Brewin *et al.*, 1989) are also likely to play a significant part in the development of these disorders, although the case for this was probably overstated in earlier studies (Duncan-Jones *et al.*, 1990).

Recovery from psychiatric disorder, such as clinical depression, is significantly predicted by levels of social support assessed during illness (Brugha *et al.*, 1987b, 1990a; Jablensky *et al.*, 1992). However, there is now some experimental evidence for the social support hypothesis in groups at high risk of depression who are not clinic attenders (Price *et al.*, 1992). It is also quite possible that different aspects of support are important at different times and for different groups of people (Brugha *et al.*, 1990a, 1991b and final chapter; Miller *et al.*, 1987). Whilst perceived deficits in social support are particularly associated with a negative course and outcome, it appears that other aspects of social relationships that are not necessarily perceived as deficient have a significant influence on future levels of clinically significant symptoms (Brugha *et al.*, 1990a). Successful prediction appears to apply to shorter follow-up periods, measured in months rather than years.

In this chapter we have not focused on the *supporters* themselves, the burden they have to bear (MacCarthy, 1988), and the growing evidence that working with families living in the community produces benefits for them and for patients (Kuipers & Westall, 1992). Some aspects of this important topic are covered alsewhere in this volume by Kuipers. The role and participation of natural supporters will also be taken up in the final chapter, in discussing the design of support interventions.

A growing number of randomised controlled trials (RCT), which aim to test the social support hypothesis explicitly, have been conducted in recent times. Although these have not included samples of psychiatric patients, in many of these trials individuals at high risk of possible psychiatric disorder have been studied. Although, in general, psychological functioning and health have benefited, expected changes in social support networks have been less obvious. Much can be learnt from a detailed review of the processes involved in such studies – hence the inclusion in this volume of contributions by two groups of psychiatrists and their colleagues (Barnett & Parker, and Dalgard *et al.*) who have pioneered such work. Many other contributors also discuss influences on social support networks and on the perception of support from others. Both individual and environmental aspects may need to be modified if deficits in social support are to be reduced through active interventions.

In the final chapter on intervention, there will be a discussion of the availability of social and psychological therapies, including individual *psychotherapy*, marital therapy and family work, which may produce at least part of their beneficial effects through alterations in social support levels. This is a potentially promising growth area for research on social support which has not been covered in this initial chapter. Nevertheless, the striking lack of clinical trial data on clearly identified patients seeking psychiatric treatment is a deficit in our knowledge that remains difficult to explain and justify. This is particularly so when faced with the growing evidence that deficits in social support in those who are currently ill predict a poorer outcome, even when, as in the case of clinical depression, concurrent physical treatment has been taken into account (Brugha *et al.*, 1991*b*), and bearing in mind the high personal, social and economic costs of continuing ill health.

In the final chapter the service planning, management, evaluation and possible public health implications of our present level of knowledge will be discussed also.

References

Alloway, R. & Bebbington, P. (1987). The buffer theory of social support: a review of the literature. *Psychological Medicine*, **17**, 91–108.

American Journal of Community Psychology (1991). Support interventions issue. *American Journal of Community Psychology*, **19**, 1–167.

American Psychiatric Association. Committee on Nomenclature and Statistics. (1980). *Diagnostic and Statistical Manual of Mental Disorders*, 3rd edn, DSM-III. Washington, DC: APA.

Andreasson, S., Allbeck, P., Engstrom, A., Rydberg, U. (1987). Cannabis and schizophrenia. *Lancet*, **ii**, 1483–5.

Arrindell, W. A., Sanderman, R., Hageman, W. J. J. M., Pickersgill, M. J. & Kwee, M. G. T. (1990). Correlates of assertiveness in normal and clinical samples: a multidimensional approach. *Advances in Behavior Research and Therapy*, **12**, 153–282.

Barrera, M. (1986). Distinctions between social support concepts, measures and models. *American Journal of Community Psychology*, **14**, 413–45.

Barrera, M. & Garrison-Jones, C. (1992). Family and peer social support as specific correlates of adolescent depressive symptoms. *Journal of Abnormal Child Psychology*, **20**, 1–16.

Beck, A. T., Rush, A. J., Shaw, B. F. & Emery, G. (1979). *Cognitive Therapy of Depression*. Chichester: Wiley.

Belsher, G. & Costello, C. G. (1991). Do confidants of depressed women provide less social support than confidants of nondepressed women? *Journal of Abnormal Psychology* **100**, 516–25.

Benum, K., Anstorp, T., Dalgard, O. S. & Sørensen, T. (1987). Social network stimulation: health promotion in a high risk group of middle-aged women. *Acta Psychiatrica Scandinavica Supplement 337*, **76**, 33–41.

Bergeman, C. S., Plomin, R., Pedersen, N. L., McClearn, G. E. & Nesselroade, J. R. (1990). Genetic and environmental influences on social support: the Swedish adoption/twin study of aging. *Journal of Gerontology: Psychological Sciences*, **3**, 101–6.

Bergeman, C. S., Plomin, R., Pedersen, N. L. *et al.* (1991). Genetic mediation of the relationship between social support and psychological wellbeing. *Psychology and Ageing*, **6**, 640–6.

Billings, A. & Moos, R. H. (1984). Chronic and non-chronic unipolar depression: the differential role of environmental stressors and resources. *Journal of Nervous and Mental Disease*, **172**, 65–75.

Birtchnell, J. (1991). Negative modes of relating, marital quality and depression. *British Journal of Psychiatry*, **158**, 648–57.

Birtchnell, J., Falkowski, J. & Steffert, B. (1992). The negative relating of depressed patients: a new approach. *Journal of Affective Disorders*, **24**, 165–76.

Blazer, D., Hughes, D. C. & George, L. K. (1992). Age and impaired subjective support: predictors of depressive symptoms at one year follow-up. *Journal of Nervous and Mental Disease*, **180**, 172–8.

Bowers, C. A. & Geston, E. L. (1986). Social support as a buffer of anxiety: an experimental analogue. *American Journal of Community Psychology*, **14**, 447–51.

Bowlby, J. (1969). *Attachment and Loss, Vol. 1, Attachment*. Harmondsworth: Penguin.

Bowlby, J. (1977). The making and breaking of affectional bonds. I. Aetiology and psychopathology in the light of attachment theory. *British Journal of Psychiatry*, **130**, 201–10.

Brewin, C. R. & Bradley, C. (1989). Patient preferences and randomised clinical trials. *British Medical Journal*, **299**, 313–15.

Brewin, C. R., MacCarthy, B. & Furnham, A. (1989). Social support in the face of adversity: the role of cognitive appraisal. *Journal of Research in Personality*, **23**, 354–72.

32   T. S. BRUGHA

Brown, G. & Rutter, M. (1966). The measurement of family activities and
    relationships. *Human Relations*, **19**, 241–63.
Brown, G. W. & Harris, T. O. (1978). *Social Origins of Depression*. London:
    Tavistock.
Brown, G. W., Andrews, B., Harris, T., Adler, Z., & Bridge, L. (1986). Social
    support, self-esteem and depression. *Psychological Medicine*, **16**, 813–31.
Brugha, T. S. (1984). Personal losses and deficiencies in social networks. *Social
    Psychiatry*, **19**, 69–74.
Brugha, T. (1988a). Social support. *Current Opinion in Psychiatry*, **1**, 206–11.
Brugha, T. (1988b). Social psychiatry. In *The Instruments of Psychiatric Research*,
    ed. C. Thompson, pp. 253–70. Chichester: Wiley.
Brugha, T. (1990). Social networks and support. *Current Opinion in Psychiatry*,
    3, 264–8.
Brugha, T. S. (1991a). Support and personal relationships. In *Community
    Psychiatry: The Principles*, ed. D. H. Bennett & H. L. Freeman, pp. 115–89.
    Edinburgh: Churchill Livingstone.
Brugha, T. (1991b). A prospective study of adversity in the course of clinical
    depression. Paper presented at the Annual Scientific Meeting of the Royal
    College of Psychiatrists, Brighton, UK.
Brugha, T. S. (1993). Social support networks. In *Principles of Social Psychiatry*,
    ed. D. Bhugra & J. Leff, pp. 502–16. Oxford: Blackwell Scientific.
Brugha, T. S. & Britto, D. J. (1992). Social support, environmental and
    conditional associations. *Current Opinion in Psychiatry*, **5**, 305–8.
Brugha, T., Conroy, R., Walsh, N., Delaney, W., O'Hanlon, J., Dondero, E.,
    Daly, L. Hickey, N. & Bourke, G. (1982). Social networks, attachments
    and support in minor affective disorders: a replication. *British Journal of
    Psychiatry*, **141**, 249–55.
Brugha, T., Sturt, E., MacCarthy, B., Potter, J., Wykes, T. & Bebbington, P.
    E. (1987a). The Interview Measure of Social Relationships: the description
    and evaluation of a survey instrument for measuring personal social
    resources. *Social Psychiatry*, **22**, 123–8.
Brugha, T., Bebbington, P., MacCarthy, B., Sturt, E., Wykes, T. & Potter, J.
    (1987b). Social networks social support and the type of depressive illness.
    Acta Psychiatrica Scandinavica, **76**, 664–73.
Brugha, T. S. Wing, J. K., Brewin, C. R. MacCarthy, B., Mangen, S.,
    LeSage, A. & Mumford, J. (1988). The problems of people in long-term
    psychiatric care: an introduction to the Camberwell High Contact Survey.
    Psychological Medicine, **18**, 443–56.
Brugha, T. S., Bebbington, P. E., MacCarthy, B., Sturt, E., Wykes, T. &
    Potter, J. (1990a). Gender, social support and recovery from depressive
    disorders: a prospective clinical study. *Psychological Medicine*, **20**, 147–56.
Brugha, T. S., Sturt, E., MacCarthy, B., Wykes, T. & Bebbington, P. E.
    (1990b). The relation between life events and social support network in a
    clinically depressed cohort. *Social Psychiatry and Psychiatric Epidemiology*, **25**,
    308–13.
Brugha, T. S., Wing, J. K., Brewin, C. R., MacCarthy, B. & Lesage, A.
    (1993). The relationship of social network deficits with deficits in social
    functioning in long-term psychiatric disorders. *Social Psychiatry and Psychiatric
    Epidemiology*, **28**, 218–24.
Burton, R. (1621). *The Anatomy of Melancholy*, vol. 1. (Reissued (1932) by
    Everyman's Library, Dent, London.)

Buunk, B. P. & Hoorens, V. (1992). Social support and stress: the role of social comparison and social exchange processes. *British Journal of Clinical Psychology*, **31**, 445–57.

Caplan, G. (1974). Support systems. *Support Systems and Community Mental Health*, ed. G. Caplan. New York: Basic Books.

Cassel, J. (1976). The contribution of the social environment to host resistance. *American Journal of Epidemiology*, **104**, 107–23.

Champion, L. (1990). The relationship between social vulnerability and the occurrence of severely threatening life events. *Psychological Medicine*, **20**, 157–61.

Cobb, S. (1976). Social support as a moderator of life stress. *Psychosomatic Medicine*, **38**, 300–14.

Coyne, J. C. (1976). Toward an interactional description of depression. *Psychiatry*, **39**, 28–40.

Coyne, J. C. & Downey, G. (1991). Social factors and psychopathology: stress, social support, and coping processes. *Annual Review of Psychology*, **42**, 401–25.

Cutrona, C. E. (1989). Ratings of social support by adolescents and adult informants: degree of correspondence and prediction of depressive symptoms. *Journal of Personal and Social Psychology*, **57**, 723–30.

Dalgard, O. S., Anstoup, T., Benum, K., Sørensen, T. & Moum, T. (1986). Social psychiatric field studies in Oslo: some preliminary results. Paper read at Second International Kurt Lewin Conference, Philadelphia.

Delini-Stula, A. & Vassout, A. (1981). The effects of antidepressants on aggressiveness induced by social deprivation in mice. *Pharmacology, Biochemistry and Behaviour*, **14**, 33–41.

Dohrenwend, B. S. & Dohrenwend, B. P. (1974). Overview and prospects for research on stressful life events. ed. B. S. Dohrenwend & B. P. Dohrenwend, *Stressful Life Events: Their Nature and Effects*, New York: Wiley.

Duncan-Jones, P., Fergusson, D. M., Ormel, J. & Horwood, L. J. (1990). A model of stability and change in minor psychiatric symptoms: results from three longitudinal studies. *Psychological Medicine*, Monograph Supplement, **18**, 1–28.

Dunn, J. & Plomin, R. (1991). Why are siblings so different? The significance of differences in sibling experiences with the family. *Family Process*, **30**, 271–83.

Elliott, T. & Gramling, S. (1990). Personal assertiveness and the effects of social support among college students. *Journal of Counselling Psychology*, **37**, 427–36.

Elliott, T. R., Herrick, S. M., Patti, A. M., Witty, T. E. Godshall, F. J. et al. (1991). Assertiveness, social support, and psychological adjustment following spinal cord injury. *Behaviour Research and Therapy*, **29**, 485–93.

Eysenck, H. J. & Eysenck, S. B. G. (1975). *Manual of the Eysenck Personality Inventory*. London: Hodder and Stoughton.

Frith, U. (1991). *Autism and Asperger Syndrome*. Cambridge: Cambridge University Press.

Geller, P. A. & Hobfoll, S. E. (1993). Gender differences in preference to offer social support to assertive men and women. *Sex Roles*, **28**, 419–32.

George, L. K., Blazer, D. G., Hughes, D. C. & Fowler, N. (1989). Social support and the outcome of major depression. *British Journal of Psychiatry*, **154**, 478–85.

Gilbert, P. (1992). *Depression: The Evolution of Powerlessness*. Hove: Lawrence Erlbaum Associates.

Goering, P. N., Lance, W. J. & Freeman, S. J. J. (1992). Marital support and recovery from depression. *British Journal of Psychiatry*, **160**, 76–82.

Goldberg, D. P. (1972). *The Detection of Psychiatric Illness by Questionnaire*. Oxford: Oxford University Press.

Goldberg, D., Bridges, K., Cook, D., Evans, B. & Grayson, D. (1990). The influence of social factors on common mental disorders: destabilisation and restitution. *British Journal of Psychiatry*, **156**, 704–13.

Goodall, J. Van L. (1973). The behaviour of chimpanzees in their natural habitat. *American Journal of Psychiatry*, **130**, 1–12.

Gotlib, I. H. & Hammen, C. L. (Eds.) (1992). *Psychological Aspects of Depression: Toward a Cognitive–Interpersonal Integration*. Chichester: Wiley.

Hahlweg, K., Revenstorf, D. & Schindler, L. (1984). The effects of behavioural marital therapy on couples' communication and problem solving skills. *Journal of Consulting and Clinical Psychology*, **52**, 553–66.

Hahlweg, K., Doane, J. A., Goldstein, M. J., Nuechterlein, K. H., Magana, A. B., Mintz, J., Miklowitz, D. J. & Snyder, K. S. (1989). Expressed emotion and patient–relative interaction in families of recent onset schizophrenics. *Journal of Consulting and Clinical Psychology*, **57**, 11–8.

Harlow, H. F. (1960). Primary affectional patterns in primates. *American Journal of Orthopsychiatry*, **30**, 678–84.

Heller, K., Thompson, M. G., Vlachosweber, I., Steffen, A. M. & Trueba, P. E. (1991). Support interventions for older adults: confidante relationships, perceived family support and meaningful role activity. *American Journal of Community Psychology*, **19**, 139–46.

Henderson, A. S. (1991). Social support and depression. In *The Meaning and Measurement of Social Support*, ed. H. Veil & U. Baumann, pp. 85–92. Washington, DC: Hemisphere.

Henderson, A. S., Byrne, D. G. & Duncan-Jones, P. (1981). *Neurosis and the Social Environment*. Sydney: Sydney Academic Press.

Henderson, S. (1977). The social network, support and neurosis, *British Journal of Psychiatry*, **131**, 185–91.

Henderson, S. (1980). Personal networks and the schizophrenias. *Australian and New Zealand Journal of Psychiatry*, **14**, 255–9.

Henderson, S. (1981). Social relationships, adversity and neurosis: an analysis of prospective observations. *British Journal of Psychiatry*, **138**, 391–8.

Henderson, S. & Bostock, F. T. (1977). Coping behaviour after shipwreck. *British Journal of Psychiatry*, **131**, 13–20.

Henderson, S. Duncan-Jones, P., McAuley, H. & Ritchie, K. (1978). The patient's primary group. *British Journal of Psychiatry*, **132**, 74–86.

Henderson, S., Byrne, D. G. Duncan-Jones, P., Scott, R. & Adcock, S. (1980). Social relationships, adversity and neurosis: a study of associations in a general population sample. *British Journal of Psychiatry*, **136**, 574–83.

Henderson, S., Byrne, D. G. & Duncan-Jones, P. (1981). *Neurosis in the Social Environment*. Sydney: Academic Press.

Hinde, R. A. (1979). *Towards Understanding Relationships*. London: Academic Press.

Hogg, J. R. & Heller, K. (1990). A measure of relational competence for community-dwelling elderly. *Psychology and Ageing*, 5, 58–588.

Holahan, C. J. & Moos, R. H. (1991). Life stressors, personal and social resources, and depression: a 4-year structural model. *Journal of Abnormal Psychology*, 100, 31–8.

House, J. S., Landis, K. R. & Umberson, D. (1988). Social relationship and health. *Science*, 241, 540–5.

Husaini, B. A. & Von Frank, A. (1983). Life events, coping resources and depression: a longitudinal study of direct, buffering and reciprocal effects. Unpublished report.

Jablensky, A., Sartorius, N., Ernberg, G., Anker, M., Korten, A., Cooper, J. E. Day, R. & Bertelsen, A. (1992). Schizophrenia: manifestations, incidence and course in different cultures. A World Health Organization ten-country study. *Psychological Medicine, Monograph Supplement*, 20, 91–7.

Kiecolt-Glaser, J. K. & Greenberg, B. (1984). Social support as moderator of the after effect of stress in female psychiatric inpatients. *Journal of Abnormal Psychology*, 93, 192–9.

Kessler, R. C., Kendler, K. S., Heath, A. & Neale, M. C. (1992). Social support, depressed mood, and adjustment to stress: a genetic epidemiological investigation. *Journal of Personal and Social Psychology*, 62, 257–72.

Kessler, R. R., Kendler, K. S., Heath, A., Neale, M. C. & Eaves, L. J. (1994). Perceived support and adjustment to stress in a general population sample of female twins. *Psychological Medicine*, 24, 317–34.

Klerman, G. L., Weissman, M. M., Rounsaville, B. J. & Chevron, E. S. (1984). *Interpersonal Psychotherapy of Depression*. New York: Basic Books.

Kuipers, L. & Westall, J. (1992). The role of facilitated relatives' groups and voluntary self-help groups. In *Principles of Social Psychiatry*, ed. D. Bhugra & J. Leff, pp. 562–71. Oxford: Blackwell Scientific.

Lakey, B. & Heller, K. (1988). Social support from a friend, perceived support, and social problem solving. *American Journal of Community Psychology*, 16, 811–24.

Lam, D. H. & Power, M. (1991). A questionnaire designed to assess roles and goals: a preliminary study. *British Journal of Medical Psychology*, 64, 359–73.

Landerman, R., George, L. K., Campbell, R. T. & Blazer, D. G. (1989). Alternative models of the stress buffering hypothesis. *American Journal of Community Psychology*, 17, 625–42.

Lane, C. & Hobfoll, E. (1992). How loss affects anger and alienates potential supporters. *Journal of Consulting and Clinical Psychology*, 60, 935–42.

Lewinsohn, P. M., Hoberman, H. M. & Rosenbaum, M. (1988). A prospective study of risk factors for unipolar depression. *Journal of Abnormal Psychology*, 97, 251–64.

Lin, N. & Dean, A. (1984). Social support and depression: a panel study. *Social Psychiatry*, 19, 83–91.

MacCarthy, B. (1988). The role of relatives. In *Community Care in Practice*, ed. A. Lavender & F. Holloway, pp. 207–30. Chichester: Wiley.

MacCarthy, B., Brewin, C. R., LeSage, A., Brugha, T. S., Mangen, S. & Wing, J. K. (1989). Needs for care among the relatives of long-term users of day care: a report from the Camberwell High Contact Survey. *Psychological Medicine*, 19, 725–36.

McLeod, J. D. Kessler, R. C. & Landis, K. R. (1992). Speed of recovery from major depressive episodes in a community sample of married men and women. *Journal of Abnormal Psychology*, **101**, 277–86.

Meltzer, H., Gill, B. & Petticrew, M. (1994). *OPCS Surveys of Psychiatric Morbidity in Great Britain. Bulletin No. 1.* The prevalence of psychiatric morbidity among adults aged 16–64, living in private households, in Great Britain. London: Office of Population Censuses and Surveys.

Miller, P. & Lloyd, C. (1991). Social support and its interactions with personality and childhood background as predictors of psychiatric symptoms in Scottish and American medical students. *Social Psychiatry and Psychaitric Epidemiology*, **26**, 171–7.

Miller, P. Mc., Ingham, J. G., Kreitman, N. B., Surtees, P. G. & Sashidarhan, S. P. (1987). Life events and other factors implicated in onset and in remission of psychiatric illness in women. *Journal of Affective Disorders*, **12**, 73–88.

Miller, P., Kreitman, N., Ingham, J. & Sashidharan, S. (1989). Self esteem, life stress and psychiatric disorder. *Journal of Affective Disorders*, **17**, 65–75.

Mitchell, J. C. (1969). The concept and use of social networks. In *Social Networks in Urban Situations*, ed. J. C. Mitchell. Manchester: Manchester University Press.

Monroe, S. M. & Steiner, S. C. (1986). Social support and psychopathology: interrelations with pre-existing disorder, stress and personality. *Journal of Abnormal Psychology*, **95**, 29–39.

Montgomery, R. J. V. & Borgatta, E. F. (1989). The effects of alternative support strategies on family caregiving. *Gerontologist*, **29**, 457–64.

Newcomb, M. D. & Chon, C. (1989). Social support among young adults: latent variable models of quantity and satisfaction within six life areas. *Multivariate Behavioural Research*, **24**, 237–56.

O'Connor, P. & Brown, G. W. (1984). Supportive relationships: fact or fancy? *Journal of Personal and Social Relationships*, **1**, 159–75.

O'Leary, K. D. & Beach, S. R. H. (1990). Marital therapy: a viable treatment for depression and marital discord. *American Journal of Psychiatry*, **147**, 183–6.

Olds, D. L., Henderson, C. R. & Tatelbaum, R. (1988). Improving the life-course development of socially disadvantaged mothers: a randomised trial of nurse home visitation. *American Journal of Public Health*, **78**, 1436–45.

Orth-Gomér, K., Rosengren, A. & Wilhelmsen, L. (1993). Lack of social support and incidence of coronary heart disease in middle-aged Swedish men. *Psychosomatic Medicine*, **55**, 37–43.

Parker, G. & Barnett, B. (1987). A test of the social support hypothesis. *British Journal of Psychiatry*, **150**, 72–7.

Parker, G. & Barnett, B. (1988). Perceptions of parenting in childhood and social support in adulthood. *American Journal of Psychiatry*, **145**, 479–82.

Parry, G. (1988). Mobilizing social support networks. In *New Developments in Clinical Psychology*, Vol. 2, pp. 83–104. ed. F. N. Watts. Chichester: Wiley.

Plomin, R. (1990). The role of inheritance in behaviour. *Science*, **248**, 183–8.

Plomin, R., DeFries, J. C. & McClearn, G. E. (1990). *Behavioural Genetics.* New York: Freeman.

President's Commission on Mental Health (1978). Report of the Task Panel on Community Support Systems. In *Task Panel Reports;* submitted to the President's Commission on Mental Health. Washington, DC: US Government Printing Office.

Price, R. H. Vanryn, M. & Vinokur, A. D. (1992). Impact of a preventive job search intervention on the likelihood of depression among the unemployed. *Journal of Health and Social Behaviour,* **33,** 158–67.

Rakos, R. F. (1991). *Assertive Behaviour: Theory, Research and Training.* London: Routledge.

Raleigh, M. J., McGuire, M. T., Brammer, G. L., Pollack, D. B. & Yuwiler, A. (1991). Serotonergic mechanisms promote dominance acquisition in adult male vervet monkeys. *Brain Research,* **559,** 181–90.

Repetti, R. (1987). Individual and common components of the social environment at work and psychological well-being. *Journal of Personal and Social Psychology,* **52,** 710–20.

Romans, S. E. & McPherson, M. (1992). The social networks of bipolar affective disorder patients. *Journal of Affective Disorders,* **25,** 221–8.

Rosenberg, C. (1992). *Explaining Epidemics and Other Studies in the History of Medicine.* Cambridge: Cambridge University Press.

Rutter, M. &. Quinton, D. (1984). Long-term follow-up of women institutionalised in childhood: factors promoting good functioning in adult life. *British Journal of Developmental Psychology,* **2,** 191–204.

Sarason, I. G. & Sarason, B. R. (1986). Experimentally provided social support. *Journal of Personal and Social Psychology,* **50,** 1222–5.

Sarason, B. R., Sarason, I. G., Hacker, T. A. & Bacham, R. (1985). Concomitants of social support: social skills, physical attractiveness and gender. *Journal of Personality and Social Psychology,* **49,** 469–80.

Schaefer, C., Coyne, J. C. & Lazarus, R. S. (1982). The health related functions of social support. *Journal of Behavioural Medicine,* **4,** 381–406.

Schuster, T. L., Kessler, R. C. & Aseltine, R. U. (1990). Supportive interactions, negative interactions and depressed mood. *American Journal of Community Psychology,* **18,** 423–38.

Segal, S. P. &. Holschuh, M. S. W. (1991). Effects of sheltered care environments and resident characteristics on the development of social networks. *Hospital and Community Psychiatry,* **42,** 1125–31.

Shumaker, S. A. &. Hill, D. R. (1991). Gender differences in social support and physical health. *Health Psychology,* **10,** 102–11.

Simonoff, E. A. & Heath, A. C. (1989). A model fitting approach to the estimation of genetic and environmental factors from twin data. *International Review of Psychiatry,* **1,** 297–305.

Sims, A. C. P., Heard, D. H., Rowe, C. E., Gill, M. M. P. & Maddock, V. (1993). Neurosis and the personal environment: the effects of a time-limited course of intensive day care. *British Journal of Psychiatry,* **162,** 369–74.

Spielberger, C. D., Gorsuch, R. L. & Lushene, R. E. (1970). *Manual for the State-Trait Anxiety Inventory (Self-Evaluation Questionnaire).* Palo Alto, California: Consulting Psychologists Press.

Spitzer, R. L., Endicott, J. & Robins, E. (1978). Research diagnostic criteria: rationale and reliability. *Archives of General Psychiatry,* **35,** 773–82.

Steinglass, P., Weisstub, E. & Denoar, A. K. (1988). Perceived personal networks as mediators of stress reactions. *American Journal of Psychiatry,* **145,** 1259–64.

38   T. S. BRUGHA

Sullivan, C. M., Tan, C., Basta, J., Rumptz, M. & Davidson, W. S. (1992). An advocacy intervention program for women with abusive partners. *American Journal of Community Psychology*, **20**, 309–32.

Suomi, S. J., Seaman, S. F., Lewis, J. K., De Lizio, R. D. & McKinney, W. T. (1978). Effects of imipramine treatment of separation-induced social disorders in rhesus monkeys. *Archives of General Psychiatry*, **35**, 321–5.

Swindle, R. W., Cronkite, R. C. & Moos, R. H. (1989). Life stressors, social resources, coping and the 4 year course of unipolar depression. *Journal of Abnormal Psychology*, **98**, 468–77.

Thoits, P. A. (1986). Support as coping assistance. *Journal of Consulting and Clinical Psychology*, **54**, 416–23.

Thompson, C. (1988). *The Instruments of Psychiatric Research*. Chichester: Wiley.

Tolsdorf, C. C. (1976). Social networks, support and coping: an exploratory study. *Family Process*, **15**, 407–17.

Toseland, R. W., Rossiter, C. M. & Labrecque, M. S. (1989). The effectiveness of peer-led and professionally led groups to support family caregivers. *Gerontologist*, **29**, 465–71.

van Praag, H. M. (1986). Affective disorders and aggression disorders: evidence for a common biological mechanism. *Suicide and Life-Threatening Behaviour*, **16**, 21–50.

Weiss, R. S. (1974). The provisions of social relationships. In *Doing Unto Others*, ed. Z. Rubin. Englewood Cliffs, NJ: Prentice Hall.

Wellman, B. (1981). Applying network analysis to the problem of support. In *Social Networks and Social Support*, ed. B. H. Gottlieb, pp. 171–200. London: Sage Publications.

West, M., Lively, W. J., Reiffer, L. & Sheldon, A. (1986). The place of attachment in the life events model of stress and illness. *Canadian Journal of Psychiatry*, **31**, 202–7.

West, M., Sheldon, A. & Reiffer, L. (1987). An approach to the delineating of adult attachment: scale development and reliability. *Journal of Nervous and Mental Disease*, **175**, 738–41.

Wing, J. K., Cooper, J. E. & Sartorius, N. (1974). *Measurement and Classification of Psychiatric Symptoms*. Cambridge: Cambridge University Press.

Zeiss, A. M. & Lewinsohn, P. M. (1988). Enduring deficits after remissions of depression: a test of the scar hypothesis. *Behaviour Research and Therapy*, **26**, 151–8.

PART I

CONCEPTS AND ORIGINS OF
SOCIAL SUPPORT

2

Understanding social support within the context of theory and research on the relationship of life stress and mental health

CAMILLE LLOYD

In the last two decades there has been a prolific amount of research aimed at investigating the relationship between stressful life experiences and psychological well-being. In Chapter 1 a multi-causal model of the stress–psychological distress relationship has been introduced. In sum, one can best understand this aetiological process in psychiatric disorder by taking into account the personality vulnerabilities/strengths of an individual, the stressors to which he or she is exposed, and the resources which he or she can call upon to help him or her respond to the stressors, be these social resources or coping resources/strategies.

Parallel developments in the life stress and social support research domains

I shall identify in this chapter several parallel themes which have occurred within the subdomains of stress, social support, personality and coping. In identifying some of these parallel developments, new areas of research might be suggested; additionally, I would like to attempt to integrate some of the findings from these various areas, since in doing so I think we can begin to develop a better understanding of how stress exerts its negative effects on psychological functioning and of how social support and these other factors also affect psychological functioning. I will emphasise first some parallel developments in the stress and social support domains, since social support factors are the focus of this book.

Concerns about conceptualisation and measurement of the variables

The first parallel in the stress and the social support domains is the proper conceptualisation and measurement of the concepts. In the stress literature, for example, one controversy has centred around identifying

41

what is the nature of the relevant 'stress'. Various conceptualisations/
definitions of stress probably have merit, and 'stress' is most probably a
multidimensional rather than a unidimensional phenomenon, which
includes adjustment to change (Holmes & Rahe, 1967), role strains
(Pearlin, 1983) and daily 'hassles' (Kanner et al., 1981; Monroe, 1983a).
A second controversy centred around a concern about whether stress was
best conceptualised as objective, external events (Dohrenwend et al.,
1984; Dohrenwend & Shrout, 1985) or as the subjective reaction of a
person to these events or to the discrepancy between events and the
personal capability of adapting to them (Lazarus & Folkman, 1984;
Lazarus et al., 1985). A third controversy centred around deciding upon
the most salient aspect of stressful events. Lubin & Rubio (1985)
reported findings suggesting that salient event qualities were their
undesirability, unexpectedness, amount of pressure and adjustment
required, and their perceived uncontrollability. For a good overall
review of the conceptual and measurement controversies in the life event
literature, see Zimmerman (1983).

It appears that the conceptualisation of social support has followed a
similar path: the probable multidimensional nature of social support;
controversy regarding the subjective versus objective nature of social
support; and an interest in identifying the most salient aspects of social
support.

Cobb (1976) defined social support as 'information that one belongs
to a socially coherent community and that one is loved and esteemed'.
In this early definition, two (or three) different aspects of support are
implied. The first emphasises belonging to a socially coherent community and may be similar to Veiel's (1985) later concept of social
integration or everyday support. The second aspect, that of receiving
information that one is loved and valued, may overlap with later
conceptualisations of support emphasising emotional or psychological
benefits or reassurance of self-worth that are frequently provided in the
face of stress or crisis. Kaplan et al., (1977) defined social support in
terms of the degree to which a person's social needs are satisfied
through interaction with others. Brown & Harris (1978), in their
important work studying social support and depression, defined it as
the presence of an intimate other in whom one could confide. Berkman
& Syme (1979) emphasised social participation, characterised for
example by marriage, friendships, church activities and group mem-
berships. House (1981) defined it as an interpersonal transaction
involving concern, aid and information about oneself and the environment. He also drew distinctions between emotional support, appraisal
support (affirmation and feedback), informational support and instrumental support. Instrumental support involves practical assistance,
such as in lending money or taking a friend to the airport, whereas

expressive support involves sharing of problems, spending time together, etc. (Dean *et al.*, 1981). Cohen & Wills (1985) differentiated among four types of support: esteem support, informational support (defined as providing help in defining and coping with problematic events), social companionship and instrumental support.

Veiel (1985) also pointed to three controversies in the conceptualisation of social support. He called attention to the controversies about whether social support really acts as a 'buffer' or 'moderator' of stress, about whether support is best characterised as objective support or as subjective (perceived) support, and about whether support is best seen as being derived from intimate, confiding relationships or from more casual ties and relationships. Veiel pointed out that empirical research can be found to support each side of each of these three controversies. Veiel also concluded that the assumption that social support is a single commodity or unitary concept is fallacious and that a multidimensional conceptualisation of social support would be needed to advance the field. Veiel proposed that social support could be categorised as either 'instrumental' or 'psychological'. Psychological support is aimed at changing intrapsychic dimensions such as moods, attitudes or cognitive processes, and could be further categorised as providing either emotional or informational aspects of support. Veiel also draw a distinction between everyday support (social integration), and crisis support which is mobilised in response to specific stressors.

Barrera (1986), in a review of the conceptualisation of social support, also concluded that a global (unidimensional) model of social support should be abandoned in favour of more precise concepts. He thought that social support was insufficiently specific as a research concept, and that more precise conceptualisation (and measurement) would be needed in order to illuminate inconsistent research findings. Barrera further proposed that existing conceptualisations of social support could be divided into three broad categories: (1) social embeddedness, (2) perceived social support, and (3) enacted social support. Social embeddedness emphasises connections and ties a person has to the social environment and is opposite to the notion of social isolation or alienation. Concepts of social embeddedness draw on the theoretical work of Mitchell (1969) describing social network morphology and on the properties of social networks listed by Kaplan *et al.* (1977). Perceived social support emphasises the cognitive appraisal or perception of the availability and adequacy of support, or satisfaction with support. Enacted support refers to the actions that others perform when they render assistance to a person, i.e. enacted support involves what individuals actually *do* to provide support.

Thus one can see that the conceptualisation of social support, like the conceptualisation of stress, has moved in the direction of being defined and studied as a multidimensional concept. And, like the stress research area, one of the controversies has centred around whether conceptualisation should emphasise the objective or the subjective nature of the concept. In both fields there has been an acknowledgement that once subjective concepts are used, there is a potential for overlap with other personality variables.

Concern about the overlap of independent and dependent variables

A second parallel is also evident. In the life event literature, considerable interest emerged in establishing that the relationship between life event stress and psychological distress was not due to a simple overlap of the two constructs. Specifically, one early measure of life stress included in its domain questions about changes in sleeping and eating habits; however, changes in these functions often occur in depressive disorders and hence are enquired about in measures of psychological distress. One had to rule out, therefore, the possibility that the relationship between the two concepts was not simply due to their overlap (Dohrenwend & Dohrenwend, 1978). This question has also been raised in the social support literature. For example, Monroe (1983b) and Monroe & Steiner (1986, pp. 30–1) discussed the problem of potential overlap between social support and symptoms or disorder. Social withdrawal, for example, can be seen as a symptom of depression.

Concern about spurious relationships

In a similar vein, there has been a concern that the relationship between stress and psychological distress may be a spurious one. Life event researchers, for example, have worried that the association between life event stress and distress might simply be due to a third variable, such as a plaintiff set. In this case, a person who is characterised by a negative cognitive set may simply by more likely both to recall negative events or circumstances (not actually experience them) and to admit to more depressive symptoms. There is also an additional concern about a mood-related cognitive set, where the depressed individual is more likely than the non-depressed person to remember stressful events. There has been a concern too that the depressed individual may also engage in 'a search after meaning' in which he or she is driven to find a reason or explanation for the depression or distress, and so may be motivated to search for an explanatory stressor.

In the social support literature there has also been a concern that depressed mood may affect the perception of the social network, so that a mood-related pessimism might lead to a negatively biased assessment of the social support provided or available to the individual (Monroe & Steiner, 1986, p. 31; Alloway & Bebbington, 1987, pp. 95–6).

Several investigators have also raised the possibility of a second manner in which the relationship between social support and psychological distress could be a spurious one. Personality factors could represent a possible third variable accounting for both support deficits and psychological distress. Among the personality dimensions that have been mentioned in this regard are introversion–extraversion and neuroticism–stability (Monroe & Steiner, 1986, p. 35). Social competence might also account for both deficits in social support and distress (Henderson *et al.*, 1981; Heller & Swindle, 1983; Cohen & Wills, 1985, p. 383). One recent study investigated this possibility, however, and reported data suggesting that the support buffering effects were not related to social skills (Cohen *et al.*, 1986). They did mention, though, that it is still possible that social support serves as a proxy for some other stable personality characteristic of import such as introversion, low assertiveness or negativistic attitudes (towards people, life, etc.).

Concern about the direction of causality

A fourth parallel also emerges. This parallel addresses the issue of causal direction. In the life event research area, investigators were concerned that the life events could follow rather than precede the illness or distress. For example, investigators were concerned that a depressed person might begin to function more poorly at work and consequently bring about his or her own job dismissal. In this case, then, the stressful event of being fired did not precede or cause the depression, but rather the depression was the cause of the stressful event of being fired. To address this issue, stress researchers were forced either to study independent events, i.e. events that could be argued to be clearly independent of the person's influences (see Paykel, 1974, for an illustrative study) or to document very carefully the time of event occurrence and the time of onset of disorder so that it could be shown that events clearly preceded in time the onset of disorder (e.g. see Brown & Harris, 1978).

In the social support literature there has been a corresponding concern that the causal direction might be the opposite of that originally supposed. It would seem possible that psychological distress might affect a person's ability to develop or utilise a social support network. Individuals who become depressed may withdraw from other people, for example, because they are embarrassed by their depressive symptoms or because they do not want to burden others with their lowered mood. In this case, the psychological distress would actually lead to the diminished social network rather than the diminished network contributing to the psychological distress. In addition, persons suffering psychological distress might receive less support because their deteriorating condition might create interpersonal tensions that alienate other people (Henderson & Morgan, 1983). Some researchers have been particularly aware of this causal direction dilemma, and so have attempted to unravel the issue by careful longitudinal study (see Krause *et al.*, 1989, and Monroe *et al.*, 1986, for examples). In fact, in both the stress and the social support lines of research, investigators have eventually been willing to acknowledge that the relationship of stress and distress as well as the relationship of social support and distress may well be bidirectional. Coyne & Delongis (1986), for example, state that 'there are undoubtedly profound connections between having good relationships and well-being, but they are likely to be complex, reciprocal and contingent'.

Interest in identifying the mechanism of action of the relevant psychosocial variable

A fifth and final parallel is that in both the life event and the social support literature the question emerges as to *how* stress or *how* social support actually exert their effects on psychological outcome. That is to say, an obvious question arising at the end of the many associational studies is that surrounding the identification of the mechanisms that underlie the associations. It is interesting that in this one respect the social support literature may actually have moved slightly ahead of the stress literature. There appears to be more discussion in the social support literature concerning the need to establish how social support directly or indirectly positively affects mental health. I shall look first at the social support literature and then at the life stress literature.

Thoits (1986) has offered an explanation of how social support affects psychological functioning that is based on the notion that social support provides coping assistance. She reviews earlier works by Pearlin *et al.* (1981), Brown (1979) and Brown & Harris (1978) suggesting that social support operates by bolstering self-esteem and a sense of environmental mastery. Thoits goes on to point out that significant others can suggest techniques of stress management, or can directly participate in coping efforts – and as coping is effective, there is a bolstering of self-esteem and a sense of environmental mastery. Heller *et al.* (1986) also concur with the proposition that social support provides stress-related interpersonal aid. They further note that esteem-enhancing appraisals from others are used to enhance one's own self-esteem and that this mechanism is one of the ways in which social support operates to protect health. They also point to the need to investigate further the mechanisms by which social support exerts it beneficial effects. Krause (1987) provided some empirical support for the proposition that social support helps to reduce the deleterious effects of stress on emotional functioning by bolstering self-esteem. However, he too notes that additional mechanisms may also be operating, citing a study by Caplan (1981) indicating that social support may increase feelings of personal control.

Cohen & Wills (1985) proposed that social support could have a beneficial effect on well-being through two different processes. First, it might exert a generalised beneficial effect because effective social networks provide the individual with regular positive experiences and a set of stable, socially rewarding roles in the community. Secondly, social support could 'buffer' or protect the individual from the potentially pathogenic influences of stress at either of two points in the causal process: it could intervene between the stressful event and a stress reaction by attenuating the appraisal process, or it could intervene between the stressful event and the onset of a negative outcome by reducing or eliminating the stress reaction or by directly influencing physiological processes.

Many emphasise social support as a mediating variable. Other theorists, however, have instead emphasised that social relationships are essential to human existence. Henderson (1977), for example, has written that 'social bonds, having become a valuable component of the primate and human behavioural repertoire, are now necessary for persons to maintain a reasonable degree of affective comfort'. Elsewhere in this book, Gilbert has explored the role and function of social support from an evolutionary perspective. In Chapter 5 Gilbert develops the theme that social relating is necessary for survival, and that human beings have innate biosocial goals of forming attachments between offspring and parents, of being able to attract and maintain a mate, and of being able to form alliances or establish rank/status in order to ensure access to necessary resources. These authors thus emphasise that social support is not just important in helping individuals to cope with specific crises or demands, but is essential to human survival and happiness.

Despite the voluminous literature establishing the deleterious effect of life stress on psychological functioning, relatively little attention has been directed to understanding how this effect occurs. Given the close tie of this literature to the early stress notions of homeostasis and change and physiological adaptation, there may have been an implicit assumption that the mechanisms of action would be identified by those studying the physiological mechanisms of stress. As notions of the conceptualisation of stress most relevant to mental health outcomes broadened or changed from their focus of simple changes to a focus on factors such as 'undesirability' or 'loss' or to a conceptualisation of stress that emphasised the appraisal process, the need for the identification of psychological as well as physiological mechanisms of action grew.

There is still a need for development of a biological or physiological model of how stress exerts its negative effects on mental health. Harris (1987) called attention to the relevance of the work by Henry & Stephens (1977). These authors discussed two physiological stress reactions, one being the pituitary-adrenocortical system and the other being the sympatho-adreno-medullary system; they also related the former to notions of conservation–withdrawal and the latter to the fight–flight response. The relevance of this work to psychological functioning, however, would need further elucidation. Post (1992) has also very recently reported a model of affective disorder where psychosocial stressors involving losses and threats of loss play an important pathophysiological role in the triggering of an affective episode, but also, because of the neurobiological encoding of memory-like functions related to these stressors, provide a long-term vulnerability to subsequent recurrences and perhaps a mechanism for retriggering of episodes with lesser degrees of psychosocial stress.

Brown (1979) was one of the first to try to develop a psychological model of how stressful events might exert their negative effects on mental health. Brown argued that stressful events and conditions could exert their negative effects by adversely affecting the self-concept of the exposed individual through actual or threatened loss of self-esteem and by invoking feelings of hopelessness. Several other investigators have also proposed that stress may exert its negative effects through adversely affecting self-esteem (Mechanic, 1978; Lazarus & Folkman, 1984; Thoits, 1983, 1985). Thoits (1983, pp. 80–87) also attempted a preliminary model of how life stress exerts its negative effects, arguing that events tend to generate ongoing strains (i.e. may have a number of consequences for the individual) and that these ongoing strains or consequences may be the more significant phenomenon. She also posited that the ongoing strains may decrease self-regard either by decreasing a sense of mastery or control over life, or by causing loss of a valued social role. She assumed that the maintenance or enhancement of self-regard is a fundamental human need and has important implications for an individual's psychological state.

The lack of understanding regarding just how stress exerts its negative effects on psychological functioning contributes to the difficulty in identifying how social support might provide a protective or buffering effect. Progress made in one area of research will benefit the other in developing an understanding of the mechanism of effects.

Having explored how the social support research field has proceeded along the same path as that taken by researchers emphasising stressful events and conditions, a very brief review of the other stress-related domains of mediating personality factors and coping can be undertaken.

Personality factors that may mediate the stress–distress relationship

Investigators have also examined how personality traits may interact with life stressors to determine mental health consequences. It has been suggested that individuals who prefer high levels of stimulation (high in sensation-seeking) may be less prone to the adverse effects of life stress than those who prefer low levels of stimulation (Smith *et al.*, 1978). Locus of control has also been studied as a mediating variable in the stress–distress relationship. Johnson & Sarason (1978) found some support for the notion that individuals who experience life events as something over which they can exert some influence or control are less distressed by events than are individuals who tend to experience events and happenings as being foisted on them and out of their control. Similarly, Kobasa (1979) identified a set of personality traits, termed 'hardiness', that can also serve as a protective influence in the face of life stress. 'Hardy' individuals were thought to evidence three characteristics: (1) the belief that they can control or influence their life experiences, (2) an ability to feel deeply involved in or committed to their life activities, and (3) an ability to anticipate change as an exciting challenge to their development. Subsequent studies of the hardy personality continued to provide evidence for a health-protective influence of this personality style, although the outcome measures reflected health/illness in general, rather than mental health or illness specifically (Kobasa *et al.*, 1981, 1982; Kobasa & Puccetti, 1983).

Self-esteem has also recently received some attention as a personality trait that might play an important mediating role in the stress–distress relationship. For example, Brown and his colleagues studied self-esteem as a mediating variable in a longitudinal study of working-class women living in Islington, north London. They found that self-esteem, when conceptualised and measured in terms of a negative evaluation of the self, acted as a vulnerability factor in the development of depression once a severely threatening event had occurred (Brown *et al.*, 1986, 1990*a*). In a further evaluation of the results of this study, additional findings suggested that positive self-evaluation could also play a protective role in some limited circumstances (Brown *et al.*, 1990*b*). A second study, by Ingham *et al.* (1987), also reported some limited evidence that self-esteem could serve as a predictor of depressive onset. In their study of women in north Edinburgh, they found that low self-esteem (as indicated by a willingness to endorse negative statements on the Rosenberg Self-Esteem Scale) could predict depressive onset, but only in women who had reported previous episodes of psychological illness for which they had sought medical help. In a subsequent additional analysis of this study sample it was reported that onset of a major depressive disorder could be predicted by an interaction between low self-esteem and high levels of total stress (Miller *et al.*, 1989).

In an interesting article by Chan (1977), several personality and attitudinal constructs were proposed as having some potential to explain reactional differences observed among individuals under stress. Among the variables mentioned were self-esteem, internality–externality, learned helplessness, a potent sense of hope and efficacy, and anxiety.

More recently, there has been an attempt to match individuals with the type of stress that would be most salient for them. For example, Beck (1983) described two personality characteristics, labelled sociotropy and autonomy, that he thought were important factors in depressive illness. Sociotropy emphasised beliefs, attitudes and goals that orient a person towards obtaining assistance from others in meeting that person's own needs. Autonomy refers to an individual's self-investment, and efforts to develop his or her own interests and capacities to achieve success. Beck suggested that each of these two sets of characteristics might serve as vulnerabilities to depression in response to specific congruent types of events. For example, individuals with a high level of sociotropy might display a psychological vulnerability to events associated with perceived social loss or rejection, whereas individuals with a high level of autonomy might display a particular vulnerability to events perceived as indicating personal failure or loss of control over the environment. The notion here is that events have different meanings to different individuals, and that the meaning of events relative to the sense of self is important. Oatley & Bolton (1965), for example, theorised that depression occurs when events disrupt roles by which people define their self-worth.

Some empirical support has emerged to support these theoretical positions. Robins & Block (1988) provided evidence for the utility of looking at the matching of events with personality styles reflecting the valuing or meaning of these events. They found that dependent or sociotropic persons were more affected by social failures, although persons high in autonomy were not found to be more affected by achievement failures. Hammen *et al.* (1985), using different measures of personally meaningful functional domains, found that 'dependent' college students were likely to become depressed when faced with negative interpersonal events but not negative achievement events. To a lesser extent, 'self-critical' persons demonstrated the reverse pattern of being more negatively affected by achievement events. Hammen *et al.* (1989) also reported that among unipolar depressives, patients displayed specific vulnerability to stressful life events that matched their relative orientation towards affiliation or autonomous achievement.

In the research literature, less attention has been directed so far towards examining the possible interaction of social support and personality variables in affecting psychological outcomes. On a hypothetical basis, it would certainly seem plausible that there could be individual differences in the amount, type or source of social support that was preferred or found to be most protective. Henderson (1984) also made the point that individuals do not all require the same amount of social support, and that variations exist in the need for supportive social contact. Miller & Lloyd (1991) provided some empirical evidence for an interaction of personality and social support on psychological functioning. They showed that for students who tended to be suspicious or reserved and shy, the costs of social relationships seemed sometimes to outweigh the benefits.

Interest in studying coping and coping styles

As in the life stress and the social support literature, there has been considerable interest in the coping literature in trying to understand just how coping can best be conceptualised or defined and measured. Lazarus & Folkman (1984), for example, defined coping as 'constantly changing cognitive and behavioral efforts to manage specific external and/or internal demands that are appraised as taxing or exceeding the resources of the person'. These theorists also discussed the importance of making a distinction between problem-focused coping and emotion-focused coping. Problem-focused coping is directed at managing or altering the problem causing the distress. Emotion-focused coping is directed at regulating the emotional response to the problem; it may be comprised of affect regulation, emotional discharge and the seeking of emotional support (the latter action, of course, reflects the seeking of social support). It can also be noted that the distinction between problem-focused and emotion-focused coping parallels the distinction between instrumental and expressive support reported in the social support literature.

An earlier approach to studying coping centred around the investigation of the maturity of ego defences used to cope in the face of threat. Ego mechanisms of defence are inferred psychological processes that function to allow the individual to cope with stressful environmental stimuli. Vaillant and his colleagues proposed a hierarchical system for classifying ego defences ranging from the least to the most mature (Vaillant, 1976; Vaillant et al., 1986). In defining coping as the adaptive application of defence mechanisms, these investigators have reported results indicating that maturity of defences is a good indicator of adult mental health and of upward social mobility. While the maturity of defensive coping style would seem to hold some promise as a mediating variable, most of the studies to date seem to have examined it only as an independent contributor to psychological functioning. One exception to this is a study by Andrews *et al.* (1978) in which the maturity of the habitually used ego defensive coping style was studied in combination with life stress and social support for its relationship to psychological symptoms. However, their data indicated a main effect for defensive style rather than a buffering effect.

It is possible to argue that there is an overlap between the domains of personality and coping, insofar as certain personality types or traits may be associated with preferred styles of coping. Coping style refers to the usual or habitual cognitions or behaviours that an individual uses to minimise the adverse impact of stressful circumstances (Billings *et al.*, 1983; Pearlin & Schooler, 1978). Nevertheless, it would appear to be useful to try to separate out coping processes from personality traits by emphasising the specific cognitions or behaviours that occur in response to particular stressors, because there is most probably variability as well as stability in the coping used by individuals. Lazarus & Folkman (1984, pp. 128–30), for example, argued that trait conceptualisations and measures of coping underestimate the complexity and variability of actual coping efforts. It would appear to be useful to study both typical coping styles and specific coping processes.

Towards an integration of possible mechanisms of action

In order to try to integrate some of the theoretical work and to bring about a greater integration of the findings from the various domains of stress, social support, personality and coping, it is helpful to highlight some of the consistencies that can be found across domains. Such an integration might lead to more systematic theory and might provide useful information for those who wish to begin applying knowledge in the stress field in order to conduct attempts at prevention and treatment.

The more physiological roots of stress theory would seem to lead to various possibilities regarding biological mechanisms of effect (Henry & Stevens, 1977), but these would seem to have more relevance for physical than for psychological disorder. Proposed biological mechanisms underlying the experience of traumatic stress and the development of post-traumatic stress disorder (Kolb, 1987), as well as mechanisms proposed to explain the development of affective disorder (Post, 1992), may provide a useful example of how a model could be developed.

Efforts at explaining how social support may mediate or mitigate the effects of stress have also produced both physiological and psychological mechanisms of effect. It has been proposed that the mere presence of other people in stressful situations serves to decrease various measures of physiological arousal. The psychological mechanisms of action of social support proposed so far seem to centre around one of four notions: First, some investigators have proposed a general (independent?) effect of social support, noting that effective networks provide the individual with frequent rewarding experiences and with satisfying roles. Mediating effects have been proposed to operate through at least three other possible mechanisms, including propositions that social support exerts its mitigating effects by: (1) directly or indirectly enhancing coping efforts so that potential threats may be minimised or eliminated (e.g. see Thoits, 1986), (2) supporting or bolstering self-esteem (e.g. see Krause, 1987), and (3) supporting one's sense of control (Caplan, 1981).

Personality variables that may mediate the stress–distress relationship that are thought to be important are: (1) hardiness as reflected in commitment, control and challenge, (2) self-esteem, (3) locus of control, and (4) sensation-seeking. Some potential overlap can be seen between the challenge dimension of hardiness and the sensation-seeking dimension in that both may reflect a favourable disposition towards stimulation or change. Potential overlap can also be seen between the control dimension of hardiness and the work arising out of the locus of control concept, in that both of these may reflect an individual's disposition to believe that he or she has a reasonable amount of influence or control over the direction of their life. Kobasa (1979) herself noted these similarities. Eliminating these redundancies leaves four variables of importance: commitment, self-esteem, sense of control and challenge/change.

Let us suppose for a moment that we take what is known about these personality variables and view them instead as process variables. That is to say, perhaps personality variables act as moderators of stress because they are closely related to process variables. We can consider the notion of commitment as our first example. Perhaps adverse events or conditions affect psychological functioning when they decrease an individual's commitment to the self, that is to say, when they decrease that individual's ability to believe in the meaning or purpose of life. To the extent that an individual has a general disposition to find life meaningful, he or she is also less likely to lose that sense of meaning in the face of a specific stressor. Thus the personality disposition is relevant because it affects the process by which events can exert negative impacts.

Taking as a second example the sense of control, perhaps events can also exert a negative impact by decreasing the individual's ability to believe that he or she can influence or control life's outcomes. Giving up and demoralisation follows, which may be related to notions of learned helplessness or to the 'giving-up' complex as described by researchers studying the effects of severe illness on patients. To the extent that a person has a general disposition towards assuming that he or she can control life outcomes, then again in the face of a specific stressor that individual may be less likely to experience a decrease in the sense of personal control.

Taking as a third example self-esteem, we can postulate that a stressful event or condition can exert a negative impact by decreasing self-esteem (Brown & Harris, 1978). Perhaps the person high in self-esteem is more able to place a specific failure or disappointment in a larger perspective or has sufficiently good feelings about the self to compensate for a disappointment in one area, and hence the self-esteem is less compromised as a result. Thus self-esteem compromise is one mechanism of action. Self-esteem as a personality disposition serves to mediate the relationship by rendering the individual less susceptible to the process of self-esteem compromise.

The personal disposition to regard change as stimulating or challenging presents more difficulties in being accepted as a process variable. Perhaps events or conditions can exert a negative impact when they aggregate to the point of overwhelming the individual's sense of coherence or meaning, sense of stable identity and worth or, indeed, the individual's physiological capacities to adapt. In this sense, these stressors affect the person negatively not so much because of the meaning of the event but because of the sheer strain of physiological processes of adaptation – more relevant perhaps, for the development of physical than psychological disorder.

Thus social support and personality dispositions may mediate the effects of life events to the extent that they (1) support the individual's ability to maintain a sense of meaning and purpose in life, (2) support the individual in the belief that he or she can influence the course of life, (3) support or bolster the individual's feelings of self-worth and self-esteem, and (4) support the individual's ability to adapt or cope with changes so that he or she does not feel overwhelmed by the amount or pace of change. Social support and personality might also have direct or main effects on psychological functioning to the extent that they contribute directly to the ability to find meaning in life, to develop a sense of control over life, and to develop a healthy self-esteem.

In evaluating the potential worth of this more theoretically derived model of stress processes, one might turn to a study by Taylor (1983) in which she attempted to derive a more empirically based model of the process of adjustment to stress. Taylor (1983) reported on her detailed observations of the adjustment processes that women and their families evidenced when faced with the knowledge that the women had breast cancer. These processes included a search for meaning in the experience, an effort to gain mastery, and an attempt to enhance the self.

Many of these women tried to understand why they developed cancer and many made specific attributions regarding the cause of their cancer. The women told of thinking about what the implications of the cancer were, and of reordering their priorities in life to ensure that they obtained the greatest possible satisfaction (meaning?) from it. Taylor also observed the need to regain a sense of control over the threatening illness. Many women developed a belief, for example, that they could keep the cancer from coming back, whether through their own efforts or through the efforts of the doctors. Taylor also described how patients would struggle with the issue of self-concept or self-esteem. She observed how the women would make downward comparisons rather than upward comparisons, thus appearing to select their comparison person to enhance their own self-esteem, a point taken up elsewhere in this volume by Gilbert and by Brewin. For example, older women considered themselves better off than the younger women, married women pitied the single women, etc.

In evaluating this model of stress and how it leads to detrimental psychological effects, it might also be noted that the model appears to be amenable to testing or verification. For example, to proceed with testing the model, a sample of individuals could be selected who are undergoing a potentially threatening event such as the break-up of a marriage (divorce). Each individual could then be asked, as they face this event, to indicate to what extent the divorce has increased or decreased: (1) their ability to find meaning and purpose in life, (2) their ability to believe that they could control the direction and course of their life, and (3) their feelings of self-worth and self-esteem. These individuals could then be followed up some time later to see to what extent they were evidencing negative psychological effects after the divorce (and perhaps positive effects as well). The model would predict that the individuals who developed the more negative effects or symptoms would be those whose marital break-up led to a decreased sense of meaning in life, a decreased sense of control over life, and a decreased self-esteem. Such a model would account for the possibility that some individuals might actually improve in mental health after a divorce while others would demonstrate a clear deterioration. For example, given a situation where a woman decides to take the initiative to get out of an unsatisfactory marriage, the divorce might actually enhance her sense of control in life, enhance her self-esteem as she sees herself as a more assertive person, and create an opportunity to find more meaning in life by pursuing a more satisfying relationship with someone else or by creating more time for finding alternative satisfying activities. In contrast, if the woman was satisfied with her marriage but her husband decided to end the marriage to seek a relationship with someone else, there would be much more potential for her to experience a decreased sense of meaning and purpose to her life, to feel as though life events and outcomes were out of her control, and to question her own sense of worth or value. Perhaps the biggest difficulty in testing this model would be to rule out the possibility that these changes in cognitions about the meaning of her life, the ability to control life events and the self, are an epiphenomenon of the psychological disorder. Careful longitudinal studies will help to rule out these competing explanations.

While these notions of stress processes await validation, for those who would like to move forward with intervention efforts, the following tentative guidelines might be suggested. First, individuals should be encouraged to recognise that potentially detrimental psychological effects can occur when an individual is exposed to high levels of stress. Events or conditions are particularly stressful if they involve a threatened or actual loss of significant others. The practical application of this knowledge is that individuals should titrate the amount of negative change or adaptive demands made upon them when possible. Individuals should also be encouraged to engage in coping activities aimed at helping them to maintain a sense of meaning and purpose in life as well as to maintain or enhance a sense of control over their lives. They should also be encouraged to engage in coping activities that will help them to maintain or restore their sense of identity and self-worth. If social support interventions are to be implemented, they should also seek to assist the individual in finding meaning and purpose in life, in believing and approaching the world as though one can affect life outcomes, and in supporting and enhancing the individual's self-worth.

References

Alloway, R. & Bebbington, P. (1987). The buffer theory of social support: a review of the literature. *Psychological Medicine*, **17**, 91–108.

Andrews, G., Tennant, C., Hewson, D. M. & Vaillant, G. E. (1978). Life event stress, social support, coping style and risk of psychological impairment. *Journal of Nervous and Mental Disease*, **166**, 307–16.

Barrera, M. Jr (1986). Distinctions between social support concepts, measures, and models. *American Journal of Community Psychology*, **14**, 413–45.

Beck, A. T. (1983). Cognitive therapy of depression: new perspectives. In *Treatment of Depression: Old Controversies and New Approaches*, ed. P. J. Clayton & J. E. Barrett, pp. 265–90. New York: Raven Press.

Berkman, L. F. & Syme, L. (1979). Social networks, host resistance and mortality: a nine-year follow-up of Alameda County residents. *American Journal of Epidemiology*, **109**, 186–204.

Billings, A. G., Cronkite, R. C. & Moos, R. H. (1983). Social environmental factors in unipolar depression: comparisons of depressed patients and non-depressed controls. *Journal of Abnormal Psychology*, **92**, 119–33.

Brown, G. W. (1979). A three-factor causal model of depression. In *Stress and Mental Disorder* ed. J. E. Barrett, pp. 111–29. New York: Raven Press.

Brown, G. W. & Harris, T. (1978). *The Social Origins of Depression*. New York: Free Press.

Brown, G. W., Andrews, B., Harris, T. O., Adler, Z. & Bridge, L. (1986). Social support, self-esteem and depression. *Psychological Medicine*, **16**, 813–31.

Brown, G. W., Andrews, B., Bifulco, A. & Veiel, H. (1990*a*). Self-esteem and depression: measurement issues and prediction of onset. *Social Psychiatry and Psychiatric Epidemiology*, **25**, 200–9.

Brown, G. W., Bifulco, A. & Andrews, B. (1990*b*). Self-esteem and depression: aetiological issues. *Social Psychiatry and Psychiatric Epidemiology*, **25**, 235–43.

Caplan, G. (1981). Mastery of stress: psychosocial aspects. *American Journal of Psychiatry*, **138**, 413–20.

Cassel, J. (1976). The contribution of the social environment to host resistance. *American Journal of Epidemiology*, **104**, 107–23.

Chan, K. B. (1977). Individual differences in reactions to stress and their personality and situational determinants: some implications for community mental health. *Social Science and Medicine*, **11**, 89–103.

Cobb, S. (1976). Social support as a moderator of life stress. *Psychosomatic Medicine*, **38**, 300–14.

Cohen, S. & Wills, T. A. (1985). Stress, social support, and the buffering hypothesis. *Psychological Bulletin*, **98**, 310–57.

Cohen, S., Sherrod, D. & Clark, M. (1986). Social skills and the stress-protective role of social support. *Journal of Personality and Social Psychology*, **50**, 963–73.

Coyne, J. C. & Delongis, A. (1986). Going beyond social support: the role of social relationships in adaptation. *Journal of Consulting and Clinical Psychology*, **54**, 457–60.

Dean, A., Lin, N. & Ensel, W. M. (1981). The epidemiological significance of social support systems in depression. *Research in Community Mental Health*, **2**, 77–109.

Dohrenwend, B. S. & Dohrenwend, B. P. (1978). Some issues in research on stressful life events. *Journal of Nervous and Mental Disease*, **166**, 7–15.

Dohrenwend, B. P. & Schrout, P. E. (1985). 'Hassles' in the conceptualization and measurement of life stress variables. *American Psychologist*, **40**, 780–5.

Dohrenwend, B. S., Dodson, M., Dohrenwend, B. P. & Schrout, P. E. (1984). Symptoms, hassles, social supports, and life events: problem of confounded measures. *Journal of Abnormal Psychology*, **93**, 222–30.

Hammen, C. L., Marks, T., Mayol, A. & de Mayo, R. (1985). Depressive self-schemas, life stress and vulnerability to depression. *Journal of Abnormal Psychology*, **94**, 308–19.

Hammen, C., Elliott, A., Gitlin, M. & Jamison, K. R. (1989). Sociotropy/autonomy and vulnerability to specific life events in patients with unipolar depression and bipolar disorder. *Journal of Abnormal Psychology*, **98**, 154–60.

Harris, T. (1987). Recent developments in the study of life events in relation to psychiatric and physical disorders. In *Psychiatric Epidemiology*, ed. B. Cooper, pp. 81–102. London: Croom Helm.

Heller, K. & Swindle, R. W. (1983). Social networks, perceived social support and coping with stress. In *Preventive Psychology, Research and Practice in Community Intervention*, ed. R. D. Felner, L. A. Jason, J. Moritsugu & S. S. Farber, pp. 87–103. New York: Pergamon Press.

Heller, K., Swindle, R. W. Jr & Dusenbury, L. (1986). Component social support processes: comments and integration. *Journal of Consulting and Clinical Psychology*, **54**, 466–70.

Henderson, A. S. (1984). Interpreting the evidence on social support. *Social Psychiatry*, **19**, 49–52.

Henderson, S. (1977). The social network, support and neurosis: the function of attachment in adult life. *British Journal of Psychiatry*, **131**, 185–91.

Henderson, A. S. & Morgan, P. (1983). Social relationships during the onset and remission of neurotic symptoms: a prospective community study. *British Journal of Psychiatry*, **143**, 467–72.

Henderson, S., Byrne, D. G. & Duncan-Jones, P. (1981). *Neurosis and the Social Environment*. Sydney: Academic Press.

Henry, J. P. & Stephens, P. M. (1977). *Stress, Health, and the Social Environment: A Sociobiological Approach to Medicine.* New York: Springer-Verlag.

Holmes, T. H. &. Rahe, R. H. (1967). The social readjustment rating scale. *Journal of Psychosomatic Research*, **11**, 213–18.

House, J. S. (1981). *Work Stress and Social Support.* Reading, Massachusetts: Addison-Wesley.

Ingham, J. G., Kreitman, N. B., Miller, P.McC., Sashidharan, S. P. & Surtees, P. (1987). Self-appraisal, anxiety and depression in women: a prospective enquiry. *British Journal of Psychiatry*, **151**, 643–51.

Johnson, J. H. & Sarason, I. G. (1978). Life stress, depression, and anxiety: internal–external control as a moderator variable. *Journal of Psychosomatic Research*, **22**, 205–8.

Kanner, A. D., Coyne, J. D., Schaefer, C. & Lazarus, R. S. (1981). Comparison of two modes of stress measurement: daily hassles and uplifts versus major life events. *Journal of Behavioral Medicine*, **4**, 1–39.

Kaplan, B. H., Cassell, J. C. & Gore, S. S. (1977). Social support and health. *Medical Care*, **15**, 47–58.

Kobasa, S. C. (1979). Stressful life events, personality, and health: an inquiry into hardiness. *Journal of Personality and Social Psychology*, **37**, 1–11.

Kobasa, S. C. & Puccetti, M. C. (1983). Personality and social resources in stress resistance. *Journal of Personality and Social Psychology*, **45**, 839–50.

Kobasa, S. C., Maddi, S. R. & Courington, S. (1981). Personality and constitution as mediators in the stress–illness relationship. *Journal of Health and Social Behavior*, **22**, 368–78.

Kobasa, S. C., Maddi, S. R. & Kahn, S. (1982). Hardiness and health: a prospective study. *Journal of Personality and Social Psychology*, **42**, 168–77.

Kolb, L. C. (1987). A neuropsychological hypothesis explaining posttraumatic stress disorders. *American Journal of Psychiatry*, **144**, 989–95.

Krause, N. (1987). Life stress, social support, and self-esteem in an elderly population. *Psychology and Aging*, **2**, 349–56.

Krause, N., Liang, J. & Yatoni, N. (1989). Satisfaction with social support and depressive symptoms: a panel analysis. *Psychology and Aging*, **4**, 88–97.

Lazarus, R. S. & Folkman, S. (1984). *Stress, Appraisal and Coping.* New York: Springer-Verlag.

Lazarus, R. S., DeLongis, A., Folkman, S. & Gruen, R. (1985). Stress and adaptational outcomes: the problem of confounded measures. *American Psychologist*, **40**, 770–9.

Lubin, B. & Rubio, C. T. (1985). Strain-producing aspects of life events. *Psychological Reports*, **57**, 259–62.

Mechanic, D. (1978). *Students under Stress: A Study in the Social Psychology of Adaptation.* Madison: University of Wisconsin Press.

Miller, P. McC. & Lloyd, C. (1991). Social support and its interaction with personality and childhood background as predictors of psychiatric symptoms in Scottish and American medical students. *Social Psychiatry and Psychiatric Epidemiology*, **26**, 171–7.

Miller, P. McC., Kreitman, N. B., Ingham, J. G. & Sashidharan, S. P. (1989). Self-esteem, life stress and psychiatric disorder. *Journal of Affective Disorder*, **17**, 65–75.

Mitchell, J. C. (ed.) (1969). *Social Networks and Urban Situations.* Manchester: Manchester University Press.

Monroe, S. M. (1983a). Major and minor life events as predictors of psychological distress: further issues and findings. *Journal of Behavioral Medicine*, **6**, 189–205.

Monroe, S. M. (1983b). Social support and disorder: toward an untangling of cause and effect. *American Journal of Community Psychology*, **11**, 81–97.

Monroe, S. M. & Steiner, S. C. (1986). Social support and psychopathology: interrelationships with pre-existing disorder, stress, and personality. *Journal of Abnormal Psychology*, **95**, 29–39.

Monroe, S. M., Bromet, E. J., Connell, M. M. & Steiner, S. C. (1986). Social support, life events, and depressive symptoms: a 1-year prospective study. *Journal of Consulting and Clinical Psychology*, **54**, 424–31.

Oatley, K. & Bolton, W. (1965). A social-cognitive theory of depression in reaction to life events. *Psychological Review*, **92**, 372–88.

Paykel, E. S. (1974). Life stress and psychiatric disorder: application of the clinical approach. In *Stressful Life Events: Their Nature and Effects*, ed. B. S. Dohrenwend & B. P. Dohrenwend, pp. 135–49. New York: Wiley.

Pearlin, L. I. (1983). Role strains and personal stress. In *Psychosocial Stress: Trends in Theory and Research*, ed. H. B. Kaplan, pp. 3–32. New York: Academic Press.

Pearlin, L. I. & Schooler, C. (1978). The structure of coping. *Journal of Health and Social Behavior*, **19**, 2–21.

Pearlin, L. I., Lieberman, M. S., Menagham, E. G. & Mullen, J. T. (1981). The stress process. *Journal of Health and Social Behavior*, **22**, 337–56.

Post, R. M. (1992). Transduction of psychosocial stress into the neurobiology of recurrent affective disorder. *American Journal of Psychiatry*, **149**, 999–1010.

Robins, C. J. (1990). Congruence of personality and life events in depression. *Journal of Abnormal Psychology*, **99**, 393–7.

Robins, C. J. & Block, P. (1988). Personal vulnerability, life events, and depressive symptoms: a test of a specific interactional model. *Journal of Personality and Social Psychology*, **54**, 847–52.

Smith, R. E., Johnson, J. H. & Sarason, I. G. (1978). Life change, the sensation seeking motive, and psychological distress. *Journal of Consulting and Clinical Psychology*, **46**, 348–9.

Snarey, J. R. & Vaillant, G. E. (1985). How lower- and working-class youth become middle-class adults: the association between ego defense mechanisms and upward social mobility. *Child Development*, **56**, 899–910.

Taylor, S. E. (1983). Adjustment to threatening events: a theory of cognitive adaptation. *American Psychologist*, **38**, 1161–73.

Thoits, P. A. (1983). Dimensions of life events that influence psychological

60   C. LLOYD

distress: an evaluation and synthesis of the literature. *Psychosocial Stress*, ed. H. B. Kaplan, pp. 33–103. New York: Academic Press.

Thoits, P. A. (1985). Social support and psychological well-being: theoretical possibilities. In *Social Support: Theory, Research and Application*, ed. I. G. Sarason & B. R. Sarason, pp. 51–72. The Hague: Martinus Nijhof.

Thoits, P. A. (1986). Social support as coping assistance. *Journal of Consulting and Clinical Psychology*, **59**, 416–23.

Vaillant, G. E. (1976). Natural history of male psychological health: V. The relation of choice of ego mechanisms of defense to adult adjustment. *Archives of General Psychiatry*, **33**, 535–45.

Vaillant, G. E., Bond, M. & Vaillant, C. O. (1986). An empirically validated hierarchy of defense mechanisms. *Archives of General Psychiatry*, **43**, 786–94.

Veiel, H. O. F. (1985). Dimensions of social support: a conceptual framework for research. *Social Psychiatry*, **20**, 156–62.

Zimmerman, M. (1983). Methodological issues in the assessment of life events: a review of the issues and research. *Clinical Psychology Review*, **3**, 339–70.

3

A developmental perspective on social support networks

LORNA CHAMPION

Despite the enormous amount of interest in the links between mental health and social support, a developmental perspective is sadly lacking. Most of the attention has been focused on cross-sectional associations at one point in time or, at best, longitudinal studies confined to a short period in one life stage. Adulthood has received the most attention, and indeed it will be the focus of this book; however, adulthood itself is a life stage in which development occurs. Too often the adult years are studied as though they were a uniform period where the myriad of crucial transitions between 18 and 60 are not considered.

This chapter will consider how supportive relationships develop from birth through to the adult years, focusing on how experiences in each preceding life stage influence what happens next. In this sense we will be concerned with social pathways through the life course. The aim is to consider social support as a developmental phenomenon in the hope that this can promote more effective understanding of the topic and facilitate better clinical research and intervention in the mental health field.

Social support from a developmental perspective: the individual, the environment and the interaction

The aim of this chapter is to take a life-span developmental perspective on the study of social support in all its aspects (Schulz & Rau, 1985; Thompson & Lamb, 1986; Baltes et al., 1980). The first task is to say something about what is meant by the concept of social support from this perspective. Definitions of social support are provided earlier in this volume. Within the context of a life-span developmental approach social support must be seen as having two major components which interact constantly throughout the life-span. The first component concerns the individual's own inner resources and characteristics which include both his or her physical characteristics and biological predisposition, and also

61

the cognitive capacity to acquire and organise a knowledge of self and others.

The individual's own internal representations or working models of relationships which are proposed to develop from birth onwards (Bowlby, 1988) are of importance here. At any one point in development these inner representations of experience are proposed to have the potential to guide the individual's future experience of relationships and influence the perception of those people encountered in his or her social world. The cognitive processes involved are discussed in the following chapter by Brewin.

The second component concerns the individual's external social environments; in other words, who is out there in the environment for them to meet and form potentially supportive relationships with. This external aspect will also include the vast range of actual experiences the individual has which involve other people. It is useful to think of this range of experiences as life events of both a normative and non-normative kind (Sugarman, 1986). Normative events are those which typically characterise a life stage, and although they may be stressful they are not necessarily negative; these events can also be called transitions (Hultsch & Deutsch, 1981). Examples in childhood would be birth of a sibling and starting school; in adulthood leaving home, marriage and becoming a parent are common examples. Non-normative events can be distinguished from normative events as being events that are not expected to happen when they do; they are often stressful and upsetting experiences (e.g. Brown & Harris, 1978). Examples of these events would be death of a parent in childhood, divorce and redundancy. Many events will involve the comings and goings of significant others in the social world. Some non-normative events such as the early loss or death of a parent may have a severe and long-lasting impact on subsequent experience. Alternatively, more normative events, such as starting school, can provide a welcome opportunity to make new friends. Each life stage will include a range of both normative and non-normative events and long-term experiences involving relationships. Our task in thinking about social support from a developmental perspective is to consider the impact of these experiences on the individual's social world and the likely risk of lasting change for the better or worse.

The interaction which takes place between the internal and external aspects outlined above will produce the level of social support that is assessed or measured at any one point in time. Because the focus of this chapter is on how social support develops and changes from birth through to adulthood, the challenge is to consider how internal representations of relationships, formed at an earlier stage, can go on to influence the external environment and, in turn, how the environment itself can influence the individual's view of relationships. The extent to which internal representations of relationships can be modified by later experience, both positive and negative, is a worthwhile topic for study and one which has considerable implications for therapeutic intervention; the reader is encouraged to consider this issue in relation to each life stage addressed in this chapter.

The importance of broad influences: sex, race, culture and class

Because of the importance of both individual predisposition and the external environment for the study of social support, its study presents a special challenge to the mental health researcher and practitioner. This challenge demands that the broad social influences on the development of social life are considered; these include sex, race, culture and class. We cannot ignore these influences in our assessment of how an individual's knowledge and experience of others operate to produce his or her own social support network. These broad influences are particularly important in the context of a developmental approach.

We need to consider where social support comes from. Different life domains will be important at different life stages and what these domains are will be influenced by the sex, culture and class of the individual or group we are concerned with. For example, Cohen & Wills (1985), in their review of the literature, conclude that women derive satisfaction from intimate, confiding relationships whereas men find satisfaction from relationships that involve taking part in social activities and accomplishing tasks. Asher *et al.* (1994) present some studies which indicate when such differential patterns may begin to emerge in children's peer relationships.

For adults, work is likely to be an important domain for men and for many women, depending on their life stage. Research has shown that work outside the home can offer protection against depression for women under stress (Brown & Harris, 1978; Warr & Parry, 1982). This finding may be due in part to the positive effect of work on social support.

For children and adolescents school will be an important domain to assess, while the family and peer relationships are likely to be important at all life stages and for both sexes. The relative emphasis placed on family as opposed to friends is likely to be greatly influenced by culture and class.

When social support is assessed in an adult the earlier influences of class, culture or race may not be obvious to a clinician or researcher. A person may have experienced much change and disruption in his or her social network. For example, there may have been a change of culture or a conflict of culture in the family; alternatively there may have been much upward or downward social mobility. Perhaps even more likely is that the person is from a social world which has expectations and patterns of relationships of which the observer has no knowledge or experience.

What is desirable and acceptable as social support is not uniform across social groups. If we ignore these differences we run the risk of offering intervention programmes which are doomed to failure because they are not acceptable to the group they set out to serve.

Attachment

In the spirit of a truly developmental approach, we must begin at the beginning with a consideration of the earliest relationships the infant develops. Attachment theory (e.g. Bowlby, 1980) and its recent developments (Bretherton, 1991) provide a rich and complex area to explore the origins of adaptive social functioning in later life. Indeed it was the impact of early family experience on later character development which provided the impetus for Bowlby's work in this area (Bretherton, 1991). Bowlby was highly critical of the trend in psychoanalysis at this time to focus exclusively on the patient's fantasy and ignore his or her real experiences in the social environment. He went to great lengths to emphasise the importance of the interactions between the organism and the environment. His idea that internal working models of relationships were built up by the infant from the earliest experience with the mother or primary caretaker was a major contribution. This idea, which has been developed by Bretherton (see Bretherton & Waters, 1985), provided the link between the internal and external worlds of the individual.

At the heart of attachment theory is the idea that the earliest attachment formed to the mother is the basis of all later intimate relationships (Bowlby, 1988). If this idea is correct then its implications for a developmental perspective on the adequacy of social support networks are enormous. At their most extreme the proponents of this view would argue that the first 2 years of life are the most important in determining the quality of later social relationships. Research taking a life-span perspective informs us that change for better or worse is always possible (Bowlby, 1988); what is essential is to look critically at what is meant by security of attachment and how this may manifest itself at different points in the life course.

Security of attachment is assessed using the Strange Situations Test. In this laboratory situation an infant (usually between the ages of 1 and 2 years) is left for about 3 minutes on two occasions with an unfamiliar person. How the child behaves during the separation periods and on reunion with the mother when she returns to the room is observed and assessed. The infant's security of attachment is then classified into one of three groups as follows.

Secure (group B). The infant shows signs of missing the parent on departure, seeks proximity upon reunion, and then returns to play. This pattern was associated with maternal sensitivity to infant signals and communications.

Insecure–avoidant (group A). The infant shows few or no signs of missing the mother and actively ignores her upon reunion. This pattern was associated with insensitivity to infant signals and rejection of attachment behaviour.

Insecure–ambivalent (group C). The infant is distressed and highly focused on the parent but cannot be settled by the parent on reunion; often anger is expressed and the infant fails to return to play. This pattern was found to be associated with maternal insensitivity and unpredictability of maternal responsiveness (Ainsworth *et al.*, 1978).

(A fourth insecure group (D) has recently been added to cover disorganised behaviour previously considered unclassifiable; see Main, 1991).

Longitudinal studies which examine the effects of the security of attachment on later functioning usually involve follow-up periods that are disappointingly short if a life-span perspective is required.

Thompson & Lamb (1986) review a range of studies indicating that secure attachment is generally associated with better social functioning in the preschool period. A range of outcome measures have been used including, for example, ego resiliency, sociability with peers, and dependency. Research by the Grossmanns in Germany (e.g. Grossmann & Grossmann, 1991) showed that secure attachment to both parents was a strong predictor of good peer relationships at age 5 years. Their research also showed that early security was reflected at age 10 years in a general confidence in oneself, one's friends and in potential supporters. They also point out that securely attached children were more likely to seek help and comfort, whereas avoidant children were more likely to get on on their own. Also, avoidant and insecurely attached children had fewer friends and more problems with being ridiculed and excluded by others in their peer group.

In this research attachment patterns were stable for over 80% of their sample over a 5 to 10 year period. The authors attribute this stability to the durability of cognitive structures established in the first year. They state that very early on cognitive structures are established on the basis of experience whereby the child learns which goals are worthy of pursuit; the Grossmanns argue that these structures, which can be termed inner working models, persist unchanged and are therefore not retested against experience. A mechanism is established whereby most expectation and social interaction produces experiences which are essentially self-fulfilling prophecies and thus serve merely to increase the stability of these mental models.

If such mental models are persistent, this research has enormous implications for understanding the picture of inadequate social support so prevalent among a psychiatric population. However, the Grossmanns point out that their data come from normal, fairly well adjusted, largely stable families. It is important to recognise that such samples are very different from the at-risk clinical groups that are of interest to us here; when children come from stable environments it is impossible to tease out the impact of early attachment experience from more recent positive experience. Furthermore, Kagan (1989) states that some investigators do not find stability of the attachment classification over the second year of life. In some studies, about one half of the children change their attachment classification during the second year (e.g. Thompson et al., 1982). This statement means that the concept of security of attachment and its measurement using the strange situation requires careful evaluation. It is premature to conclude that the foundation of a supportive social network is a secure attachment to parents in infancy.

Issues in assessing the impact of patterns of attachment on later social support networks

Thompson & Lamb (1986) also report that security of attachment is likely to vary with the degree of stress in the form of life events occurring in the infant's family; a higher level of stress is associated with a move from secure to insecure classifications. It is important to note that such high stress levels are much more common in socioeconomically disadvantaged families than in middle-class, stable families with two parents (e.g. Brown & Harris, 1978). Care must therefore be taken when generalising from the findings of studies using samples of stable, largely middle-class, educated, two-parent families.

We also need to consider the exact nature of the events the infant experiences and the likely effects on that particular individual. For example, Kagan (1989) reports that security of attachment can be affected by mothers returning to work and by the degree of psychopathology in the mother. It is of interest that Thompson et al. (1982) found that mothers returning to work and the introduction of non-maternal care were associated with bidirectional changes in attachment status; some infants shifted from securely to insecurely attached whereas others changes in the opposite direction. This finding draws attention to the need to consider the infant's actual day-to-day experience of care and who looks after them. It is not sufficient simply to assume that the mother is the caretaker.

Rutter has consistently pointed out since 1972 (e.g. Rutter, 1981) that it is the quality of care that a child receives that is important in determining the long-term effects on functioning. The long-term effects on the child of the presence or absence of the mother herself or any stress or separation that is experienced by the child will largely depend on how this stress is handled and how much disruption and discord the child is actually exposed to.

A retrospective study which aimed to explore the effects of early loss of mother on the risks for depression in women in adult life showed that it was not the experience of loss *per se* that determined the risk, but instead the quality of care that was received following the loss. It was the experience of lack of care that was the crucial factor in creating later risk for psychiatric disorder (Harris, *et al.*, 1986, 1987; Harris & Bifulco, 1991). How a child understands experiences of loss, disruption and conflict is therefore of great importance, and such understanding is likely to depend on the abilities and resilience of *both* the child and those who are in the role of carer to the child. As Thompson & Lamb (1986) conclude, 'it seems to be a combination of early attachment status in interaction with the quality and consistency of the caregiving environment over time that contributes to the prediction of later socioemotional behaviours' (p. 28).

Attachment studies have also been criticised in a number of other ways. For example, Kagan (1989) has drawn attention to the importance of temperament and socialisation practices in determining how an infant responds in the strange situation. He argues that both temperament and how a child has been socialised can have an effect on how the child copes in the strange situation, aside from the issues of attachment *per se*.

To address the issue of temperament first, Kagan (1989) points out that there are differences from birth between infants with regard to how they cope with frustration and the extent to which they react to change and stimulation. These temperamental differences have been shown to affect how the infants are classified on the strange situation test. The data available are at least suggestive of the hypothesis that the temperamental characteristics involving ease and the quality of arousal to unfamiliar events make some contribution to the classification of secure and insecure attachment. However, not all investigators would support this view (e.g. Sroufe, 1985).

Second, there is considerable evidence that infants from different cultural groups show different proportions in the three attachment categories and these differences can be linked to culturally different child rearing practices in the different groups (see Thompson & Lamb, 1986, for a review). We need to ask to what extent the infant's parents have encouraged self-reliance and the control of anxiety. If self-reliance has been encouraged, an avoidant classification is more likely.

Third, studies of the security of attachment in infancy have not paid attention to caretakers other than the parents – usually the mother. Ainsworth (1989, 1991) states that we know little about the role of parental surrogates, older siblings, grandparents, nannies, teachers and priests regarding their potential role in the development of internal working models of attachment. She states that this issue requires research and is likely to be especially important in at-risk groups who are less likely to have good relationships with parents. Some research evidence is suggestive of this effect in those at risk as a result of institutional care in childhood (see the Quinton and Rutter in-care study on positive school experiences described in the section on longitudinal studies, p. 83). One area of particular interest is the extent to which a good relationship with a father or significant other can compensate for a poor relationship with the mother. How much time the child is actually spending in the care of the mother herself should be considered. We know that a large proportion of mothers in the United Kingdom work, and that children are cared for by grandparents, other relatives, childminders and nannies for a large proportion of their waking hours. There have of course been historical changes in the extent of this practice, and to what extent and in what way it takes place will be influenced by the social class and culture of the individual concerned.

It is all these issues that the clinician or researcher should bear in mind when considering the development of social support networks over the life span in assessing the likely impact of experience on the individual or group of interest. It is indeed naive to assume that out of the myriad of experiences an infant or child can potentially receive from caretakers and significant others, it will internalise only that which is experienced with the mother. Further research is required to assess the validity of the assumptions made here. The implications for our understanding of how adequate social support develops and how it may be possible to influence this development by treatment or more naturalistic intervention are enormous.

For example, psychotherapy, via the importance of the relationship with the psychotherapist, has been assumed to provide an attachment-type relationship, possibly by providing a secure base (Ainsworth, 1991). However, it is unclear to what extent such psychotherapy may work to modify existing mental models of attachment relationships or to what extent new and different models are established. A major question relates to how powerful and enduring such hypothesised changes in mental models may be. Does it depend on the individual's life stage when the psychotherapy is received? How impervious are such changes to external stressors? Perhaps it is in this area that we shoud look to assess the effectiveness of psychotherapy and other treatment programmes. To state the aim more explicitly: To what extent do these treatments affect individuals' perceptions of their close relationships and their capacity to establish new relationships? How is any potential effect of the treatment demonstrated in an assessment of social support at a later point in the life course?

The issue of whether maladaptive mental models can be altered by later good experiences also poses the question of how other, more normative, non-professional relationships can have similar beneficial effects. Research we shall examine later (see the section on longitudinal studies, p. 81) certainly suggests the benefits of later good relationships in preventing continuities between poor relationships in childhood and poor relationships in adulthood.

The points that the reader should consider in pursuing further research or intervention studies on the long-term effects of attachment patterns can be summarised as follows:

1 The assessment of early attachment should include measures of the infant/child's social, physical and material environment as well as the attachment classification with mother and father.
2 The role and relative importance of other key caretakers apart from the parents should be considered.
3 Major stresses and changes which the infant and/or the family have been exposed to during the period of interest should be assessed for their impact on the infant/child.
4 Our knowledge of critical periods is at present inadequate. There is an assumption that working mental models laid down in the first year of life are more enduring and have greater implications for later functioning than models which may be established later on. This assertion requires more research.

Before moving away from studies of attachment we will consider research on intergenerational continuities in attachment patterns.

Studies of attachment and intergenerational continuities

The interest in patterns of attachment and the development of internal working models has led to an interest in the intergenerational transmission of relationship difficulties. According to attachment theory, parenting a child is likely to evoke problems in the parent's own childhood which have remained unresolved. How the parent deals with this difficult experience and understands it will determine the experience the new child receives. Indeed this whole area has produced research linking mothers' attachment patterns with those of their infants. There is now some evidence that how a mother describes her own relationships with her parents is related to the pattern of attachment her child has with her (Main & Goldwyn, 1984; Main *et al.*, 1985).

The development of the Adult Attachment Interview (AAI) (Main, 1991) has provided an instrument to examine adults' internal working models of attachment relationships. Links with the individual's parenting have been made. Recent research using a prospective study design has shown that first-time mothers' responses on the AAI predict patterns of attachment in their own infants when they are 1 year old (Fonagy et al., 1991). Similar results were also found for fathers when the infants were 18 months old. The authors claim that the observed concordance between the parents' security and the infant's security was due, at least in part, to the capacity for self-reflection in the parents.

It is most important to point out at this stage that this work is not suggesting that a straightforward relationship exists between the parents' experience in their own childhood and their infant's experience a generation later. Instead, what is of greater importance is how the parents have understood their experience as a child and been able to integrate this understanding into a working model of relationships which can, in turn, benefit them in their interactions with their own infant. This point is important because these researchers, along with others who have conducted similar work, have found that good functioning on the AAI indicating security of attachment is not always associated with good experiences of care in childhood (Main, 1991; Fonagy et al., 1991). What is more important is the individual's capacity to reflect on his or her experience and talk openly and coherently about it. At present we know little about what factors contribute to this capacity and this is likely to be an important area of future research.

Studies that have examined the links between attachment in childhood and the quality of social support in adult life

A range of studies have addressed the association between attachment problems in childhood and the quality of social support in adult life (see Parker et al., 1992, for a review). While there appears to be some relationship, the links are by no means straightforward. Most studies have assessed childhood attachment retrospectively using the Parental Bonding Instrument (Parker et al., 1979; Wilhelm & Parker, 1988). This instrument is a 25 item self-report questionnnaire asking subjects to rate their parents as they remembered them in their first 16 years. Although the instrument has good reliability and validity, the retrospective nature of the data obtained does present a problem regarding a general negative response bias. It is nevertheless of interest that in several normal samples of adults links were found between poor relationships in childhood and the quality of current intimate relationships (Flaherty & Richman, 1986; Parker & Barnett, 1988).

One interesting study examined the links between scores on the

Parental Bonding Instrument and the quality of the marital relationship in a sample of Canadian adults attending a health centre (Truant *et al.*, 1987). They found that poor marital quality was linked with low care ratings on the Parental Bonding Instrument in the case of the 'least caring parent' as defined by the respondent (50% fathers, 40% mothers, 10% others). This finding applied most clearly for female respondents even when neurotic symptoms were controlled for; in fact the association between childhood experience and adult marital dissatisfaction was stronger for those who had not had psychiatric disorder or a previously broken marriage. Flaherty & Richman (1986) also examined the effects of major separations in childhood and found that it was in the group of females who had experienced such separations that the associations between the quality of childhood relationships and adult marriage were the strongest (correlations of 0.7 and 0.8 were obtained). They concluded that negative experiences in childhood such as separation may have more potent effects on adult functioning in marriage than coexisting good experiences in childhood. However, this rather pessimistic conclusion requires further research on larger and more representative samples, preferably using prospective rather than retrospective designs.

This study also suggests that one hypothesis worthy of further investigation is that poor relationships with parents in childhood are most likely to exert an effect on later marital quality when there has also been childhood adversity such as parental separation.

It is clear that the links between childhood experiences of parenting and patterns of attachment in adult life are not straightforward. All studies that rely on retrospective recall are likely to be difficult to interpret, although there is perhaps reason to regard retrospective reports as more reliable than was previously thought (see Brewin *et al.*, 1993, for a review).

Before moving on from the significance of early attachment for later functioning, one study worthy of special consideration will be outlined. This prospective study involved a long-term follow-up spanning almost 40 years on 62 men and women studied from infancy as part of the Berkeley Guidance Study (Skolnick, 1986). The original sample of 124 included every third child born in Berkeley, California, in 1928 and 1929. Security of attachment to the mother was assessed for the 21 to 30 month age period. The assessment was based on detailed transcripts of interviews and extensive observation in the subject's home. In addition careful assessment was made of the subject's peer relationships in early childhood (ages 6–8 years), late childhood (9–11 years), early adolescence (12–14 years), and late adolescence (15–18 years). The subjects were then assessed in adulthood (age 30 and 40 years) to assess sociability, marital satisfaction and psychological health (see Skolnick, 1986, for details).

The results showed that security of attachment in infancy was significantly correlated with the quality of peer relationships in childhood in girls and with adult sociability in men. Security of attachment was not correlated with the quality of peer relationships in adolescence, nor with marital satisfaction and psychological health in adulthood for either sex.

Skolnick (1986) also analysed the data by charting each individual on a series of paths across the four life periods assessed (infancy, childhood, adolescence and adulthood). It is of interest that the two most common paths were those denoting all positive (+ + + +) or all negative (− − − −) assessments. However, the third most common path was − + + +, namely a negative rating on attachment in infancy and then positive ratings from childhood onwards. This study does seem to indicate that early attachment is not the only indicator of adaptive social functioning throughout the life span but, in addition, that childhood peer relations may be an equally or possibly more appropriate focus for future study and intervention.

Childhood

The study by Skolnick (1986) outlined in the previous section has already indicated the likely importance of childhood peer relationships as an indicator of good social support in adulthood. She found that the quality of childhood peer relationships predicted adult psychological health in the total sample. Also the quality of childhood peer relationships strongly predicted adolescent peer relationships for both males and females, which in turn predicted psychological health and the quality of social relationships in adulthood, including marital satisfaction.

Ainsworth (1989) has also drawn attention to the importance of childhood peer relationships. She speculates about the extent to which friends can provide attachment-type relationships, especially in early childhood. We know that some early friendships are enduring and have the quality of attachment relationships, but we do not know why or how some relationships develop in this way and others do not. Ainsworth (1989) states that in view of the fact that most 4-year-olds have developed sufficient capacity for cognitive perspective taking and communication to establish goal-corrected partnerships with attachment figures, it is interesting that 6- to 8-year-olds are apparently unable to do this with friends. She goes on to say that such a capacity may be masked by the fact that metacognitive ability is not sufficiently developed in children under the age of about 12 years to enable them to reflect about relationships in an interview situation, nor to articulate subtle feelings and attitudes that have been implicit from a much younger age.

Asher et al. (1994) note that it is possible to observe the affective functions of these early friends although these functions cannot be verbalised. Perhaps the lesson to learn from this is that it is easy to underestimate the importance of children's friendships in promoting adaptive working models of supportive social relationships. Once again it is important to bear in mind the possibility that for certain socially deprived or disadvantaged children peers may replace what most children obtain from parents or close relatives.

It is important to think about where we might start in considering the development of adaptive friendships. As early as age 2 years co-operative play is apparent: there is more turn taking and complementary and reciprocal behaviour. Also, imitation appears to be a major strategy for learning how to interact with peers before the development of language (Asher *et al.*, 1994).

So far in our consideration of the early development of the capacity to form satisfactory relationships we have not considered the importance of support functions (introduced in earlier chapters). Most of the work on attachment is generally assumed to relate to the capacity to form intimate relationships which would include confiding. Such relationships are most often formed with a partner, usually of the opposite sex. However, much of the work on social support in adult life, especially in relation to psychiatric disorder, has examined the importance of a range of support functions, which are based on the original work of Robert Weiss (e.g. Weiss, 1974). In this scheme intimacy is usually referred to as *emotional support*. While this is a key support function and one that is likely to be particularly crucial in protecting against the effects of stress in those vulnerable to psychiatric disorder, it is not the only function of importance (Wills, 1985; Champion & Goodall, 1994).

The other support functions that need to be considered are: *instrumental support*, also called practical support, and *social companionship*, which is the experience of being with known others while engaging in an activity, often for pleasure. In addition to these three 'core' functions Wills (1985) has drawn attention to *informational support* and *motivational support*. Informational support involves the provision of information, advice and guidance and, of course, specialist knowledge which may be crucial to enable an individual to function in a particular peer group. Motivational support includes the provision of encouragement to pursue a certain goal, to take one course of action rather than another and to sustain an activity in the face of difficulty or resistance.

Once we move into the realm of childhood friendships the provision of each of these functions begins to assume its place. From early childhood *peer relationships* have the potential to provide all of these functions. The extent to which each is more or less important will vary according to the age and sex of the child (see Asher *et al.*, 1994, for a review). We know that children learn to both offer and receive each of the support functions outlined above with their friends. In childhood, friends, rather than family, are more likely to emphasise the need for reciprocity in the distribution of rewards and obligation (Newcomb *et al.*, 1979). We know that in adult social relationships the presence of 'caring debts' in which reciprocity has not been possible can be a major source of stress (Pearlin, 1985). Such a situation is particularly likely to occur for those individuals who are not in a good position to reciprocate (such as the psychiatrically ill) and may be particularly likely to occur with a professional involved in their care over an extended period. Parry (1988) points out that the low self-esteem of depressed patients may lead them to focus excessively on the negative aspects of receiving support. These negative aspects are likely to include an assumption that they will be unable to repay any caring debts that accumulate. If a depressed patient thinks in this way, it is likely to interfere adversely with his or her ability to mobilise support or accept the support that is offered.

To consider when in an individual's life such a negative set of beliefs develops and in what way, would be a valuable source of information for prevention and intervention. What we know little about is how children develop the skills necessary to form relationships with their peers which are adaptive and satisfying to them, such as the skills involved in acquiring reciprocity in a relationship. Also we know little about how these early experiences of friendships influence the quality of social support received at later life stages such as adolescence and adulthood.

Simple questions that can be asked about the importance of childhood peer relationships for later social support could include the following:

Are those children who have very limited opportunity to form peer relationships adversely affected by this lack of opportunity in their ability to form relationships in adult life?

Is an early start, for example, extensive preschool experience of peers, an advantage in influencing the quality of social support in adult life, especially in those at risk?

To what extent can good peer relationships substitute for the lack of support functions from parents and family and, conversely, to what extent can family, such as siblings, substitute for the lack of peer relationships?

Do patterns of relating persist from childhood into adulthood? For example, if a child has been unsuccessful in forming satisfying peer relationships in childhood, does this pattern persist in adulthood?

It would seem likely that the reason for the lack of successful peer relationships would be crucial in determining whether the pattern persists, but this is a question for further research. Parker & Asher (1987) suggest that children who are actively rejected rather than neglected by their peers are most at risk for adult dysfunction. Asher *et al.* (1994)

review a range of studies which indicate that the type of peer relationship difficulty experienced in childhood may determine the particular pathway observed in terms of adult functioning. For example, the experience of loneliness without aggression or active rejection from peers may be associated with 'internalising difficulties' such as depression and anxiety. In contrast, more aggressive children who experience rejection by their peers are less likely to report loneliness but instead tend towards a pathway characterised by conduct disorder, delinquency and crime; in other words 'externalising' difficulties (Parker & Asher, 1987; Kupersmidt *et al.*, 1990; Rubin *et al.*, 1990).

Some studies have addressed directly the relationship between children's peer relationships and later functioning. Asher *et al.* (1994) report on a range of studies which show that poor acceptance by peers is strongly associated with dropping out of school early (Parker & Asher, 1987; Asher & Parker, 1989). Also mental health problems in adulthood are associated with a higher incidence of poor peer relationships in childhood. However, it is misleading to suggest that there is a consistent or simple relationship between poor peer relationships in childhood and later problems. While most adults showing difficulties in adulthood had peer relationship difficulties in childhood, many of those children who show poor peer relationships in childhood do not show later problems. We do not know what factors determine which pathway a child will take.

The lack of continuity for some children could be a result of the intervention of more positive experiences in the normal life course. For others it may have more to do with the inner development of the individual towards either greater health or greater disorder.

There is a great deal of interesting research on how children develop social skills and competencies to lead to either greater acceptance or rejection by their peers (Asher *et al.*, 1994). There is not space here to consider this literature, but it is likely to be invaluable to those concerned with elucidating the development of processes by which individuals come to have satisfying or unsatisfying social networks in adult life. For example, Asher *et al.* (1994) present evidence from a range of studies which indicate that better-accepted children demonstrate the capacity to coordinate multiple goals which may at times conflict with each other. Other behaviours demonstrated by such children include more prosocial and co-operative play and more active interactions which are longer in duration (they are less likely to terminate interactions and when they experience ambiguous provocation by a peer they are more likely to respond by asking the peer for clarification). Better-accepted children are also more likely to exhibit mastery-orientated responses when they face social disappointment.

Research which focuses on the social cognitive processes that may determine behavioural differences observed in children who are well accepted by their peers compared with those who are not may also be valuable to researchers interested in taking a developmental perspective on social support in adulthood. One aspect of this research, which may be particularly interesting to pursue in intervention studies, relates to the finding of Dodge (1980) that low-accepted aggressive children tend to attribute hostility to their peers. Asher *et al.* (1994) relate this finding to attribution theory; they state that the attribution a child makes for another's intention will affect his or her expectation of the other's behaviour and their own behaviour. However, it is also possible to relate this finding to the psychoanalytic mechanism of projection and in so doing place the mechanism in a developmental context.

The argument here would be that internalised aspects of self and significant others are the basis for understanding others (cf. Bowlby, 1988). Hence, these internalised aspects are projected onto others as a means of understanding the other's expected and actual behaviour. The consequence of this process is that if a child's understanding of others is dominated by an aggressive internal model this will be the way they will understand others and determine their expectation of those others. Conversely, if a child has internalised a more co-operative, less threatening view of others, possibly as a result of more positive early experiences of relationships, then that child will, in turn, expect peers to behave in a more cooperative, less aggressive way. It is not difficult to see how the projection of such a view could lead to all relationships conforming to the original pattern, either by selecting out certain individuals or by evoking a certain type of response from others. While these ideas will be familiar to those who work within dynamic psychotherapy (e.g. Brown & Peddar, 1991), they have yet to gain a place in our understanding of the literature on social support.

Our goal here is to examine social support developmentally, so if we consider intervention studies in childhood to enable low-accepted children to make more appropriate attributions for the behaviour of their peers, we need to think about how these problems may manifest themselves later on in adult life. In other words, is the intervention likely to have lasting effects and if so why? Intervention studies which aim to help vulnerable adults to form satisfying relationships will need to address the internal working models of their clients that have served to create, at least in part, the interpersonal patterns that may have been a problem throughout much of their life. One crucial aspect which is likely to have implications through the life course relates to how individuals come to form appropriate interpersonal goals and plans and how they can pursue these effectively. Such processes will relate not only to how an individual forms an understanding of others but also to how they set about finding suitable others and focusing their attention on pursuing goals with one peer as opposed to another. The issue of choice of peers assumes even greater importance in adolescence. However, the consideration of childhood peer relationships presented here should have highlighted that this process starts early on.

A number of studies have indicated that in middle childhood children already show differences in the types of interpersonal goal to which they give priority. For example, Renshaw & Asher (1983) found that low-accepted 8- to 11-year-old children proposed fewer prosocial goals in hypothetical situations (e.g. entering a group) than their better-accepted peers. Wentzel (1991) examined the goals of children (aged 11–12) of various levels of acceptance by asking them how often they tried to pursue a range of prosocial goals (e.g. 'How often do you try to help other kids when they have a problem?') and social interaction goals (e.g. 'How often do you try to be with other kids rather than by yourself?'). Better-accepted children reported trying to achieve social interaction and prosocial goals significantly more often than did the low-accepted children. These results suggest that better-accepted children place higher priority on relationship-orientated goals, given that they appear to pursue such goals with greater frequency, whereas low-accepted children give relationship-orientated goals relatively lower priority (Asher *et al.*, 1994).

These findings may be useful regarding the apparent importance of planning for relationships in at-risk groups (see the Quinton & Rutter study outlined in the section on longitudinal studies, p. 83). At present we know very little about when and how children learn to plan. Adolescence is likely to be a crucial period for the study of planning for relationships, because at this life stage an individual's peer group has been shown to be particularly influential in determining what behaviour that individual engages in. For example, research in criminality has consistently demonstrated that peers play an influential role in causing an individual to engage in delinquent behaviour and that breaks with a delinquent peer group may markedly reduce offending (Farrington, 1986; West, 1982).

Adolescence

The importance of adolescence as a bridge between childhood and adulthood has already been referred to in several places in this chapter. The results from the study by Skolnick (1986) outlined in the section on attachment above suggest that the quality of relationships in adolescence is likely to indicate the quality of relationships in adulthood. This result suggests that adolescence may be a good time to target intervention studies which address the formation of adaptive and positive social relationships. This is clearly a question which research on social support needs to address. It has already been established that the links between relationship problems in childhood and adulthood are not straightforward. Indeed, much research has demonstrated that determining continuities and discontinuities in development is a highly complex task and that pathways can be straight or highly devious (see Robins & Rutter, 1990). There is not space here to review all the literature on social support in adolescence. Instead this life stage will be considered in relation to its likely effects on the pathway between childhood and adulthood.

Adolescence can be regarded as the second normal individuation, or major task in establishing the self, that needs to take place for normal development to proceed (Blos, 1967). The first individuation occurs between the second and third year of life when there is the attainment of a separation in perception between the self and other. Blos argues that both periods have in common a heightened vulnerability of the personality organisation, and a common urgency for change in which a maturational surge forward takes place. This conceptualisation is useful to us here as we can consider how this process is likely to affect the social support an individual has and the likely consequences for adult social networks. If we accept Blos's notion, then one of the main tasks of adolescence is to disengage from the parents as the main objects with which to identify and to establish new, namely extrafamilial love objects in the outside world. To put this in more everyday terms, the task is to establish one's own identity as distinct or different from the parents.

A principal task of adolescence is not merely to substitute or replicate what one has had before with the parents, but instead to establish a new, unique self or ego. This process will produce vulnerability because it necessitates giving up the parental ego which, until now, has been a legitimate extension of the child's own ego (Blos, 1967). While establishing one's own identity will touch on many areas of life, relationships usually occupy centre stage for the adolescent. Peer relationships are likely to assume greater importance, hence the peer group in which an individual exists or selects himself or herself into is likely to have an effect on the individual's subsequent development and choices – as has been demonstrated by many investigators (e.g. Magnusson et al., 1986; West, 1982).

However, some changes in peer group and social affiliation in adolescence may only be temporary, rather like experiments carried out to see what happens, rather than choices which produce lasting change. But, conversely, such changes in peer group or behaviour can lead to more lasting change where choices are reduced and the route out proves too demanding for the individual to follow successfully (teenage pregnancy is one such example). It is, therefore, important to consider not only the individual's peer group but also the other resources available to him or her. Such resources could include his or her own inner capacity to cope with stress, and the support he or she may or may not have from the family. Can such resources help the individual if adolescent 'experiments' cause too much anxiety or potentially negative consequences such as a drug overdose, an unwanted pregnancy or dropping out of school? For an individual who has good support from the family or other social network members such situations may not present any long-term disadvantages. When considering the inner resources of the individual it may be helpful to look back at experiences in infancy and childhood. Blos (1967) puts it thus: 'When the psychological navel cord has to be cut in adolescence, children with early ego damage fall back on a defective psychic structure that is totally inadequate to the task of the adolescent individuation process' (p. 176). Unfortunately, research tells us that it is those least able to cope with stress as a result of adverse childhood experience who are likely to receive more than their fair share of it. At this point some research findings from studies that have focused their interest on adolescence will be considered.

Magnusson *et al.* (1986) conducted a longitudinal study to examine the effect of early puberty on later social adjustment in adulthood. The sample consisted of a complete school year cohort in a Swedish town where less than 1% of children did not attend the ordinary school system. The results of this study showed that while the early-maturing girls did violate norms significantly more often than late-maturing girls, this effect was mediated entirely through the peer group. Early-maturing girls had an older peer group. For those girls who reported having no older friends, there was no significant difference in norm-breaking among the menarcheal groups of girls. When the cohort was followed up when aged 26 years no difference was found in alcohol use between the early- and late-maturing girls. Although the early-maturing girls had started drinking earlier, the late-maturers had caught up. However, there was a significant difference between the two groups regarding educational attainment in adulthood. The early-maturing girls were less likely to have pursued any further education beyond compulsory schooling than the late-maturing girls, despite there being no difference between the two groups in general intelligence or their parents' educational status. Magnusson *et al.* (1986) stated that:

> the lower educational level among the menarcheal groups of girls at adulthood can be seen in part as a function of the greater influence of the peer culture (especially older peers) on the early-developed girls in the adolescent years. Devoting more time to steady contacts with boys and to more intimate relations (sexual intercourse), viewing themselves as more mature and wanting to bring up their own children, the early developed girls are more likely to engage in activities such as family life than to aspire to higher education compared to the late-maturing girls. (p. 168)

This study is informative in that it demonstrates well the interaction between the individual's own internal characteristics and the environment at a variety of points in the life course, and how this interaction can affect what is observed. However, it is important to point out that this study did not directly address the links between the quality of social support in the two groups in adolescence and adulthood. In contrast to the psychiatric samples which are of most interest to us here, this sample was a normal cohort of girls. It is possible to speculate that in a more deprived sample with fewer economic and social resources early norm-breaking, earlier entry into family life and fewer formal educational qualifications could increase the risk of depression and inadequate social support so often seen in psychiatric services (Cohen & Wills, 1985). However, the study emphasises the importance of peer influences on the experiences an adolescent has and how these experiences can influence what happens next to that individual.

Another study worthy of consideration here was conducted by Kandel & Davies (1986). In this study the sequelae of depressed mood and the quality of family relationships were examined in a sample of New York school children when they were aged 15–16 years and again 9 years later when they were 24–25 years old. The results showed that the adolescents who were distant from their parents became those young adults who were distant from their spouses or partners. Kandel & Davies stated:

> There appeared to be a carryover or transfer phenomenon, with individuals reproducing within the marital family the types of interactions they experienced with their parents and especially parents of the opposite sex. The phenomenon was exacerbated if distance from the opposite-sex parent was accompanied by dysphoria. These data provide some evidence for the basic psychoanalytic tenet that individuals reproduce in their important interpersonal relationships patterns of behaviour they first learned from their parents. (p. 261)

Unfortunately for our purposes here the results presented provided little information on the links between quality of peer relationships in adolescence and adulthood, although measures were taken. The authors do state that adolescent depressive affect did not seem to affect the individual's ability to maintain a circle of male and female close friends, although there is no mention of the quality of these relationships. A later report on this study (Kandel et al., 1990) presents a detailed analysis of homophily, or the extent to which individuals pair with others like themselves, in relationships in both adolescence and adulthood in this sample. The results showed that individuals in intimate relationships tend to share certain characteristics and attitudes. For example, ethnicity, education, drug use, religion, closeness of relationships to parents, peer orientation and leisure activities all showed concordance in adolescence and in adulthood. However, the results also demonstrated that individuals vary in the extent to which they seek to affiliate with others like themselves. This variation in the degree of homophily is fairly consistent between adolescence and adulthood.

The authors state that a tolerance for others similar to or different from oneself or lack of such tolerance is a stable trait. However, it is important to recognise that homophily as measured in this study contains two components that cannot be estimated separately: dyads form because of similarity, and dyads may grow more similar over time. The continuity from adolescence to adulthood reflects both processes. When considering the social support networks of adults, especially those with psychiatric disorder, it may be useful to consider first the extent to which they have sought out or are attracted to others like themselves, and second what their explanation of this may be. Information such as this may be very useful when considering what advice or intervention would be most suitable. For example, an intervention study set up to improve the social networks of isolated depressed mothers in a new town found that there was considerable variation amongst the women with regard to whether they wished to be placed in a self-help group with other women like themselves. Some women welcomed this opportunity while others did not. Those who were keen on being with others like themselves were, not surprisingly, able to benefit more from the intervention than those who were not keen. For these latter women individual treatment was more appropriate (Champion, 1985). However, this generalisation and use of the data presented above could be harmful for some individuals. The negative consequence of a tendency to seek others like oneself on certain characteristics must be considered. If an adolescent has difficulties in relating to others, tends towards aggressive behaviour, or has other serious problems, the tendency to seek out similar others is likely only to create further stress for the individual concerned. For someone like this an intervention which aimed to address the possible negative effects of tending to seek out others with similar problems may be the most helpful course. In addition any life change, naturally occurring or imposed by treatment, which serves to break the individual's links with a peer group in which negative traits and behaviour (e.g. see Kirke, this volume) are perpetuated is likely to be helpful. We will examine a range of studies that have addressed this issue in the next section.

Longitudinal studies that have indirectly addressed social support across the life span and their implications for future research

Research studies that examine social relationships across the life span, including assessments in both childhood and adulthood, are rare. Even

rarer are studies that have directly addressed social support and drawn
on the modern conceptualisations presented in this volume and elsewhere
(e.g. Champion & Goodall, 1994). The study of social support and its
relation to psychiatric disorder is relatively recent, beginning in the
1970s. Thus if longitudinal studies are prospective, the early phases of
data collection are likely to have preceded the beginning of a serious
interest in this topic. However, in spite of this problem longitudinal
research on mental health does seem to have ignored social support. A
recent and highly influential volume (Robins & Rutter, 1990) on
research addressing the links between adaptive functioning in childhood
and adult life makes no direct references to social support; the term does
not even appear in the index. The aim of this section is to draw the
reader's attention to some influential studies that take a life-span
perspective on adaptive functioning in adulthood and to consider what
they tell us about social support from a developmental perspective. This
task has already been attempted elsewhere in the context of the transition
to early adult life (Maughan & Champion, 1990).

One rich data set which has already been referred to in the section on
attachment above (Skolnick, 1986) has also been examined in a variety of
different ways by a number of other investigators. For example, Elder (e.g.
1979, 1986) combined data from two cohorts of individuals (the Berkeley
and Oakland cohorts) born in the 1920s just 8 years apart. One aim of this
research was to demonstrate the impact of historical events, in this case the
great depression of the 1930s, on individual life histories. Because the two
cohorts were of different ages, they experienced the stressful impact of the
depression at different points in the life course. The younger Berkeley
cohort experienced the worst stress while still in childhood, whereas the
older Oakland cohort had by this time reached adolescence. What is of
interest to us here is how relationships emerged as crucial in moderating
the impact of the stress experienced and how this effect depended on the
life stage of the sample in question when the stress occurred. One
important finding was that a good relationship with the parent of the same
sex in childhood prior to the impact of the stress of economic hardship
protected against the negative effects on adolescent functioning. A poor
father–son relationship seemed to be particularly important in determining
an incompetent self in adolescence amongst boys, regardless of economic
deprivation. The importance of the same-sex parent as a role model for this
younger cohort was emphasised by Elder (1979). In contrast the older
cohort seemed less adversely affected by such relationships, but instead the
impact on their functioning was determined by the role they were able to
take within the family and perhaps more generally. Unfortunately the role
of peers was not assessed, but our assessment of research on adolescence
suggests that for this older group peer influences may have become more
important than parental role models.

Elder (1986) also found that many of the younger boys who appeared passive and indecisive in adolescence had achieved the highest level of self-competence by the age of 40 years. This discontinuity was attributed by Elder (1986) to the importance of military service for this vulnerable group. A high proportion of the deprived boys took this opportunity and most had done so by the age of 21. For this group military service was a way to break with the family and offered a whole range of new opportunities including the increased chance of a college education. However, one aspect which should not be overlooked is the potential this opportunity provided to alter the individual's social support network by providing a new set of positive role models and a wider range of peers to choose from with a range of different expectations and aspirations (Elder, 1986). What this research suggests is that later positive experiences can reverse apparently negative pathways between childhood and adulthood. To what extent this is due to the environment providing a wide choice of peers or role models and to what extent it depends on the individual's inner capacity to exploit the opportunities made available is an important question for future research.

Another prospective study addressed a group at risk as a result of extended periods of institutional care in childhood. A central concern was to assess the implications of an institutional upbringing for the women's own later skills as a parent; however, a broad range of outcome measures were used including functioning in a range of relationships (Quinton & Rutter, 1988; Quinton *et al.*, 1984). Females and males were also compared with a control group brought up in their own families who came from the same part of inner London as the institution-reared group (Rutter *et al.*, 1990). The individuals in this study had been placed in care as children because of parenting breakdown or because they were being reared in severely disrupted families. Many of the sample entered institutional care before the age of 2 years and remained in care until at least the age of 16 years. These children often experienced more than 50 different caretakers during their time in care. Although social support *per se* was not a focus of this study, it is clear that family relationships were likely to have been poor for this institution-reared group; there was little or no opportunity for stable relationships to form.

In early adult life the ex-care group showed a lower level of functioning on a range of psychosocial measures: the quality and availability of love relationships, marriage and friendships. The ex-care group also showed significantly more psychiatric disorder, criminality, poorer performance in the domain of work and in their independent living conditions (see Rutter *et al.*, 1990, for details). However, for both men and women, just over a fifth of the ex-care group showed good functioning.

Factors associated with good outcome in the ex-care group will now be considered in turn. Good marital support from a non-deviant spouse stood out as the factor associated with a powerful protective effect for both men and women in the ex-care group. Although in the accounts of this research marital support is not termed social support, the terms can be regarded as equivalent. Marital support included the presence of a harmonious marital relationship with demonstrated warmth and definite confiding. Indeed this definition would classify as good emotional support in a more traditional social support framework (Champion & Goodall, 1993).

How did some members of this at-risk group come to have this good supportive relationship in the first place? Quinton & Rutter point to the importance of two other factors: positive school experiences and planning for relationships and, to a lesser extent, planning for work. For the ex-care group those who had positive school experiences were more likely to plan for their transition into marriage and were consequently more likely to end up with a non-deviant, supportive spouse. The effect here was much clearer for women than for men. Rutter *et al.* (1990) concluded that the women may have been more important in the processes leading to selection of a marital partner. This conclusion was drawn because the ex-care men were less likely than the ex-care women to marry a deviant spouse, and their own planning style seemed to play a lesser role in marital choice. It is important to note that in this study positive school experiences, planning and a supportive partner all exerted an independent effect in producing a more positive outcome for the ex-care group but not for the control group. The explanation presented for this differential effect between the ex-care group and the controls was that the controls already had a range of alternative sources of self-worth whereas for the ex-care group a positive school experience may have been the factor that made the crucial difference in determining whether an individual felt able then to influence what happened next for him or her and so avoid the likelihood of a negative outcome.

There seems little doubt that the control group had what would be regarded as a better and more protective social support network around them. Most of this group were living in relatively stable families and many would have had the benefit of help from older siblings and relatives outside the immediate family. One of the most important findings from this research is how those who were raised in care were then, on leaving care, likely to return to discordant families and to have little or no social support. Indeed all the support functions, both emotional and practical, likely to be important in helping with the demanding transition to adult life, were likely to be lacking for this group. The research also shows that those whose parenting was disrupted in the first 2 years of life showed the worst outcomes in adulthood. Rutter *et al.* (1990) suggest that this was because secure parent–child attachments were not formed in this group. Similarly, a longitudinal study by Hodges & Tizard (1989), which examined the long-term effects of early institutional rearing, showed that the adverse effects on relationship formation and satisfaction persisted to some extent even when the children spent the later years of their childhoods in stable, supportive and harmonious families.

An important point from considering the results of the Quinton & Rutter study is the extent to which good social support in one domain may have the potential to offset disadvantage in those at risk. Positive school experiences and the capacity to plan may well have resulted from the presence of one or more positive relationships at school or the presence of a positive role model in the form of a teacher or peer – a potentially fruitful avenue for future research. Indeed, such a research effort could be extended to adults at risk, such as those recovering from mental illness, who embark on further education or job training.

The issue of pregnancy in women at risk needs to be addressed also. A range of research studies have shown that those women who are at risk as a result of early disruption in relationships are more likely to get pregnant early. Rutter & Quinton point out that an unwanted pregnancy for the ex-care women was often the reason for marrying a deviant spouse and so ending up with an unsupportive marital relationship. A similar pattern was observed in a retrospective study of a group of working-class women who had experienced lack of adequate parental care in childhood (Harris *et al.*, 1986, 1987; Harris & Bifulco, 1991). Those women who had experienced lack of adequate parental care following loss of mother due to death or separation were much more likely to experience a premarital pregnancy, to go on to have an unsupportive marital relationship and to become clinically depressed. This pattern of a continued chain of adversity was much more common in working-class than middle-class women in this sample. Harris *et al.* (1986) present a model to explain their findings which includes a consideration both of how the inner resources of the individual are depleted by the early lack of care and how the external environment also continues to be adverse and stressful as a result of this lack of care. In adulthood, with the occurrence of a premarital pregnancy and marriage to an unsupportive partner, the two strands, inner and outer, become inextricably linked to result in the pattern of clinical depression so often seen in working-class women with young children at home (cf. Brown & Harris, 1978).

Another way of explaining this and other findings would be in terms of the adequacy of the individual's social network. Poor-quality relationships in childhood predispose to poor-quality relationships later on in the life span. As already suggested above, both the inner resources of the individual and the properties of the external environment are likely to be involved in the genesis of this state of affairs (Maughan & Champion,

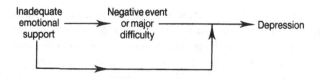

Figure 3.1. The effect of inadequate social support both on the occurrence of negative events and difficulties and on depression.

1990). The prospective follow-up study of adolescence conducted by Kandel & Davies (1986) already outlined above produced the interesting finding that those adolescent females in the sample who were depressed went on to have more children by the age of 25 years than the non-depressed adolescents. The authors point out that this result suggests that the cause of the depression so often seen in young women with children may not be due mainly to current stress, as has been suggested by many investigators (e.g. Brown & Harris, 1978). Instead it could be a result of earlier depression, which in some way contributed to the stress that is observed. They suggest that children may represent an attempt by depressed young women to increase their sense of connectedness to and intimacy with others in their social network.

These findings indicate that stress and social support are linked in a complex interrelationship throughout the life span. The linking of the two concepts in this way, where a lack of support generates stress and stress in turn reduces support, can easily be overlooked in cross-sectional studies. For example, the finding that good emotional support from a partner is protective against the onset of depression in women in the face of a severely threatening life event (e.g. Brown & Harris, 1978) has been replicated in many similar studies (see Brown & Harris, 1986). However, an alternative model in which the lack of support also contributes to the presence of the stressor in the first place has also been shown to be valid by a re-analysis of the data from the studies demonstrating the link between stress and the onset of depression (Champion, 1990). This more complex model is shown in Fig. 3.1.

Other studies that have examined the issue of intergenerational continuities in styles of relating have demonstrated well how both stress and inadequacies in social support can be passed from one generation to the next as well as from one life stage to the next (Caspi et al., 1987, 1990; Elder et al., 1986). The processes underlying such continuity are likely to be linked to the finding reported by McGuffin et al. (1988) that the rates of threatening life events were higher in the relatives of depressed patients, suggesting that patterns of stress run in families. The evidence for intergenerational continuities suggests that the concept of social vulnerability should also address generations.

The relation between the quality of social relationships in childhood and early adult life

Before leaving the issue of continuity in the quality of social support networks in childhood and adulthood, some preliminary findings from a 20 year prospective follow-up study to assess this will be outlined (Champion *et al.*, 1995). This study involved a sample of London school children first studied when they were aged 10 years by Rutter and his colleagues in 1970 (Rutter *et al.*, 1975*a*, *b*; Maughan, 1989). The results reported here are based on findings from 228 individuals; approximately half of these had behaviour problems at school at age 10 years and the rest were a randomly selected control group from the same school population. Detailed interviews were conducted with the parents when the children were aged 10 and interviewer-based assessments were made of a range of relationships within the child's family and of the child's relationships with peers. A follow-up in their late twenties assessed the individuals using both a detailed semi-structued interview that directly measured social support and a questionnaire measure of current social support, the Significant Others Scale (SOS: Power *et al.*, 1988). The version of this questionnaire used assessed the availability and perceived adequacy of the six most important individuals in the subject's current social network (Power & Champion, 1992). The questionnaire assessed the availability and perceived adequacy of both emotional support and practical support.

Preliminary analysis from examining the correlations between childhood relationship measures and scores on the SOS nearly 20 years later revealed some striking associations (Table 3.1; Champion *et al.*, unpublished data). Taking the sample as a whole the quality of the relationship the child had with the mother at age 10 years showed a significant association with both the availability and perceived adequacy of emotional and practical support 20 years later from the six most important people in their current social network. The results were all in the expected direction: that is, a poor relationship with mother was associated with a lower availability of emotional and practical support and a greater discrepancy between the actual support received from significant others and that ideally required. A similar pattern of results was also obtained for the quality of the relationship with father in childhood.

The importance of childhood peer relationship difficulties in predisposing to later problems in obtaining an adequate social support network were also suggested by this preliminary analysis (Table 3.1). Problems in peer relationships in childhood showed a significant association with perceived adequacy of both emotional and practical support in adulthood.

Table 3.1. *The significance of correlation between the quality of social relationships in childhood (age 10 years) and in early adult life (age 30 years) as assessed by the Significant Others Scale (SOS)*

	Adult measures (age 30 years)				
Childhood measures (age 10 years)	AEM	APR	DEM	DPR	DBF
Relationship with mother	***	*	***	*	**
Relationship with father	*	*	***	*	
Peer relationships			***	*	***
Quality of parental marriage	**	**	**	*	**

Significance of Pearson r correlation: $*p \leq 0.05$; $**p \leq 0.01$; $***p \leq 0.001$.
SOS measures: AEM, actual emotional support; APR, actual practical support; DEM, discrepancy on emotional support; DPR, discrepancy on practical support; DBF, discrepancy on relationship with best friend.

The presence of peer relationship difficulties in childhood was associated with a higher level of discrepancy between actual and ideal support for the six most important people rated on the SOS when respondents were in their late twenties.

Another set of consistent findings from this preliminary analysis revealed that the quality of the parents' marriage as assessed by the interviewers in 1970 showed a highly significant association with the availability and perceived adequacy of both emotional and practical support for the respondents in early adulthood (Table 3.1). A significant association was also found between a poor parental marriage and a perceived inadequacy in the respondent's current best friend. This finding suggests that early experiences of the parental relationship may have lasting effects on the ability to form satisfying friendships in adulthood.

These preliminary findings confirm the view that we can learn a great deal about what contributes to inadequate social networks in adult life by examining relationship difficulties and their causes in childhood. Although continuities do exist there is also clear evidence of much discontinuity. Although the correlations found were statistically significant they were still of modest proportions. Other analyses of this data set have shown that, as in the Quinton & Rutter study, planning for relationships is likely to be protective for those at risk as a result of childhood difficulties. Those who plan their transitions to cohabitation or marriage are much more likely to end up with good emotional support and less severely upsetting or unpleasant life events in early adult life than those at risk who do not plan. As Robins & Rutter (1990) point out

Broad influences			
Sex	**Race**	**Class**	**Culture**

INFANCY	CHILDHOOD	ADOLESCENCE	ADULTHOOD
Domains	*Domains*	*Domains*	*Domains*
Mother	Family	Family	Love relationships
Father	Peers	Peers	Family
Other carers	School	Other interests/hobbies	Work
		School/college	Independent living
			Other interests
Transitions	*Transitions*	*Transitions*	*Transitions*
Separations	Starting school	First sexual relationship	Starting work
	Birth of sibling	Leaving school	Promotion
		First work experience	Becoming a parent
			Leaving home
			Marriage

Figure 3.2. Life stages, domains and transitions.

it is through the detailed study of these individuals who defy the pattern of continuity that we can learn about both environments and skills or personality traits which are potentially protective. If these environments and skills can then be cultivated or taught for those at risk, they can constitute the basis of interventions likely to succeed.

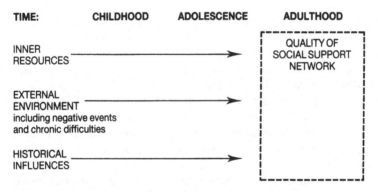

Figure 3.3. A model for conceptualising social support from a developmental perspective.

A model for conceptualising social support from a developmental perspective

A developmental perspective of social support and its impact on mental health can be expressed in a model which should be helpful to the clinician and researcher. The main aspects of this model are outlined below (Figs. 3.2, 3.3).

First, the model incorporates the concept of life stages. Here we have considered four: infancy, childhood, adolescence and adulthood. Each life stage of interest needs to be defined and the key domains, transitions or tasks for each stage outlined. This is important as the consideration of domains will show whether any are missing for an individual or whether some are overvalued at the expense of others (Lam & Power, 1991). An assessment of the normative events or tasks in each life stage will indicate points of risk for losses or gains in social support.

Second, the role of broad social influences such as sex, culture and class have been shown to be crucial to our understanding of an individual's social pathway through the life course. These influences must be considered in assessing social support at each life stage. At this point the concept of historical time also needs to be addressed. The importance of this concept was emphasised by Elder's work outlined above. The impact of changes in economic climate, social and political changes in opinion need to be considered for their impact on social relationships (Fig. 3.3).

Third, the inner resources of the individual that are expected to relate to effective social functioning must be considered. How these are defined will depend on the interest and theoretical orientation of the clinician or researcher. Here we have considered a wide range, including biological factors, self-esteem, ego strength, mental models, intelligence, and the ability to plan (Fig. 3.3).

Fourth, the external environment has been shown to be most important, especially the actual experiences the individual has with others. A plea has been made to consider the external environment within a life stress framework, assessing both life events and more chronic difficulties within each life stage of interest. This suggestion is made because of the considerable evidence that negative life events are associated with the onset of psychiatric disorder. Thus, identifying events, especially those involving interpersonal relationships, is likely to be highly informative for our understanding of social support and its development.

Finally, the interaction between the individual's internal resources and the external environment must be addressed within a developmental framework; at each point of interest the likely impact of one upon the other should be considered. Assessing the interaction and relative contribution of the internal and external aspects is especially important when addressing the need for intervention and whether this should be targeted mainly at manipulating the environment or altering some internal aspect of the individual.

References

Ainsworth, M. D. (1989). Attachments beyond infancy. *American Psychologist*, **44**, 709–16.

Ainsworth, M. D. (1991). Attachments and other affectional bonds across the life cycle. In *Attachment Across the Life Cycle*, ed. C. M. Parkes, J. Stevenson-Hinde & P. Marris, pp. 33–51. London: Routledge.

Ainsworth, M. D., Blehar, M. C., Waters, E. & Wall, S. (1978). *Patterns of Attachment*. Hillsdale, N.J.: Lawrence Erlbaum.

Asher, S. R. & Parker, J. G. (1989). The significance of peer relationship problems in childhood. In *Social Competence in Developmental Perspective*, ed. B. H. Schneider, G. Attili, J. Nadel & R. P. Weissberg, pp. 5–23. Amsterdam: Kluwer Academic.

Asher, S. R., Erdley, C. A. & Gabriel, S. W. (1994). Peer relations. In *Development Through Life: A Handbook for Clinicians*, ed. M. Rutter & D. Hay. Oxford: Blackwell Scientific.

Baltes, P. B., Reese, H. W. & Lipsett, L. P. (1980). Life-span developmental psychology. *Annual Review of Psychology*, **31**, 65–110.

Blos, P. (1967). The second individuation process of adolescence. *Psychoanalytic Study of the Child*, **22**, 162–86.

Bowlby, J. (1980). *Attachment and Loss*, Vol. 3, *Loss: Sadness and Depression*. London: Hogarth.

Bowlby, J. (1988). *A Secure Base: Clinical Applications of Attachment Theory*. London: Routledge.

Bretherton, I. (1985). Attachment theory: retrospect and prospect. In *Growing Points of Attachment Theory and Research*, ed. I. Bretherton & E. Waters, *Monograph of the Society for Research in Child Development 50* (1-2, serial no. 209).

Bretherton, I. (1991). The roots and growing points of attachment theory. In *Attachment Across the Life Cycle*, ed. C. M. Parkes, J. Stevenson-Hinde & P. Marris, pp. 9–32. London: Routledge.

Bretherton, I. & Waters, E. (eds.) (1985). *Growing Points of Attachment Theory and Research, Monograph of the Society for Research in Child Development 50* (1-2, serial no. 209).

Brewin, C. R., Andrews, B. & Gotlib, I. H. (1993). Psychopathology and early experience: a reappraisal of retrospective reports. *Psychological Bulletin*, **113**, 82–98.

Brown, G. W. & Harris, T. (1978). *The Social Origins of Depression: A Study of Psychiatric Disorder in Women*. London: Tavistock.

Brown, G. W. & Harris, T. (1986). Establishing causal links: the Bedford College Studies of depression. In *Life Events and Psychiatric Disorder: Controversial Issues*, ed. H. Katschnig, pp. 107–87. Cambridge: Cambridge University Press.

Brown, D. & Peddar, J. (1991). *Introduction to Psychotherapy: An Outline of Psychodynamic Principles and Practice*, 2nd edn. London: Tavistock.

Caspi, A., Elder, G. H. Jr & Bem, D. J. (1987). Moving against the world: life-course patterns of explosive children. *Developmental Psychology*, **33**, 308–13.

Caspi, A., Elder, G. H. Jr & Herbener, E. S. (1991). Childhood personality and the prediction of life-course patterns. In *Straight and Devious Pathways from Childhood to Adulthood*, ed. L. Robins & M. Rutter, pp. 13–35. Cambridge: Cambridge University Press.

Champion, L. A. (1985). A psychosocial approach to the mental health of women: depression, social support and self help on a new housing estate. PhD thesis, University of Birmingham.

Champion, L. A. (1990). The relationship between social vulnerability and the occurrence of severely threatening life events. *Psychological Medicine*, **20**, 157–61.

Champion, L. A. & Goodall, G. (1994). Social support: positive and negative aspects. In *Seminars in Psychology and the Social Sciences*, ed. D. Tantam & M. Birchwood, London: Gaskell Press.

Champion, L. A., Goodall, G. M. & Rutter, M. (1995). Behaviour problems in childhood and acute and chronic stressors in early adult life: I. a twenty year follow-up study. *Psychological Medicine* (in press).

Cohen, S. & Wills, T. A. (1985). Social support and the buffering hypothesis. *Psychological Bulletin*, **98**, 310–57.

Dodge, K. A. (1980). Social cognition and children's aggressive behaviour. *Child Development*, **51**, 162–70.

Elder, G. H. Jr (1979). Historical change in life patterns and personality. In *Life Span Development and Behaviour*, vol. 2, ed. P. B. Baltes & O. G. Brim, pp. 118–59. New York: Academic Press.

Elder, G. H. Jr (1986). Military turning points in men's lives. *Developmental Psychology*, **22**, 233–45.

Elder, G. H. Jr, Caspi, A. & Downey, G. (1986). Problem behaviour and family relationships. In *Human Development and the Life Course: Multidisciplinary Perspectives*, ed. A. B. Sorensen, F. E. Weinert & L. R. Sherrod, pp. 293–340. London: Lawrence Erlbaum.

Farrington, D. P. (1986). Stepping stones to adult criminal careers. In *Development of Antisocial and Prosocial Behaviour*, ed. D. Olweus, J. Block & M. Radke-Yarrow, pp. 335–56. New York: Academic Press.

Flaherty, J. A. & Richman, J. A. (1986). Effects of childhood relationships on the adult's capacity to form social supports. *American Journal of Psychiatry*, **143**, 851–5.

Fonagy, P., Steele, M., Steele, H., Moran, G. S. & Higgit, A. C. (1991). The capacity for understanding mental states: the reflective self in parent and child and its significance for security of attachment. *Infant Mental Health*, **13**, 200–16.

Grossman, K. E. & Grossman, K. (1991). Attachment quality as an organizer of emotional and behavioural responses in a longitudinal perspective. In *Attachment Across the Life Cycle*, ed. C. M. Parkes, J. Stevenson-Hinde & P. Marris, pp. 93–114. London: Routledge.

Harris, T. & Bifulco, A. (1991). Loss of parent in childhood, attachment style and depression in adulthood. In *Attachment Across the Life Cycle*, ed. C. M. Parkes, J. Stevenson-Hinde & P. Marris, pp. 234–67. London: Routledge.

Harris, T., Brown, G. W. & Bifulco, A. (1986). Loss of parent in childhood and adult psychiatric disorder: the role of lack of adequate parental care. *Psychological Medicine*, **16**, 641–59.

Harris, T., Brown, G. W. & Bifulco, A. (1987). Loss of parent in childhood and adult psychiatric disorder: the role of social class position. *Psychological Medicine*, **17**, 163–83.

Hodges, J. & Tizard, B. (1989). Social and family relationships of ex-institutional adolescents. *Journal of Child Psychology and Psychiatry*, **30**, 77–97.

Hultsch, A. S. & Deutsch, F. (1981). *Adult Development and Aging: A Life-Span Perspective*. New York: McGraw-Hill.

Kagan, J. (1989). *Unstable Ideas: Temperament, Cognition and Self*. Cambridge, Mass.: Harvard University Press.

Kandel, D. B. & Davies, M. (1986). Adult sequelae of adolescent depressive symptoms. *Archives of General Psychiatry*, **43**, 225–62.

Kandel, D., Davies, M. & Baydar, N. (1990). The creation of interpersonal contexts: homophily in dyadic relationships in adolescence and young adulthood. In *Straight and Devious Pathways from Childhood to Adulthood*, ed. L. Robins & M. Rutter, pp. 221–41. Cambridge: Cambridge University Press.

Kupersmidt, J. B., Coie, J. D. & Dodge, K. A. (1990). The role of poor peer relationships in the development of disorder. In *Peer Rejection in Childhood*, ed. S. R. Asher & J. D. Coie, pp. 274–305. Cambridge: Cambridge University Press.

Lam, D. H. & Power, M. J. (1991). A questionnaire designed to assess roles and goals: a preliminary study. *British Journal of Medical Psychology*, **6**, 89–93.

Magnusson, D., Stattin, H. & Allen, V. L. (1986). Differential maturation among girls and its relation to social adjustment: a longitudinal perspective. In *Life-Span Development and Behaviour*, vol. 7, ed. P. B. Baltes, D. L. Featherman & R. M. Lerner, pp. 136–72. Hillsdale, N.J.: Lawrence Erlbaum.

Main, M. (1991). Metacognitive knowledge, metacognitive monitoring, and singular (coherent) vs. multiple (incoherent) model of attachment: findings and directions for future research. In *Attachment Across the Life Cycle*, ed. C. M. Parkes, J. Stevenson-Hinde & P. Marris, pp. 127–59. London: Routledge.

Main, M. & Goldwyn, R. (1984). Predicting rejection of her infants from mother's representation of her own experience: implications for the abused–abusing intergenerational cycle. *International Journal of Child Abuse and Neglect*, **8**, 203–17.

Main, M., Kaplan, N. & Cassidy, J. (1985). Security in infancy, childhood and adulthood: a move to the level of representation. In *Growing Points of Attachment Theory and Research*, ed. I. Bretherton & E. Waters, *Monograph of the Society for Research in Child Development 50* 1-2, serial no. 209).

Maughan, B. (1989). Growing up in the inner city: findings from the inner London longitudinal study. *Paediatric and Perinatal Epidemiology*, **3**, 195–215.

Maughan, B. & Champion, L. A. (1990). Risk and protective factors in the transition to young adulthood. In *Successful Aging: Perspectives from the Behavioral Sciences*, ed. P. B. Baltes & M. M. Baltes, pp. 296–331. Cambridge: Cambridge University Press.

McGuffin, P., Katz, R. & Bebbington, P. (1988). The Camberwell collaborative depression study. III. Depression and adversity in the relatives of depressed probands. *British Journal of Psychiatry*, **143**, 1074–87.

Newcomb, A. F., Brady, J. E. & Hartup, W. W. (1979). Friendship and

94L. CHAMPIONincentive conditions as determinants of children's task-orientated social behaviour. *Child Development*, **50**, 878–88.
Parker, J. G. & Asher, S. R. (1987). Peer relations and later personal adjustments: are low accepted children at risk? *Psychological Bulletin*, **102**, 357–89.
Parker, G. & Barnett, B. (1988). Perceptions of parenting in childhood and social support in adulthood. *American Journal of Psychiatry*, **145**, 479–82.
Parker, G., Tupling, H. & Brown, L. B. (1979). A parental bonding instrument. *British Journal of Medical Psychology*, **52**, 1–10.
Parker, G. B., Barrett, B. A. & Hickie, I. B. (1992). From nurture to network: examining links between perceptions of parenting received in childhood and social bonds in adulthood. *American Journal of Psychiatry*, **149**, 877–85.
Parry, G. (1988). Mobilizing social support. In *New Developments in Clinical Psychology*, vol. 2, ed. F. N. Watts, pp. 83–104. Chichester: Wiley.
Pearlin, L. I. (1985). Social structure and process of social support. In *Social Support and Health*, ed. S. Cohen & S. L. Syme, pp. 43–59. London: Academic Press.
Power, M. J. & Champion, L. A. (1992). The Significant Others Scale (SOS). In *Assessment: A Mental Health Portfolio*, ed. D. Milne. Windsor: NFER-Nelson.
Power, M. J., Champion, L. A. & Aris, S. J. (1988). The development of a measure of social support: the significant others scale. *British Journal of Clinical Psychology*, **26**, 349–59.
Quinton, D. & Rutter, M. (1988). *Parenting Breakdown: The Making and Breaking of Intergenerational Links*. Aldershot, UK: Avebury.
Quinton, D., Rutter, M. & Liddle, C. (1984). Institutional rearing, parenting difficulties and marital support. *Psychological Medicine*, **14**, 107–24.
Renshaw, P. D. & Asher, S. R. (1983). Children's goals and strategies for social interaction. *Merrill-Palmer Quarterly*, **29**, 553–74.
Robins, L. N. & Rutter, M. (1990). *Straight and Devious Pathways from Childhood to Adulthood*. Cambridge: Cambridge University Press.
Rubin, K. H., Lemare, L. J. & Lollis, S. (1990). Social withdrawal in childhood: developmental pathways to peer rejection. In *Peer Rejection in Childhood*, ed. S. R. Asher & J. D. Coie, pp. 217–49. Cambridge: Cambridge University Press.
Rutter, M. (1981). *Maternal Deprivation Reassessed*, 2nd edn. Harmondsworth, UK: Penguin.
Rutter, M. &. Quinton, D. (1984). Long-term follow-up of women institutionalised in childhood: factors promoting good functioning in adult life. *British Journal of Developmental Psychology*, **2**, 191–204.
Rutter, M., Cox, A., Tupling, C., *et al.* (1975a). Attainment and adjustment in two geographical areas. I. The prevalence of psychiatric disorder. *British Journal of Psychiatry*, **126**, 493–509.
Rutter, M., Yule, B., Quinton, D., *et al.* (1975b). Attainment and adjustment in two geographical areas. III. Some factors accounting for area differences. *British Journal of Psychiatry*, **126**, 520–33.
Rutter, M., Quinton, D. & Hill, J. (1990). Adult outcomes of institution-reared children: males and females compared. In *Straight and*

Devious Pathways from Childhood to Adulthood, ed. L. Robins & M. Rutter. Cambridge: Cambridge University Press.

Schultz, R. & Rau, M. T. (1985). Social support through the life course. In *Social Support and Health*, ed. S. Cohen & S. L. Syme, pp. 129–49. London: Academic Press.

Skolnick, A. (1986). Early attachment and personal relationships across the life course. In *Life-span Development and Behaviour*, vol. 7, ed. P. B. Baltes, D. L. Featherman & R. M. Lerner, pp. 174–206. Hillsdale, N.J.: Lawrence Erlbaum.

Sroufe, L. A. (1985). Attachment classification from the perspective of infant–caregiver relationships and infant temperament. *Child Development*, **56**, 1–14.

Sugarman, L. (1986). *Life-span Development: Concepts, Theories and Interventions*. London: Methuen.

Thompson, R. A. & Lamb, M. E. (1986). Infant–mother attachment: new directions for theory and research. In *Life-span Development and Behaviour*, vol. 7, ed. P. B. Baltes, D. L. Featherman & R. M. Lerner, pp. 1–42. Hillsdale, N.J.: Lawrence Erlbaum.

Thompson, R. A., Lamb, M. E. & Estes, D. (1982). Stability of infant–mother attachment and its relationship to changing life circumstances in an unselected middle-class sample. *Child Development*, **53**, 144–8.

Truant, G. S., Herscovitch, J. & Lohrenz, J. G. (1987). The relationship of childhood experiences to the quality of marriage. *Canadian Journal of Psychiatry*, **32**, 87–92.

Warr, P. & Parry, G. (1982). Paid employment and women's psychological well-being. *Psychological Bulletin*, **91**, 493–516.

Weiss, R. (1974). The provisions of social relationships. In *Doing Unto Others*, ed. Z. Rubin, pp. 17–26. New York: Prentice-Hall.

Wentzel, K. R. (1991). Social and academic goals at school: motivation and achievement in context. In *Advances in Motivation and Achievement*, vol. 7, ed. M. Maehr & A. Pintrich, pp. 185–212. Greenwich, CT: JAI Press.

West, D. J. (1982). *Delinquency: its Roots, Careers and Prospects*. London: Heinemann.

Wilhelm, K. & Parker, G. (1988). The development of a measure of intimate bonds. *Psychological Medicine*, **18**, 225–34.

Wills, T. A. (1985). Supportive functions of interpersonal relationships. In *Social Support and Health*, ed. S. Cohen & S. L. Syme, pp. 281–98. London: Academic Press.

4

Cognitive aspects of social support processes

CHRIS R. BREWIN

The study of social support is frequently described in terms of dichotomies: studies of social support as a personality trait versus a situational factor, investigations of perceived levels of support versus actual supportive transactions, studies of structure versus studies of function, etc. To some extent these dichotomies simply reflect investigators' theoretical backgrounds or the limitations of the methods they employ, but they do emphasise the exceedingly complex nature of social support processes. In the individual case support-seeking and support-giving depend upon a variety of factors, both social (such as the availability of support, or the opportunity to give it) and cognitive (such as the appraisal that support is worth seeking or will be appreciated). In this chapter I will describe how a cognitive perspective is of value in understanding some of the mechanisms that underlie these interrelated processes.

The chapter is divided into four sections. In the first I discuss social support as a personality or individual difference variable, emphasising continuities in individuals' expectations of the support they can expect to receive, and in their propensities to approach or avoid others for the purpose of obtaining support. Evidence linking these propensities to early childhood experiences will be reviewed. The second section will be concerned with the cognitive appraisal of situations and with the types of appraisal that are likely to encourage or inhibit the seeking of support. In the third section I will review studies of cognitive processes in help-givers, which may be equally crucial in determining whether support is obtained in a crisis. Finally I will consider the implications for clinical practice.

Social support and personality

There are now many indications that perceptions of social support may usefully be considered as an aspect of personality. Sarason et al. (1986) put forward this view after finding that perceived support was remarkably stable for periods of up to 3 years, even during transitional events that led to major changes in the composition of the person's support network. More recently Lakey & Cassady (1990) reported that measures of perceived support, in contrast to measures of actual support received, were highly correlated with measures of personality such as trait anxiety, dysfunctional attitudes and self-esteem. At the same time perceived support was not part of a global dimension of 'negative affectivity' (i.e. a global affective state producing the tendency to endorse any kind of negative judgement) but formed a distinct factor. Lakey & Cassady also found that people low in perceived social support interpreted novel supportive behaviours more negatively than those who felt well supported, and were less likely than them to remember instances of helpful, supportive behaviour. These data suggest that perceived support does not simply reflect some changing external reality but can also provide a more consistent framework for seeing and interpreting the world.

In what way could expectations of social support develop as an aspect of personality? The helplessness of the human infant means that it starts life totally dependent on the protection and nurturance provided by other people, and there appear to be a number of innate mechanisms that are designed to strengthen such relationships and to ensure their continuity. There is now a great deal of evidence that the success or failure of these early relationships has significant implications for later personality development and for the risk of psychopathology. The person most associated with this view is Bowlby (1973, 1980, 1982), whose theory of attachment has been described in the previous chapter by Champion. Children gradually build up internal representations or working models of themselves and of their main attachment figures, which are used to appraise and guide behaviour in new situations. Crucial elements of the adult personality, including interpersonal trust and confidence in others' ability to provide support, depend on the quality of early social interaction, and particularly on the inferences children draw about the acceptability of their negative feelings. Thus, the working model of the self is intimately connected to models of others, and confidence in the availability and responsiveness of attachment figures is gradually internalised as an important aspect of self-esteem. Working models continue to develop through infancy, childhood and adolescence, and the expectations formed about self and others are thought to persist thereafter relatively unchanged, exerting an influence on the course of subsequent adult relationships.

Bowlby's pioneering ideas were a forerunner of current thinking by researchers in the area of social cognition, who have proposed that children develop organised knowledge structures in memory that represent a synthesis of prior information. A variety of knowledge structures have been described, including prototypes, scripts and schemas (see Singer & Salovey, 1991, for a review). Whereas prototypes consist of the essential set of elements that make up a category of object or person, scripts represent knowledge about the structure of common situations, for example what happens if someone cries or asks for help. The self-schema consists of a structure or set of structures containing information about one's own capabilities, characteristics, etc. Based on direct experience and input from the social environment, it provides a frame of reference for interpreting new situations, directing the child's attention to certain features and biasing assessment of ambiguous material. Information consistent with that contained in the self-schema is processed rapidly and automatically, whereas information inconsistent with the self-schema is processed more slowly and may be ignored or have its importance minimised. Thus self-schemas not only reflect prior experience but actively shape the conscious appraisal of new experiences.

Because individuals have so many disparate and contradictory experiences, self-schemas are thought to be complex, containing dominant elements that are frequently used in assessing experience and subordinate elements that may be occasionally elicited in certain specific situations. For example, a child brought up by one very supportive and one highly critical parent would be likely to have two highly developed, contrasting sets of elements in their self-schema. It would be expected that they would be capable of very positive and very negative feelings about themselves, and that these would be elicited by interactions with critical or supportive others. In the same way, individuals are thought to have schemas that reflect their experience of close others, particularly family members. There is evidence that these schemas are easily activated and come to influence social judgements (e.g. Andersen & Cole, 1990; Baldwin & Holmes, 1987). Thus it seems likely that prior experiences, particularly within families, may help to explain why perceptions of social support have some stable, trait-like characteristics.

Empirical evidence for family influences on support

A study by East (1989) investigated the theory that family experiences lead to enduring perceptions of interpersonal risks and benefits in early adolescents. In boys, the less their fathers reported being supportive to them, the more interpersonal risks they perceived. Fathers' support of girls, on the other hand, was related to their perceiving more interpersonal benefits. In both boys and girls, perceiving greater interpersonal benefits was related to feeling better supported by family and friends. East also found that those adolescents who were lonely or had low self-esteem perceived more interpersonal risks.

In contrast, the majority of studies have investigated the importance of recalled childhood experiences in influencing the likelihood that a person will receive social support as an adult. Many of these have been conducted with late adolescent or student samples reporting their perceptions of support. Sarason *et al.* (1986) reported that scores on their Social Support Questionnaire reflecting the availability or satisfactoriness of support were correlated with reports of parenting on the Parental Bonding Inventory (PBI: Parker *et al.*, 1979). The PBI is a widely used retrospective measure with good reliability and validity on which people assess the amount of care and the amount of overprotection they received from each of their parents during their childhood. Sarason *et al.*'s results indicated that reports of parental care were positively related to perceived social support in both sexes, whereas among women students only there was a negative relation between maternal overprotection and support.

Flaherty & Richman's (1986) study of medical students also revealed that less perceived social support was associated with less parental care on the PBI (but not with more overprotection). Sarason *et al.*'s and Richman & Flaherty's findings have since been replicated a number of times. Sarason *et al.* (1991: study 1) found that lower levels of parental care as measured by the PBI were consistently related to the perception that support was less satisfactory, and that less paternal care was associated with reduced availability of support. Greater parental overprotection was also associated with reduced availability of support. In a second study Sarason *et al.* (1991) found that less perceived support was consistently correlated with less parental care and greater maternal overprotection. Similarly, Mallinckrodt (1992) reported that a measure of satisfaction with social support, the Social Provisions Scale (Cutrona & Russell, 1987), was associated with less parental care on the PBI (there were no significant correlations with overprotection).

All these studies are open to the objection that the subjects were at an age when parents would be major sources of support, leading to possible overlap between the measures. It is therefore important to consider the results found with other groups or other supporters. Sherman & Donovan (1991) studied a sample of at-risk pregnant adolescents. Their reports of having been rejected by their mother in childhood were associated with perceiving less support from a variety of sources, including the father of the baby and his relatives. Primiparous women were studied 1 week after the birth of their baby and again a year later by Parker & Barnett (1988), who interviewed them using the Interview Schedule for Social Interaction (ISSI: Henderson *et al.*, 1981). Immediately post-partum there were significant relationships between women's reports of the care they had received from their mothers and the availability of both current attachment and social integration. At 1 year greater availability of attachment and social integration correlated significantly with more maternal care and less maternal overprotection.

Finally, Mallinckrodt (1991) reported that maternal overprotection was associated with less satisfaction with social support in a sample of counselling clients. This was one of the very few studies not to find a significant link between parental care scores and perceptions of social support.

In summary, there is highly consistent evidence that perceived support is associated with reports of less parental care, and somewhat less consistent evidence for a link with reported parental overprotection. Is there any reason to discount this evidence because the effects of mood state or response bias artificially inflate the correlations? Although there is evidence that mood may affect measures of perceived social support (Cohen *et al.*, 1988), a recent review has concluded that mood state in fact has little effect on reports of parenting (Brewin *et al.*, 1993), and therefore this factor should not be a concern. Parker & Barnett (1988) attempted to control for response bias in their study by partialling out women's scores on the neuroticism scale of the Eysenck Personality Inventory from the correlation between the PBI and support. Significant relationships between maternal care and availability of attachment scores were still present at both time points. Other relevant data are provided by Sarason *et al.* (1991), who asked significant others in their subjects' social network to describe the subjects' positive and negative characteristics. Subjects' perceived support was related to these independent appraisals of approval as well as to subjects' own ratings of these relationships.

Although supportive of the proposition that childhood experiences shape future expectations of support, these studies have little to say about actual social support transactions and how they might differ in people with unsatisfactory parenting. One of the few studies to shed light on this was published by Andrews & Brown (1988). Their community study of working-class women in Islington was primarily aimed at understanding the factors that made women more prone to depression, and in the course of it they collected data on actual attempts to seek support and on the reactions women received. Andrews & Brown identified in a subset of women a pattern of 'non-optimal confiding' – a tendency to confide in people who could not or would not provide support and who either withdrew or responded in a critical way. In addition to having low self-esteem and being unlikely to receive crisis support, 'non-optimal confiders' were found to have had particularly poor parenting themselves, characterised by parental indifference, lack of control, or antipathy with mother. They tended to be unwilling to get close to people and found it difficult to solicit support. This interesting study suggests that having experienced poor parenting and consequently having low expectations of support may not simply cause people to avoid potentially supportive interactions. In addition it may prevent people from discriminating supportive and non-supportive interactions, and lead them to continue with interactions that are at best counter-productive and that at worst undermine them and further damage their confidence. Readers may also refer to the previous chapter by Champion on the relation between disrupted childhood relationships and the quality of adult relationships.

Situational appraisals and support-seeking

Lack of support is sometimes due to the failure to seek it, which may be the result of social anxiety, social withdrawal, or the belief that confiding will be of little value. Three main types of cognitive explanation are relevant to the decision not to seek support: one to do with beliefs about social competence, one that emphasises the role of social comparison processes, and one concerned with the effects on self-esteem. Although these appraisals may partly be the result of personality factors, there is also scope for the immediate social situation to affect appraisals and hence support-seeking. The various theories are not mutually exclusive, and all may be helpful in analysing the problems of a particular individual. Their different causal focus does, however, point to different kinds of intervention strategy for improving social support.

Social competence beliefs

Shyness, loneliness and social anxiety are extremely common, and in some cases social anxiety is so intense that the mere presence of other people leads to social withdrawal. Shy and lonely people tend to attribute interpersonal failures (but not necessarily other kinds of failure) to internal, stable, and uncontrollable factors such as lack of social ability (Anderson *et al.*, 1983; Teglasi & Hoffman, 1982). These kinds of attribution lead to low self-esteem and to low expectations of success or, in Bandura's (1977) term, to low self-efficacy. This in turn would be expected to reduce the amount of effort expended to initiate and persist at social encounters. Leary *et al.* (1986) have also investigated attributions for subjective feelings of nervousness, one of the factors claimed by Bandura to contribute to estimates of self-efficacy. In support of this model, Leary *et al.* showed that people who attribute their feelings of social anxiety to stable characteristics of themselves are more likely to avoid social encounters than people who attribute them to unstable characteristics of themselves or to situational factors.

The relevance of these cognitions to social behaviour has been further investigated in an elegant experiment by Anderson (1983). College students were first selected according to their tendency to make either uncontrollable, characterological attributions (character style) or controllable, behavioural attributions (behaviour style) for interpersonal failures. These two groups of subjects then took part in an interpersonal persuasion task (getting people to donate blood to a local blood bank) under one of three conditions. In one condition it was suggested that success at the task was due to abilities and personality traits, in another condition that success was due to using the right strategies and to effort, while in the third condition subjects received no prior attributional information. Anderson found that when attributions were not manipulated, behaviour style subjects had higher success expectancies, demonstrated greater motivation, and were more successful at the task than character style subjects. When attributions were manipulated, these group differences were abolished. Prior ascription of success to ability factors did not affect the character style group, but it reduced the performance of the behaviour style subjects to a level equal to that of the other group. Conversely, when the experimenter suggested in advance the importance of effort and choosing the correct strategies, there was no effect on the behaviour style subjects, but the performance of the character style group improved to a level equal to that of the behaviour style subjects. This experiment provides a convincing demonstration of the association between generalised causal beliefs and success in a novel interpersonal situation, and illustrates the potential impact on people's behaviour of changing their beliefs about the importance of various causal factors.

Social comparison

Theories based on beliefs about social competence are particularly relevant to those individuals who desire social interaction but have low expectations of being able to perform adequately. Other individuals may be socially competent, and know it, but actively avoid interaction because they have other attributes or experiences which they consider to be abnormal and of which they are embarrassed or ashamed. Goffman (1968) has described the many social difficulties experienced by stigmatised individuals who belong to a despised race or religion, or who have physical deformities or character blemishes. The adverse reactions of others may lead to a self-imposed isolation from society, as he illustrates in the following quotation from a 43-year-old unemployed mason: 'How hard and humiliating it is to bear the name of an unemployed man. When I go out, I cast down my eyes because I feel myself wholly inferior. When I go along the street, it seems to me that I can't be compared with an average citizen, that everybody is pointing at me with his finger. I instinctively avoid meeting anyone' (p. 28). More recent studies of HIV-positive men have revealed a similar pattern of withdrawal from social support systems (Donlou et al., 1985).

Goffman's analysis is largely concerned with the social rejection experienced by stigmatised people and with the strategies they employ to avoid this. He distinguishes between 'discredited' people such as paraplegic individuals, whose stigma is evident on the most casual acquaintance, and 'discreditable' people who have a secret they are trying to conceal, such as their illiteracy. In many cases, however, a process of self-stigmatisation may produce similar effects in a person who does not fall into one of Goffman's socially despised categories, and who has not experienced actual societal rejection. Ørner (1987) described these reactions in a group of British servicemen who had fought in the Falklands War 5 years previously and continued to experience the after-effects in the form of vivid memories or nightmares (post-traumatic stress disorder). According to Ørner, they felt marked out by their experiences and different from other people in an important way. In the absence of other servicemen with similar experiences, they felt unable to talk to others and chose rather to isolate themselves from society.

Other examples of stigma or self-stigma are common. The teenager who has had an abortion, the woman who sometimes feels violent towards her child, and the person who is HIV-positive are all likely to experiences some anxiety about a public revelation. Prompted by feelings of shame over some action or attribute, they must still estimate society's reaction if the secret is revealed. Expectations of censure and scorn, whether veridical or mistaken, may lead them to withdraw from social encounters. Even individuals who are obviously 'discredited' must make similar estimates. If they are to avoid social isolation they may choose to focus on some feature of which they can feel proud and which emphasises their comparability with others, as in the case of the physically handicapped who take part in sporting contests. Experimentally inducing feelings of shame and embarrassment in ordinary college students can also lead to a decreased desire for social interaction with peers (Sarnoff & Zimbardo, 1961). The fact that similar effects can be demonstrated in the laboratory with non-discredited subjects emphasises that we are dealing with an intrapersonal process as well as a societal one.

The notion of stigma involves being classified as different from and inferior to one's peers. But, in the absence of continued rejection, how does a person arrive at the conclusion that their attributes or experience make them different and inferior? The attitudes, values and behaviour of those closest to them will obviously be important, but not necessarily crucial. Social comparison theory (Festinger, 1954) was originally developed to explain how people evaluate their opinions and abilities, but it can also be applied to the evaluation of actions, feelings and experiences such as that of illness. According to Festinger, people who want to evaluate themselves first seek objective information and then turn to social comparison, preferring to compare themselves with similar others when doing so. This is because it is usually more informative to compare oneself with others who are similar on the relevant attributes than with others who are very dissimilar. The work of Schachter (1959) indicates that these affiliative tendencies increase when people are uncertain or fearful. In the following chapter Gilbert provides an evolutionary understanding of processes of social comparison, in a discussion of rank theory.

Social comparison theory therefore suggests that people with a 'problem' they are uncertain or fearful about should avoid 'normal' (i.e. dissimilar) people and seek out similar others, sharing their problem with selected friends or perhaps joining self-help groups composed of people in related situations. Receiving information that others share their problems should increase their self-esteem and reduce self-stigmatisation. Consistent with this view, Yalom (1975) has identified 'universality', or the sharing of one's experiences with similar others, as one of the most potent factors for change in therapeutic groups. But many factors may interfere with this process of gaining consensus information via direct social comparison. The 'discreditable' person may be unable to identify a group of similar others, and both 'discreditable' and 'discredited' may be prevented from mixing with their peers because of excessive shame and embarrassment, lack of social skills, etc.

A great deal will depend on the person's initial estimate of the frequency of their 'problem'. The more unusual the 'discreditable' think themselves, the more likely they are to doubt the availability of similar others, and on this basis fear social interactions in which their 'secret' might be unmasked. This process may account for the fact that depressed patients have smaller social networks than the non-depressed. The depressed believe that they are dissimilar to others and that negative experiences are more likely to happen to them than to other people (e.g. Brewin & Furnham, 1986; MacCarthy & Furnham, 1986). Brewin & Furnham suggested that these beliefs should lead the depressed to avoid others, thus restricting their access to normative or consensus information. In this way inaccurate consensus judgements would tend to persist through lack of disconfirmatory evidence, and social interaction would continue to be aversive. According to this approach, the reduced network size and relative lack of intimacy enjoyed by those prone to depression is explained by specific consensus beliefs that influence the attractiveness, and hence the probability, of social interaction.

The empirical evidence is broadly supportive of this view of the causes of avoidance. Snyder & Ingram (1983) identified women college students with either average or marked test anxiety and told them that the problem was either common or uncommon. Being told that it was common had opposite effects on the two groups. The intention to seek help for the problem was significantly decreased in those with average anxiety but was significantly increased in those with marked anxiety. Unlike Snyder & Ingram, who only asked about intentions, Brewin *et al.* (1989*a*) investigated actual reactions to homesickness in first-year university students. Homesickness was a reasonably common, albeit short-lived, phenomenon in both men and women and both sexes were equally distressed by it. Women were much more likely to cope with it by seeking cheerful company and discussing their feelings with others, but surprisingly were also more likely to regard themselves as more prone to homesickness than the majority of people they knew. This pattern of sex differences may have accounted for the finding that consensus beliefs were unrelated to support-seeking in women. In the small sample of male students, however, there were sizeable correlations between perceiving homesickness to be more likely to happen to other people and increased support-seeking.

Brewin *et al.* (1989*b*: study 1) investigated the association between subjects' attributional style, including consensus judgements, and perceived support. Individuals who tended to see negative outcomes as more likely to happen to them than to other people also perceived that social support was less available to them. In a second study Brewin *et al.* investigated appraisals of specific events that subjects had actually experienced and how they had coped with the event. Factor analysis indicated that support-seeking could be divided into three separate elements: emotional support, practical support, and social withdrawal, i.e. the tendency to avoid rather than approach family, friends and people in general. The results indicated that judgements of low consensus, internal attributions and self-blame for the event were specifically associated with more social withdrawal rather than less seeking of practical and emotional support.

One implication of Brewin *et al*'s (1989*b*) results is that individuals have different expectations of confidants, or people with expert knowledge, compared with ordinary members of their social network. Negative self-appraisal may render people much more discriminating in their choice of companions, and lead them to reject others whom they would normally tolerate. Logically there seems no reason, however, why the avoidance of marginal others, or others perceived as unhelpful, should extend to close confidants and to the possessors of valuable information. Taken together, Brewin *et al*'s (1989*b*) two studies are consistent in suggesting that negative cognitive appraisal, including consensus judgements, is related to perceiving the availability or appropriateness of seeking support through companionship, but is not necessarily related to obtaining information or to obtaining support from intimates. Homesickness may be an exceptional situation, in that by definition the person is cut off from many or all of his or her close confidants.

Threats to self-esteem

There is a strong case to be made that frequency of different kinds of social interaction, including the seeking and utilisation of social support, is linked to social comparison processes. But the relation between social comparison, social support-seeking, and negative emotions such as anxiety, depression or embarrassment is a complex one. It does seem likely that inaccurate consensus beliefs are related to negative emotions and that these in turn are related to social withdrawal. For some patients the opportunity to gain consensus information, either in written form or by actually mixing with similar others, may therefore be extremely valuable. But mixing with similar others is less likely to appeal to those who do not wish to evaluate their feelings and experiences, either because they have access to adequate expert advice or because their coping strategies depend on attending to certain kinds of information and not others. For example, patients who use the 'downward comparison' strategy of comparing themselves with others who are worse off to maintain their self-esteem may find it upsetting to meet others who are managing better than they are and who make them feel like a failure. Patients who use the 'upward comparison' strategy, on the other hand, may be uncomfortable mixing with others they perceive as worse off than themselves, since this may bring home the reality of their problem or disability.

This point is illustrated by studies of patients with chronic physical impairment such as multiple sclerosis (MS). Miles (1979) has identified two alternative coping strategies used by married couples with one partner suffering from MS. The 'normalisation' strategy involves continuing social relationships according to the pre-illness pattern and avoiding other sufferers. The 'disassociation' strategy involves withdrawing from relationships with non-sufferers, sometimes by moving house. In an investigation of the association between social contact and well-being in MS sufferers, Maybury & Brewin (1984) reported that greater self-esteem and reduced psychological distress were related to greater contact with the able-bodied. Well-being was unrelated to the amount of contact with other MS sufferers, however, suggesting that the opportunity to obtain regular consensus information was not of great value to this group. It would be interesting to know whether there are certain times, for example immediately after the diagnosis is made, when consensus information would be useful for MS sufferers.

It is evident from the above discussion that social comparison is closely linked with the maintenance of self-esteem, and several theorists have suggested that perceived threats to self-esteem are an important determinant of help-seeking. Fisher et al. (1982) noted that to seek help may be aversive because it implies inferiority, and that individuals who perceive support attempts as suggesting or confirming their inferiority will tend to withdraw. It is also possible that seeking help may draw attention to some aspect of the self which is a source of low self-esteem. For example, a recent study of HIV-positive gay men found that those with negative attitudes towards their own and others' homosexuality were more likely to avoid others and less likely to seek out social support (Nicholson & Long, 1990).

Folkman *et al.* (1986) interviewed 85 married couples and enquired about the coping strategies employed in response to different appraisals of stressful events. They reported that perceiving a threat to self-esteem was associated with more escape-avoidance and less social support. In a further analysis of these data, Dunkel-Schetter *et al.* (1987) confirmed that a perceived threat to self-esteem was consistently and inversely related to all indices of support received, including the amount of information, aid and emotional support, and the total number of sources from whom support was available. The authors commented, 'Situations that threaten self-esteem are typically ones in which a person has failed somehow, for example, on a task or in a relationship. Under these circumstances, assistance from others can be inappropriate or intrusive and might be rejected, or accepted from only a few close network members. Thus, our finding that threat to self-esteem is associated with less support and fewer providers of support may be explained speculatively, within a social-contextual perspective on the role of appraisals in social support processes' (p. 78).

It is, however, necessary to caution against an overly simplistic view of the impact of self-esteem on support-seeking. We know that self-esteem is closely bound up with the quality of intimate relationships, particularly marriage, and that support from spouses or intimate partners is of particular importance (e.g. Brown *et al.*, 1986). In some cases, therefore, rather than low self-esteem inhibiting support-seeking, lack of support and low self-esteem may stem from the same unsatisfactory intimate relationship. This is illustrated in a study by Hobfoll *et al.* (1986), who investigated a sample of women following the outcome of both normal and medically complicated pregnancies. Although self-esteem was correlated with satisfaction with support, path analysis showed that the relationship was only an indirect one. Self-esteem was in fact mainly associated with having an intimate relationship with a spouse, and this in turn was related to greater satisfaction with support.

Help-giving

For social support to be obtained, someone else must be able and willing to give it. The quality of the support may depend on a number of cognitive factors, such as the perceived threat produced in the supporter by the victim's or sufferer's condition, the supporter's uncertainties about appropriate behaviour, and the supporter's misconceptions about the coping process (Wortman & Lehman, 1985). Although there are few empirical studies directly concerned with who gives support and why, there have been many investigations of the closely related topic of help-giving. One of the most influential models of help-giving has been put forward by Weiner (1986). Weiner's cognition–emotion–action model proposes that person A's problem or distress is causally evaluated by the potential help-giver B. If B believes that the causes of A's problem are not controllable by A (or if A is not responsible, in Weiner's more recent writings), then B will feel pity or sympathy, and this in turn will lead to an increased desire to help. If B sees A's problems as controllable by A (or A is responsible), Weiner suggests that B will feel anger and will be correspondingly less likely to help. This model has been supported in a number of studies of help-giving among non-intimates, for example students lending their class notes to each other.

While the scope of Weiner's theory is wide, and applicable to many supportive interactions, it is not clear to what extent it applies to social support processes within very different contexts, for example intimate, family or professional relationships. Sharrock et al. (1990) studied attributions, emotions and preparedness to help among professional care staff working in a medium-secure unit for mentally disordered offenders. Staff were asked to make judgements about a particular target patient whom they knew well. In this context the extent to which staff perceived the patient to have control over his problems was related to their feelings of sympathy but not to their feelings of anger, and neither emotion was related to their willingness to help. Rather, helping was related to staff optimism, which in turn was associated with attributions to unstable and uncontrollable causes.

A second set of findings that are highly relevant to a cognitive analysis of help-giving concern the effect of relatives' levels of expressed emotion (EE) on patients' probability of relapse. Two major components of high EE are hostility and criticism, and these elements characterise a social environment that tends to be lacking in social support, or where support is undermined by specific negative interactions. It is now well established that depressed and schizophrenic patients are more likely to relapse when living with a high EE relative, and a recent review suggests that the adverse effects of high EE may apply equally to patients with a variety of physical and psychiatric disorders (Leff & Vaughn, 1985). Interventions with high EE relatives typically try to eliminate negative interactions in favour of positive, supportive ones (see Kuipers, this volume).

From the perspective of Weiner's theory, hostility and criticism on the part of a relative would be expected to stem from causal beliefs emphasising the patient's control over and responsibility for his or her negative behaviours. This was tested in a recent study by Brewin *et al.* (1991), who assessed attributions made spontaneously by relatives during the course of a semi-structured interview. Hostile and critical relatives were found to differ from low EE relatives in making more controllable attributions. What typified these relatives even more, however, was that they attributed the symptoms and negative behaviours to the patients' personal characteristics – that is, they saw the behaviours as reflecting the patients' character or whims rather than as manifestations of an illness that would be common to many sufferers. In contrast, emotional overinvolvement (the third component of high EE) was not related to any specific attributional pattern.

Particularly gratifying from the point of view of the attributional model was the confirmation that relatives did spontaneously make numerous attributions, did hold a wide variety of causal beliefs and were frequently engaged in a struggle to understand the origin of behaviours that to them were quite baffling. For example, one mother remarked of her 21-year-old son: 'There has been times when my husband's turned round to me and said: "Oh, he's lazy", 'cause he lays about, and I say: "No it's not, it's an illness." But he won't have it, he says: "No, he's just being idle." And I say: "It's not that at all." '

Very similar patterns of cognitions and emotions have been observed in studies of marital satisfaction. For example, Fincham *et al.* (1987) compared non-distressed couples with distressed couples seeking counselling. They found that distressed and non-distressed spouses were clearly differentiated by responsibility judgements for partners' behaviour that focused on negative intention, selfish motivation and blameworthiness. The general conclusion from a large number of studies reviewed by Bradbury & Fincham (1990) is that distressed spouses are more likely to see their partner and their relationship as the source of their difficulties. They also tend to see these causes as more global, i.e. affecting many areas of the marriage, as more blameworthy, and as more reflective of their spouse's negative attitude toward them.

Implications for clinical practice

Research on the family antecedents of perceived social support strongly suggests that, for some people, there will be deep-rooted barriers to the utilisation of existing resources. These individuals will be characterised by mistrust of supporters' motives, pessimism concerning the value of confiding, and a greater awareness of the risks rather than of the benefits of confiding. Such beliefs will almost certainly manifest themselves in the therapeutic situation as well and may impede the formation of any therapeutic alliance.

Therapists should therefore attempt an early evaluation of attitudinal constraints to receiving support, their date of origin and the extent to which mistrust and pessimism have generalised across a variety of relationships. These beliefs are likely to require longer-term therapeutic work, in either a cognitive or psychodynamic framework. One productive approach may be to make explicit the client's expectations of the therapist and of other people, and to subject these expectations wherever possible to empirical test. Expectations may be written down prior to therapeutic sessions or other interactions, and then evaluated in the light of how others actually behaved. Results disconfirming the client's expectations need to be fed back regularly and the implication for the existing belief system discussed.

Cognitive appraisals that are situationally based rather than rooted in enduring belief systems should in principle be easier to modify, and a number of examples of simple interventions have already been given (Anderson, 1983; Snyder & Ingram, 1983). Social competence beliefs that are inhibiting support-seeking may reflect veridically low estimates of social competence, and in these cases it would be wise to institute social skills training. Where beliefs in social incompetence do not reflect reality, however, some kind of cognitive restructuring is indicated. One approach is attribution therapy (e.g. Brewin, 1986, 1988), in which clients are required to identify specific instances of perceived social failure. Clients' attributions to social incompetence are questioned, and they are encouraged to generate alternative explanations for their experiences. Instructions to record their spontaneous attributions *in vivo* and to question them at the time may gradually lead to enduring cognitive change (see also Parry, this volume).

As discussed above, the presentation of normative information is frequently sufficient to reassure people about the acceptability of their feelings, symptoms or experiences, and to encourage help-seeking. Although some evidence suggests that unfavourable social comparisons are more strongly related to social withdrawal than to support-seeking from intimates or experts (Brewin *et al.*, 1989*b*), this finding does not apply to all problems. Homesick men, but not homesick women, tended to seek support when they perceived the feeling as a common reaction (Brewin *et al.*, 1989*a*), possibly because the problem was felt to be role-inappropriate only by the men. The absence of a link between social comparison and support-seeking may also not apply to particularly stigmatising conditions. For example, the increased coverage of childhood sexual abuse in the media seems, anecdotally, to have led to a greater willingness on the part of clients to disclose such experiences to professionals, often for the first time.

Another interpretation of Brewin *et al.*'s (1989*b*) data is suggested by social comparison theory. If social withdrawal is a strategy for maintaining the self-esteem of those who perceive themselves as deviant, those stigmatised by society or by themselves might find it attractive to interact with others perceived as similarly deviant, for example within the framework of a self-help group. In other words, perceiving few sources of support may be a consequence of the difficulty of finding suitable persons, rather than indicating a desire to avoid people generally. Coates & Peterson (1982) reported an experiment in which depressed and non-depressed students spoke with other students who were instructed to present themselves as either cheerful or complaining. Their depressed subjects were more pleased by conversations with complaining others, whereas their non-depressed subjects preferred the cheerful conversations.

The research reviewed has demonstrated, however, that trying to correct adverse social comparisons will not always be effective, for reasons that are generally related to self-esteem maintenance. Some conditions, such as being homosexual or HIV-positive, are still perceived as stigmatising, and are still negatively evaluated by others, even though they are recognised as common. Some individuals may have adopted coping strategies that depend on them identifying sufferers who are worse off than themselves. In these cases re-establishing the value of social support may involve focusing on related beliefs such as low self-esteem or pessimism about the future.

It is also worth considering how depression might affect both the processes involved in support-seeking and clinical recommendations. In addition to being associated with the symptom of social withdrawal, depression is known to affect a wide variety of cognitive appraisals, including the perceived risks and benefits of social interaction (East, 1989; Pietromonaco & Rook, 1987), social competence beliefs (Lewinsohn *et al.*, 1980), comparisons of self with others (Brewin & Furnham, 1986) and self-esteem (Brewin & Furnham, 1986; Brown *et al.*, 1986). All these cognitive changes are in a direction that would theoretically lead to the depressed person being less likely to utilise social support. There are considerable dangers, however, in regarding these changes simply as cognitive distortions that must be overcome if support networks are to be created or reinstated. Lewinsohn *et al.* (1980) found that depressed people's judgements about their social competence were supported by independent observers, and there is a considerable body of evidence that other people find it aversive to interact with someone who is depressed (e.g. Coyne, 1976; Gotlib & Robinson, 1983). Given the depressed person's typical sensitivity to criticism and rejection, clinicians should be exceptionally cautious in suggesting that they should seek additional support.

The work of Andrews & Brown (1988) suggests that therapists should additionally be on the lookout for instances of 'non-optimal confiding' in the depressed. In particular, it may be necessary to examine assumptions about what constitutes a supportive response, and to collect detailed descriptions of what supporters did and said. Given that negative comments from confidants can lead to increased characterological self-blame (e.g. Andrews & Brewin, 1990), part of the therapeutic work may lie as much in discouraging inappropriate confiding as in encouraging increased use of the support network.

The fact that relationships with spouses and intimate partners are of great importance in both depression and social support suggests that, instead of trying to increase general use of the support network, the most direct way of augmenting social support may be through marital or family therapy. Here it will be helpful to consider the kinds of cognitive appraisals made by family members and to modify these where appropriate. Work both with distressed couples and with the relatives of psychotic patients is strongly suggestive that judgements of controllability, intentionality and blame are precursors of the negative emotions that stand in the way of support being offered. Other cognitive components of marital conflict have been described by Epstein *et al.* (1993). They include selective attention to undesired behaviours, low expectations of the partner and of being able to resolve relationship problems, and incompatible assumptions and standards about appropriate behaviour.

There is scope for investigating and adapting existing treatment packages to focus more explicitly on these appraisals. For example, the findings of Brewin *et al.* (1991) identified hostile and critical relatives as attributing symptoms and undesirable behaviours to causes that were controllable by and idiosyncratic to the psychotic family member. It is known that relatives' critical attitudes can be modified either by family therapy or by attending a group for relatives of psychotic patients (e.g. Leff *et al.*, 1982, 1989), and it is plausible that attributional change is one of the major mechanisms underlying the success of these interventions. A follow-up study (Brewin, 1994) has found that as high EE relatives receiving an intervention became less hostile, there were commensurate changes in these personal and controllable attributions. It is interesting to note that, consistent with the specific theoretical link between attribution and anger, these interventions have been more successful at reducing hostility and criticism than at reducing emotional overinvolvement.

Summary

Cognitions enter into many aspects of help-seeking and help-giving. It may be helpful to distinguish enduring beliefs and assumptions about whether others are likely to be a reliable source of support from appraisals that are more relevant to a specific situation or class of situations. These may include beliefs about social competence, about similarity with others, and about the consequences for self-esteem. Enduring schemas about self and others may be more or less available to consciousness, and may have to be deduced from detailed questioning or repeated observations of behaviour. They are typically resistant to change and long-term therapeutic work may be necessary. Situational appraisals on the other hand are more likely to be available to consciousness and may be considerably easier to modify by an appropriate combination of behavioural social skills training and cognitive therapy. Careful note will, however, have to be taken of the implications for the client's habitual ways of maintaining self-esteem, and of potential exposure to sources of criticism, lack of empathy or rejection. Finally, it was noted that social support might best be enhanced via direct intervention with the client's family. Cognitive theories of help-giving are likely to prove of considerable value in designing more effective interventions of this kind.

Acknowledgement

I am grateful to Bernice Andrews for many discussions about the nature of social support.

References

Andersen, S. M. & Cole, S. W. (1990). 'Do I know you?': The role of significant others in general social perception. *Journal of Personality and Social Psychology*, **59**, 384–99.

Anderson, C. A. (1983). Motivational and performance deficits in interpersonal settings: the effect of attributional style. *Journal of Personality and Social Psychology*, **45**, 1136–47.

Anderson, C. A., Horowitz, L. M. & French, R. (1983). Attributional style of lonely and depressed people. *Journal of Personality and Social Psychology*, **45**, 127–36.

Andrews, B. & Brewin, C. R. (1990). Attributions of blame for marital violence: a study of antecedents and consequences. *Journal of Marriage and the Family*, **52**, 757–67.

Andrews, B. & Brown, G. W. (1988). Social support, onset of depression and personality. *Social Psychiatry and Psychiatric Epidemiology*, **23**, 99–108.

Baldwin, M. W. & Holmes, J. G. (1987). Salient private audiences and awareness of the self. *Journal of Personality and Social Psychology*, **52**, 1087–98.

Bandura, A. (1977). Self-efficacy: toward a unifying theory of behavioral change. *Psychological Review*, **84**, 191–215.

Bowlby, J. (1973). *Attachment and Loss*, vol. 2, *Separation*. London: Hogarth Press.

Bowlby, J. (1980). *Attachment and Loss*, vol. 3, *Loss, Sadness and Depression*. London: Hogarth Press.

Bowlby, J. (1982). *Attachment and Loss*, vol. 1, *Attachment*, 2nd edn. London: Hogarth Press.

Bradbury, T. N. & Fincham, F. D. (1990). Attributions in marriage: review and critique. *Psychological Bulletin*, **107**, 3–33.

Brewin, C. R. (1986). Strategies in the assessment and modification of causal attributions. In *Behavior Therapy: Beyond the Conditioning Framework*, ed. P. Eelen & O. Fontaine, pp. 234–52. Leuven: Leuven University Press/Lawrence Erlbaum.

Brewin, C. R. (1988). Attribution therapy. In *New Developments in Clinical Psychology*, vol. 2, ed. F. N. Watts, pp. 20–34. Leicester: British Psychological Society.

Brewin, C. R. (1994). Changes in attribution and expressed emotion among the relatives of patients with schizophrenia. *Psychological Medicine* **24**, 905–11.

Brewin, C. R. & Furnham, A. (1986). Attributional versus pre-attributional variables in self-esteem and depression: a comparison and test of learned helplessness theory. *Journal of Personality and Social Psychology*, **50**, 1013–20.

Brewin, C. R., Furnham, A. F. & Howes, M. (1989a). Demographic and psychological determinants of homesickness and confiding among students. *British Journal of Psychology*, **80**, 467–77.

Brewin, C. R., MacCarthy, B. & Furnham, A. F. (1989b). Social support in the face of adversity: the role of cognitive appraisal. *Journal of Research in Personality*, **23**, 354–72.

Brewin, C. R., MacCarthy, B., Duda, K. & Vaughn, C. E. (1991). Attribution and expressed emotion in the relatives of patients with schizophrenia. *Journal of Abnormal Psychology*, **100**, 546–54.

Brewin, C. R., Andrews, B. & Gotlib, I. H. (1993). Psychopathology and early experience: a reappraisal of retrospective reports. *Psychological Bulletin*, **113**, 82–98.

Brown, G. W., Andrews, B., Harris, T. D., Adler, Z. & Bridge, L. (1986). Social support, self-esteem and depression. *Psychological Medicine*, **16**, 813–31.

Coates, D. & Peterson, B. A. (1982). Depression and deviance. In *Integrations of Social and Clinical Psychology*. ed. G. Weary & H. L. Mirels, pp. 154–70. New York: Oxford University Press.

Cohen, L. H., Towbes, L. C. & Flocco, R. (1988). Effects of induced mood on self-reported life events and perceived and received social support. *Journal of Personality and Social Psychology*, **55**, 669–74.

Coyne, J. C. (1976). Depression and the response of others. *Journal of Abnormal Psychology*, **85**, 186–93.

Cutrona, C. E. & Russell, D. W. (1987). The provisions of social relationships and adaptation to stress. In *Advances in Personal Relationships*, vol. 1, ed. W. H. Jones & D. Perlman, pp. 37–67. Greenwich, Conn.: JAI Press.

Donlou, J. N., Wolcott, D. L., Gottlieb, M. S. & Landsverk, J. (1985). Psychosocial aspects of AIDS and AIDS-related complex: a pilot study. *Journal of Psychosocial Oncology*, **3**, 39–55.

Dunkel-Schetter, C., Folkman, S. & Lazarus, R. (1987). Correlates of social support receipt. *Journal of Personality and Social Psychology*, **53**, 71–80.

East, P. L. (1989). Early adolescents' perceived interpersonal risks and benefits: relations to social support and psychological functioning. *Journal of Early Adolescence*, **9**, 374–95.

Epstein, N., Baucom, D. H. & Rankin, L. A. (1993). Treatment of marital conflict: a cognitive-behavioral approach. *Clinical Psychology Review*, **13**, 45–57.

Festinger, L. (1954). A theory of social comparison processes. *Human Relations*, **7**, 117–40.

Fincham, F. D., Beach, S. & Nelson, G. (1987). Attribution processes in distressed and nondistressed couples. III. Causal and responsibility attributions of spouse behavior. *Cognitive Therapy and Research*, **11**, 71–86.

Fisher, J. D., Nadler, A. & Whitcher-Alagna, S. (1982). Recipient reactions to aid: a conceptual review. *Psychological Bulletin*, **91**, 27–54.

Flaherty, J. A. & Richman, J. A. (1986). Effects of childhood relationships on the adult's capacity to form social supports. *American Journal of Psychiatry*, **143**, 851–5.

Folkman, S., Lazarus, R. S., Dunkel-Schetter, C., DeLongis, A. & Gruen, R. (1986). Dynamics of a stressful encounter: cognitive appraisal, coping, and encounter outcomes. *Journal of Personality and Social Psychology*, **50**, 992–1003.

Goffman, E. (1968). *Stigma*. London: Penguin.

Gotlib, I. H. & Robinson, L. A. (1982). Responses to depressed individuals: discrepancies between self-report and observer-rated behavior. *Journal of Abnormal Psychology*, **91**, 231–40.

Henderson, S., Byrne, D. G. & Duncan-Jones, P. (1981). *Neurosis and the Social Environment*. New York: Academic Press.

Hobfoll, S. E., Nadler, A. & Leiberman, J. (1986). Satisfaction with social support during crisis: intimacy and self-esteem as critical determinants. *Journal of Personality and Social Psychology*, **51**, 296–304.

Lakey, B. & Cassady, P. B. (1990). Cognitive processes in perceived social support. *Journal of Personality and Social Psychology*, **59**, 337–43.

Leary, M. R., Atherton, S. C., Hill, S. & Hur, C. (1986). Attributional mediators of social avoidance and inhibition. *Journal of Personality*, **54**, 704–16.

Leff, J. & Vaughn, C. E. (1985). *Expressed Emotion in Families*. London: Guilford Press.

Leff, J., Kuipers, L., Berkowitz, R., Eberlein-Vries, R. & Sturgeon, D. (1982). A controlled trial of social intervention in the families of schizophrenic patients. *British Journal of Psychiatry*, **141**, 121–34.

Leff, J., Berkowitz, R., Shavit, N., Strachan, A., Glass, I. & Vaughn, C. E. (1989). A trial of family therapy versus a relatives group for schizophrenia. *British Journal of Psychiatry*, **154**, 58–66.

Lewinsohn, P. M., Mischel, W., Chaplin, W. & Barton, R. (1980). Social competence and depression: the role of illusory self-perceptions. *Journal of Abnormal Psychology*, **89**, 203–12.

MacCarthy, B. & Furnham, A. (1986). Patients' conceptions of psychological adjustment in the normal population. *British Journal of Clinical Psychology*, **25**, 43–50.

Mallinckrodt, B. (1991). Clients' representations of childhood emotional bonds with parents, social support, and formation of the working alliance. *Journal of Counseling Psychology*, **38**, 401–9.

Mallinckrodt, B. (1992). Childhood emotional bonds with parents, development of adult social competencies, and availability of social support. *Journal of Counseling Psychology*, **39**, 453–61.

Maybury, C. P. & Brewin, C. R. (1984). Social relationships, knowledge and

116   C. R. BREWIN

adjustment to multiple sclerosis. *Journal of Neurology, Neurosurgery, and Psychiatry*, **47**, 372–6.

Miles, A. (1979). Some psychosocial consequences of multiple sclerosis: problems of social interaction and group identity. *British Journal of Medical Psychology*, **52**, 321–31.

Nicholson, W. D. & Long, B. C. (1990). Self-esteem, social support, internalized homophobia, and coping strategies of HIV+ gay men. *Journal of Consulting and Clinical Psychology*, **58**, 873–6.

Ørner, R. J. (1987). Post-traumatic stress disorders in victims of the Falklands War: syndrome and treatment. Paper delivered at the British Psychological Society Annual Conference, Brighton.

Parker, G. & Barnett, B. (1988). Perceptions of parenting in childhood and social support in adulthood. *American Journal of Psychiatry*, **145**, 479–82.

Parker, G., Tupling, H. & Brown, L. B. (1979). A parental bonding instrument. *British Journal of Medical Psychology*, **52**, 1–10.

Pietromonaco, P. R. & Rook, K. S. (1987). Decision style in depression: the contribution of perceived risks versus benefits. *Journal of Personality and Social Psychology*, **52**, 399–408.

Sarason, I. G., Sarason, B. R. & Shearin, E. N. (1986). Social support as an individual difference variable: its stability, origins and relational aspects. *Journal of Personality and Social Psychology*, **50**, 845–55.

Sarason, B. R., Pierce, G. R., Shearin, E. N., Sarason, I. G., Waltz, J. A. & Poppe, L. (1991). Perceived social support and working models of self and actual others. *Journal of Personality and Social Psychology*, **60**, 273–87.

Sarnoff, I. & Zimbardo, P. G. (1961). Anxiety, Fear, and social affiliation. *Journal of Abnormal and Social Psychology*, **62**, 356–63.

Schachter, S. (1959). *The Psychology of Affiliation*. Stanford, California: Stanford University Press.

Sharrock, R., Day, A., Qazi, F. & Brewin, C. R. (1990). Explanations by professional care staff, optimism and helping behaviour: an application of attribution theory. *Psychological Medicine*, **20**, 849–55.

Sherman, B. R. & Donovan, B. R. (1991). Relationship of perceived maternal acceptance–rejection in childhood and social support networks of pregnant adolescents. *American Journal of Orthopsychiatry*, **61**, 103–13.

Singer, J. L. & Salovey, P. (1991). Organised knowledge structures and personality. In *Person Schemas and Maladaptive Interpersonal Patterns*, ed. M. J. Horowitz, pp. 33–79. Chicago: University of Chicago Press.

Snyder, C. R. & Ingram, R. E. (1983). 'Company motivates the miserable': the impact of consensus information on help seeking for psychological problems. *Journal of Personality and Social Psychology*, **45**, 1118–26.

Teglasi, H. & Hoffman, M. A. (1982). Causal attributions of shy subjects. *Journal of Research in Personality*, **16**, 376–85.

Weiner, B. (1986). *An Attributional Theory of Motivation and Emotion*. New York: Springer-Verlag.

Wortman, C. B. & Lehman, D. R. (1985). Reactions to victims of life crises: support attempts that fail. In *Social Support: Theory, Research and Practice*, ed. I. G. Sarason & B. R. Sarason, The Hague: Martinus Nijhoff.

Yalom, I. D. (1975). *The Theory and Practice of Group Psychotherapy*. New York: Basic Books.

5

Attachment, cooperation and rank: the evolution of the need for status and social support

PAUL GILBERT

This chapter will explore the role and function of social support from an evolutionary perspective. It is suggested that social behaviour has evolved over many millions of years and has given rise to a range of possibilities for social relating. Although in any particular interpersonal encounter many factors come into play (such as personal history, goals, emotional state (as discussed by Champion and by Brewin in this volume) and cultural values; see Hinde, 1987, 1992), it is still possible to recognise archetypal patterns of social relating. Examples are those based on attachment, cooperation and rank (e.g. dominant–subordinate). An evolutionary perspective clarifies our need for supportive relationships and offers a bridge to understanding the biological consequences of gaining and losing supportive relationships. In other words the importance of social support is very much related to the fact that we have evolved into highly social animals. A central facet of the argument developed here is that supportive relationships are reliable, should support status (the recipient feels valued) and are experienced as status-enhancing rather than opening a possibility for shaming and loss of status (Parry, 1988). This perspective also broadens the emphasis from individualistic theories of the causes and cures of psychopathology to understanding individuals in communities and their patterns of interaction.

Development

Infants are born ready to respond to other social beings. They are innately prepared to learn and take interest in the social environment (interest in faces, smiling, seeking and being reassured by physical contact, suckling, and so on). The role of touch and tactile input is of major importance (Montagu, 1986). In fact we now know that the neonate is extraordinarily talented and is born a social being (Slavin & Kriegman, 1992). Chamberlain (1987) says:

> Newborns have impressive resources for communicating actively with
> people around them. They express strong personal feelings facially and

vocally, listen with unbelievable precision, and show perceptive awareness of important changes as they scan the environment. Not only are they equipped to sense people but they respond strongly to social stimulation, prolong such stimulation, and what is more, initiate social interaction. Relationships are not static or one sided but dynamically changing, influential and reciprocal in nature. (p. 51)

From the first day of life, if attachment proceeds normally, we are held, fed, supported, encouraged, comforted, protected and cared for, and this can be a matter of life or death. Via interaction with others we build internal models of ourselves and others that will guide subsequent emotional and affectionate styles of relating; (Bowlby, 1969, 1973, 1980; Hinde, 1989; and the chapters by Champion and by Brewin in this volume). Running parallel to these facets is the fact that we are beings who are constantly looked at, scrutinised and evaluated by others. As we mature, we become increasingly aware that how we exist for others (how others see and judge us) determines their reactions to us. We learn quickly that some reactions are painful (if we are viewed negatively) while other reactions give a sense of pleasure and security. Hence one line of thought to be developed here is that recognition of our needs for support (for care, love, protection, approval and help) and our ability to elicit and utilise such support is monitored against *evaluations of how such signals will be scrutinised, judged and responded to.* Expressing our vulnerability and need for support may elicit fear of negative evaluation (e.g. we worry that others will judge it as a sign of weakness). Thus although we may be biologically prepared to be social and support-seeking animals, such behaviour is shaped via social context and values (Hinde, 1992). This will influence what is, and is not, sought out. For example, as a professional I might ask for support with a difficult clinical case but have more inhibition in seeking support for personal, depressed feelings and needs for personal reassurance (see Rippere & Williams, 1985; and Brewin, this volume). This, I shall argue, comes from our attempts to maintain status in the eyes of others and avoid evaluations that our needs mark us as inferior (Buunk & Hoorens, 1992).

   Moreover, there is growing awareness that social relations are major modulators of internal biological processes. Despite our growing understanding of the various messenger systems of the brain (neurotransmitters, receptor types, ATP, etc.) there is evidence that psychosocial stresses are key mediators of many such biological processes (Cacioppo & Berntson, 1992; Henry & Stephens, 1977; Ornstein & Swencionis, 1990; Sapolsky, 1990a, b) and that the stresses of early life can have profound long-term effects on endocrine and neurotransmitter systems with serious maturational consequences (Gabbard, 1992; Reite & Field, 1985), while new data suggest that psychosocial factors can interact with messenger RNA and DNA (Post, 1992).

Symptoms and relationships

Following the models and theories of Sullivan (1953), Leary (1957) and others, interpersonal theorists suggest there are two salient dimensions of relating. The first is concerned with *rank/status* (dominance–submission). The second is concerned with *affiliation/attachment* (closeness–distance, love–hate or friendly–hostile) (Birtchnell, 1990; Horowitz & Vitkus, 1986). In numerous studies these two dimensions of rank and affiliation have shown themselves to be robust dimensions of interpersonal behaviour (Wiggins & Broughton, 1985). Furthermore, their interaction (e.g. dominant–affiliative, dominant–hostile, subordinate–affiliative and subordinate–hostile) appear to account for variations in types of psychopathology and personality difficulties (Wiggins & Pincus, 1989). These give rise to particular forms of social relating that are either hard to do or are engaged in too much; for example, the person finds it hard to be assertive, hard to be intimate/trust, hard to be supportive, or is too aggressive, too intimate/open, etc. (Horowitz & Vitkus, 1986).

Wilhelm & Parker (1988), apparently unaware of the work by interpersonal theorists, developed a scale to measure intimate bonds. Via principal component analysis they elicited two dimensions of intimate relationships: *care* and *control*. Items from the care scale include: (my partner) is considerate of me; is a good companion; is affectionate to me. Items from the control scale include: (my partner) wants me to take his/her side in an argument; tends to try to change me; tends to criticise me in small ways. On the face of it, this research seems to be tapping into dimensions of dominance–subordination(control) and affiliation (care).

Researchers studying the biological consequences of changes in social relationships have also focused on these two dimensions of rank and attachment. Movement up and down the hierarchy is a major source of biological variation, both within (an individual animal gaining and losing rank) and between animals (comparison of low- and high-ranking animals). Biological parameters affected by rank include stress and sex hormones and monoamine activity (Henry, 1982; Sapolsky, 1989, 1990*a*, *b*). The biology of attachment and separation also shows that disruptions of social relationships have major biological effects (e.g. Reite & Field, 1985).

An evolutionary perspective

An evolutionary approach starts with the premise that our most basic social dispositions, like those of rank and attachment, are core potentials for relating and have a long-evolved history (Gilbert, 1989; Slavin & Kriegman, 1992). Core motivational systems represent the products of *selective pressure* (Buss, 1991; Trivers, 1985). Moreover the brain is not a unitary system, but consists of a set of mixed, social motivations, strategies and modular, evaluative systems that evolved to solve certain problems. Goals and strategies that increase the chances of the carrier's genes being represented in subsequent generations are passed on. This is called inclusive fitness. One central concern is phylogeny, that is the way *past* (breeding) environments have shaped evolutionarily stable social behaviours (e.g. courtship, care of offspring, altruism) over the long term and laid down gene–neural structures that underlie them (MacLean, 1985, 1990; Trivers, 1985; Gardner, 1988; Buss, 1991). All our innate potentials for social relating, such as attachment and dominance–subordination, evolved before the advent of modern society and agriculture (Barkow *et al.*, 1992).

A second concern is *ontogeny*, that is the way *current* environments amplify and/or inhibit, recruit and select from an array of (previously evolved) possible strategies. For example, ecology and social environments can vary as to how they facilitate the development of open, cooperative, mutually supportive and trusting relations, in contrast to individualistic, possessive, aggressive and distrustful relations (MacDonald, 1988; Power, 1991). Evolutionary theorists suggest that although there can be numerous variations on a theme (e.g. many different styles of attachment) and various combinations of different themes, nevertheless there are evolved stable 'cores' to our human interactions (e.g. care of offspring, mate selection) (Wenegrat, 1984; Trivers, 1985; MacDonald, 1988; Gilbert, 1989; Buss, 1991; Barkow *et al.*, 1992). Generally speaking, these core themes represent our human biosocial goals and strategies and they evolved as past solutions to problems posed by selective pressure (see Chisholm, 1988, for a good discussion). These focus on problems such as:

1 Care of offspring, together with the capability to shape the experience of offspring such that they can acquire the knowledge base necessary to live as a viable representative of that species.
2 Selecting, attracting and maintaining mates, including successful conception.
3 Selecting, attracting and maintaining alliances, including discrimination between ingroup–outgroup, or ally–non-ally.
4 Successfully negotiating social hierarchies and social place.

Social success

Successfully passing on genes (inclusive fitness) usually requires social success in the above domains (Gilbert, 1989; Nesse, 1990). For example, failing to care for offspring usually ends in their death. Importantly, many of our emotions seem connected with social success. Hence, we tend to feel good when we feel cared for and find a mate, have access to friends, have a sense of belonging within a group, gain respect and prestige. Negative emotions, in contrast, are associated with not being cared for, feeling alienated from others (an outsider), losing or failing to obtain respect, and not finding or losing a desired mate (Nesse, 1990). Affects seem set up to help us seek out and be rewarded by particular social relationship outcomes. Hence what is rewarding and threatening is not simply learnt but often relates to social success and evolutionarily meaningful goals. Such a view also leads to a theory of the evolution of human needs (e.g. for support, care, attachments, closeness, status, respect, freedom from terror: Gilbert, 1992*a*). There is now a sizeable literature showing that competent social behaviour in making friends and forming supportive intimate relations is linked to well-being and mental health (Argyle, 1987).

Evolutionary theorists currently suggest that social behaviour can be broken down into at least three basic functions: biosocial *goals*, evolved stable *strategies* and *algorithms*. Each evolved because it solved problems and gave reproductive advantage.

Biosocial goals

In general, biosocial goals turn out to be finite and relate to establishing control over resources. Goals may be experienced as something one is aiming for. Among the commonly agreed ones are:

1 *Attachment* between parent and offspring, involving the relationship of care-giving and care-eliciting.
2 *Mate selection* and sexual behaviour, involving choice, courting, conception and mate retention.
3 *Formation of alliances*, involving aggression inhibition, sharing, cooperative and reciprocal behaviour.
4 *Ranking behaviour*, involving gaining and maintaining rank/status and accommodation to those of higher rank.

Strategies

To secure any of the above biosocial goals there are a variety of potential strategies. These include aggression, deception, appeasement, altruism/helping/caring, or affiliation (or some combination). Strategies are goal serving. Thus one does not, say, deceive just for the sake of it, but to achieve some goal (e.g. gaining and enticing a mate, gaining a job, or money, maintaining status). Strategies are rewarding or punishing according to how far they move one towards a goal. Although strategies may be enacted consciously, they do not require conscious awareness but can be triggered automatically. For example, becoming angry and critical in an argument may be automatic and not the result of a conscious choice to use a coercive strategy. Indeed, on subsequent reflection we may wish we had exerted more conscious control over our anger.

Algorithms

Algorithms represent information processing routines. They influence attentional mechanisms and are the evaluative or reasoning modules; that is how information is evaluated *vis à vis* the goal that is being pursued. Typical algorithms are concerned with:

1 *Proximity–distance*. This concerns the awareness of distance–closeness to another; for example, an infant's awareness and monitoring of the availability of their caretaker. Separation, or too much distance, can activate protest (Bowlby, 1973). This algorithm may also be activated in situations where there are concerns about accessibility to supportive/ desired others (friends and confidants). Judging one is too distant from a desired lover or confidant might activate pinning and strategies to reduce the distance.

2 *Reciprocation*. This concerns judgements of give and take and evaluations that, over time, relationships are equitable (Parry, 1988). Alliance formations involve judgements of reciprocal altruism (Trivers, 1985), equity, and give and take. Negative affects can arise if one feels that one is taking more than one can repay, being obligated, a burden to others, or even fearful of being found deficient in repayment. Alternatively negative affects can arise from judging that one is giving more than is being repaid. This may include judgements of being taken advantage of, exploited or deceived (e.g. a person may say 'I always try to help others, but others are rarely there when I need them'). This can lead to anger or depressed mood. Recent research suggests that we may have specialised information processing abilities for the detection of cheating and non-reciprocation (for a review see Cosmides & Tooby, 1992).

3 *Social comparisons*. There seem to be two basic forms of social comparison: same–different (like me–not like me) and rank, inferior–superior. Comparison judgements of *same–different* seem important in defining ingroup and outgroup membership and also with whom one wishes to develop reciprocal relationships. These kinds of judgements also help to define self-identity (Brown & Lohr, 1987; Abrams *et al.*, 1990). Reciprocation, for humans, seems more likely to be established with individuals who share similar goals, attitudes and values. The other form of social comparison is not about judging how similar one is to a target group or other, but concerns one's relative rank and status position. Here the judgements are related to *inferior–superior*, stronger–weaker, etc.

Different goals, strategies and algorithms can link up in different ways. For example, in alliance formation and forming supportive networks, identifying potential allies (e.g. friends) might use the algorithms of social comparison of same–different. As noted, alliances are more likely to be developed with those seen as similar to oneself and this modifies aggression. The elicitors and forms of aggression differ according to whether they are directed at an ally/friend or non-ally (Hartup, 1989). With maturation (as we separate from parents and siblings and switch to peer group and sexual relationships) the judgements for selecting allies may change and centre on shared values (e.g. political, religious, academic, views on child-rearing). These are crucial judgements in order to avoid forming alliances with dissimilar others that might activate considerable conflict.

When the interpersonal theorists talk of 'too much or too little' (i.e. hard to be assertive, or too aggressive) they are referring to how *strategies* are being enacted, but these do not necessarily tell us what the biosocial goal is. A person may be aggressive because he or she wants to dominate and control others, or is feeling vengeful for being let down (non-reciprocated) by others, or is (mistakenly perhaps) hoping that others will recognise his or her needs and offer care/love. A person may like to ask for help but sees such requests as a mark of inferiority which would lower self-esteem (Fisher *et al.*, 1982) or cause a sense of shame–weakness (Gilbert, 1992*a*, 1993). Hence the way different individuals enact their life goals and the strategies are complex (Emmons, 1989). Because a person does not seek social support, or avoids closeness and intimacy, does not mean that they do not want it. Rather they may be distrustful, or too shame-prone to seek it (see Brewin, this volume). Buunk & Hoorens (1992) have recently outlined how social support interacts with the two social dimensions of social comparison and exchange processes, which overlap considerably with evolutionary concepts such as rank and reciprocal altruism (cooperation). Thus the degree to which gaining and giving social support is seen to raise or reduce rank/status and the degree to which it is seen as reciprocal (i.e. is part of social exchange and equity) have important effects.

Social and cultural constructions

As noted above, interpersonal researchers have repeatedly shown the importance of rank and affiliation/attachment, and their combinations. Evolution theorists might say that helping/investing in others versus coercing others are different strategies that have been associated with reproductive success (and will be used differently by males and females and directed differently at outgroup and ingroup members). However, this tells us little about their psychological organisation and great caution should be exercised in moving between innate potential and actual behaviour (Hinde, 1992). Indeed, the biggest gap in our understanding is the linkage between the evolved stable potentials of humans, laid down in gene–neural structures, and their psychosocial/ cultural modification (Barkow, 1991; Barkow *et al.*, 1992). As soon as we take into account that evolved biosocial goals and strategies are mediated through flexible developmental processes, which are sensitive to particular punishments and frustrations/deprivations, and are influenced by contextual and environmental indicators of fitness, then the old genetic determinism that sees culture and evolution as alternatives fades away (Hinde, 1987, 1989, 1992). Furthermore, it becomes possible to see that the environment (and even the ecology: Van Schaik, 1989; Power, 1991) tends to select and amplify different goals and strategies. An extreme human example is that in some cultures, some individuals may be so motivated to gain economic success (i.e. make a career and money) that they forego interest in rearing or caring for offspring.

But more salient to the area of social support is that although the evidence suggests that early humanoids were cooperative, mutually supportive and egalitarian (e.g. see Glantz & Pearce, 1989; Howells & Willis, 1989; Power, 1992), this has changed in modern industrial societies. Thus in some sections of Western culture the emphasis is on toughness, face saving, and avoidance of showing emotional distress. The avoidance of being seen as weak, especially for males, may do much to recruit individualistic focused goals, preoccupation with social status and aggressive strategies (Gilbert, 1992a, 1993; Miedzian, 1992). This style is not reflected in all cultures (Howells & Willis, 1989; Hinde & Groebel, 1991). The social construction of gender does much to encourage or dissuade males and females to confide in others and develop close emotional, supportive and affectionate relationships, or avoid them. This cultural scripting of gender affects the styles of friendship (both between and across genders), the organisation of networks, the degree of intimate confiding and sharing that takes place in supportive relationships and the areas that are shameful, and run counter to gender definitions (Nardi, 1992).

Thus we need to stress that evolutionary approaches speak of potentials rather than texts that proscribe certainties. In the next section rank and affiliation are explored in more detail.

Rank

We are now in position to take a closer look at rank. When we do this we see that rank is a description of a relationship. In humans (and probably other primates) seeking to gain rank (and thus control over resources) may utilise different strategies of coercion/aggression and affiliation/ attractiveness (Gilbert, 1990, 1992*a*, *b*; Barkow, 1991).

1. Being (seen as) powerful and making others submit or avoid challenging out of fear. This is showing one's toughness/fighting ability: the authoritarian hierarchy – one takes what one wants or enforces control. In the interpersonal approach it is called hostile-dominance. Here, higher ranks seek the submission and compliance signals of those lower in the hierarchy. Time and energy may be directed in preventing others from doing things (e.g. gaining access to mates).

2. Being seen as able and talented, desired or positively attractive. This is demonstrating attributes that are useful to others: the authoritative–affiliative hierarchy (or friendly-dominance). One entices the other to give *voluntarily* what is wanted; to be chosen, selected, sought out (Gilbert, 1992*a*). Kemper (1988, 1990) calls this eminence. Barkow (1980, 1991) refers to it as gaining prestige. The focus is on gaining status via affiliative behaviour rather than threat. I suspect that this profile involves two basic signals: (1) Demonstrating ability/talent so that one might be chosen above others (as a mate or friend) or affectionately respected – this is a status aspect; and (2) Reciprocal altruism and affiliation. Thus a complex signal is communicated which indicates both the quality of oneself and the type of relationship one is offering; e.g. 'If you choose me (as a mate, or friend/ally, etc.) I will be useful/supportive of you and your goals'.

In general, then, tactics of influence fall into two main domains as shown in Fig. 5.1.

Generally speaking, involuntarily losing rank and status has rather negative effects on mood and behaviour (Gilbert, 1990, 1992*a*; Henry, 1982). As noted above an important social evaluation for rank is *social comparison* (Suls & Wills, 1991). Research has shown this to be an important judgement in support-giving and -receiving (Buunk & Hoorens, 1992; and Brewin, this volume).

When animals, including birds and reptiles, threaten each other their behaviour and the type of social signals exchanged are not that dissimilar from those of humans. (Price, 1988; Price & Sloman, 1987). For example, in conflict situations animals will often stare at each other and pull themselves up to their full height with erect posture and tense musculature. This behaviour allows each to weigh up the other and compare their strength with the contestant. The one that evaluates itself as superior pushes home the challenge, while the one that evaluates it will lose, backs off, runs away or sends submissive signals. If you watch two boxers in a stand off, the meeting of eye gaze and standing erect are still powerful threat signals.

Competing to be recognised as attractive/desirable or wanted may lead

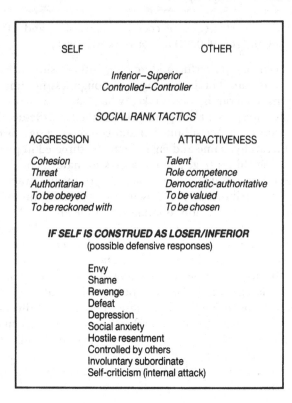

Figure 5.1. Social rank perceptions.

to exhibition of talent (e.g. to gain a prestigious job), or to be popular, or in some way exhibit qualities that others bestow interest on. Here there are more complex forms of social comparison. For example, a man may be aware, say, that his lover might prefer someone else and seeks constant reassurance: 'Do you love me more than Fred?' There is recognition that he may be in competition with Fred, and he compares himself both with Fred and what the lover says about Fred and how she acts towards him. In intimate relationships support of status comes from showing signals of preference for the partner, demonstrating that he or she is valued. This sense of being valued by others is a core dimension of social support (Parry, 1988). Rivalries and jealousies that can disrupt social bonds (intimate and social) often centre around concerns that others are gaining more prestige or attention (are seen as more attractive) than oneself.

Biological considerations

Gaining rank bestows many advantages, the most important of which is that it opens up preferential access to resources. Those higher in the rank structure usually have better access to resources compared with those of lower rank. But there are also important biological *effects* of rank. In most non-human primate studies to date subordinates show greater activation of the hypothalamic-pituitary-adrenocortical (HPAC) axis with higher levels of circulating cortisol being especially noted. However, in unstable groups dominant animals can show levels almost as high as subordinates. Sapolsky (1989, 1990*a*, *b*) suggests that low-cortisol dominant baboons tend to express various social behaviours.

1 They differentiate well between a threatening rival and other animals.
2 When threatened they initiate fights and usually win.
3 If they lose they displace aggression on to a third party.
4 They have high levels of non-sexual affiliative interactions with infants and females.

The relationship between HPAC activity and dominance is not straightforward and there are species differences (McGuire, 1988), but the data might suggest the following linkage: affiliative-dominant individuals have the lowest levels of HPAC activation, aggressive and insecure dominant males the next highest, and low ranks the highest levels.

Sapolsky's work makes clear that the biological profiles of rank are *consequences not causes of rank succession*. Sapolsky (1989, 1990*a*, *b*) in his studies of free-ranging baboons has also shown that subordinates, even in stable groups, can be dexamethasone resistant, although the reasons for this are complex. Although the linkage of HPAC activity with dominance–subordination is complex, similar findings have been found in humans (Price, 1982; Kemper, 1990). Central factors relate to control/power to influence others, predictability and affiliation. Depression and other pathologies are known to involve heightened cortisol levels, disturbance of HPAC and dexamethasone resistance (Arana *et al.*, 1985). Life event difficulties in depressed patients have also been shown to be associated with high(er) urinary free cortisol (Dolan *et al.*, 1985).

Raleigh *et al.* (1984) have found that blood levels of the neurotransmitter serotonin (5-HT) are sensitive to the rank situation. Subordinates have lower levels of blood 5-HT than dominant individuals – sometimes considerably lower. 5-HT alters according to dominant–subordinate relationships. In dominant animals 5-HT falls if subordinates are removed from the group and it falls if the dominant animals themselves are removed. Thus, it has been suggested that 5-HT is sensitive to rank relationships. As far as I know the hostile–affiliative dimension has not been controlled for, so we do not know whether the same relations arise in hostile (insecure) dominant and affiliative (secure) dominant animals. A recent study by Raleigh *et al.* (1991) found that serotonergic antidepressants (which enhance 5-HT transmission) affect behaviour that has the consequence of increasing an animal's rank. The exact mechanism of this is unknown. For example, it may be that these antidepressants reduce social fear, or reduce internal inhibition, or have general effects on defence system processing (Gilbert, 1989, 1992a).

The hormone testosterone is higher in dominant than subordinate animals, and many studies have suggested that testosterone is sensitive to rank changes (Kemper, 1990). Thus, in non-human primate and human studies, subordinates show differences in neuroendocrine state compared with the more dominant (for a review see Henry & Stephens, 1977; Henry, 1982; McGuire, 1988). But in humans these relations are complex. For example a testosterone increase may arise from winning at competitive games (e.g. tennis) but much depends on the value placed on winning; and if the winner is unhappy with the way he played, then winning fails to produce testosterone increases (Kemper, 1990). Kemper (1990) also points out that the social environment does much to set the context and opportunities for competing for status, and gives values to different types of status behaviours. These will affect whether any specific behaviour will be related to testosterone change.

Status, shame and self-presentation

For humans, self-presentation (the signals we send to others) is a central concern (Baumeister, 1982, 1986) and is clearly linked with status in the eyes of others (Gilbert, 1992a) and the avoidance of shame (Scheff, 1988; Kaufman, 1989; Broucek, 1991). Shame arises from (fear of) being seen as weak, inferior and an object of scorn, which motivates concealment and deception. It may be that there are evolved mechanisms that alert us to the fact that to be seen as weak/needy and vulnerable makes us unattractive as an ally. Rather, such social investments tend to go to those who show health, confidence and talent. Thus, one may deceive others of one's true feelings/needs/vulnerabilities and keep them hidden. Thus, fear of shame need not be solely the consequence of developmental history.

Brewin & Furnham (1986) found that depressed persons often fail to reveal to others their internal experiences for fear of scorn. Generally, self-presentation involves efforts to direct (and avoid) certain types of attention from others. We monitor our behaviour and present ourselves to others such that we try to reduce threats (e.g. loss of approval) and defend our own displays and presentations. Hence a person may not like to cry in front of others, or may deny/conceal true feelings, such as anger or emotional needs, in case this elicits counter-anger, loss of status or rejection. This takes us into the area of social prescriptions of social displays/signals that meet with approval or rejection. Support seems contingent upon sending the right signals and not those that could result in shame.

Work on gender identity, for example, suggests that men may be concerned to demonstrate their power and toughness and to play down their capacities for empathy, nurturing and affectionate intimacy (Gilbert, 1994). Miedzian (1992) notes studies where men wanted to be closer to their children but felt it was not manly. Thus, the image of themselves they were endeavouring to create for themselves and in the minds of others significantly inhibited forms of affectionate relating. Until recently women seeking support for sexual abuse or marital violence were the exception rather than the rule because to admit to this was to risk shame.

Rank judgements (which can be derived from both social comparisons and the social signals directed at the self) are salient sources of self-esteem (Robson, 1988; Gilbert, 1990, 1992*a*) and are active in social support giving and eliciting (Buunk & Hoorens, 1992). Thus, a person may label or judge him/herself and/or has judgements made by others that are not only negative but also suggest they have been allocated a low rank and/or low status. Thus, judgements such as unlovable, worthless, bad, inadequate or useless are in effect assignments of status that locate the individual in a low status position and thereby convey dramatic reductions or confinements on their eligibility to participate advantageously in social relationships and elicit helpful alliances. Sometimes this relates to feelings of how much one deserves. It is not uncommon for depressed people to suggest that they do not deserve help, support, to be loved, or other resources, because of preoccupations with low self-worth and/or guilt.

Attacks on rank/status

Attacks on rank and status involve put-down signals which can take various forms: *physical attacks/threats*, such as aggression (hitting) or ritualised aggression (shouting, screaming, intimidating); *verbal insults and symbolic threats*, such as scorn, ridicule, criticism, sarcasm, jokes and condescending verbal and non-verbal behaviour; *neglect*, such as ignoring, not listening to or taking notice of, and lack of interest; and *removal of investment signals*, such as actual withdrawal of or threats to withdraw love/attention/support/help, etc.

Getting others to submit can have positive effects for the one seeking control but will not develop the more prosocial possibilities in a *relationship* (e.g. openness, mutuality, equality, sharing, moral behaviour) and can have very serious effects on those who are the recipients of neglect, attack and put-down (Gilbert, 1992*a*). Research suggests that spouse criticism, for example, is a salient predictor of relapse into depression (Hooley & Teasdale, 1989). Some of these signals are examples of high 'expressed emotion' (e.g. see Jenkins & Karno, 1992;

and Kuipers, this volume) which is now well established as influencing relapse and recovery of certain pathologies.

Clinical experience suggests that people who do not seek or use social support fear eliciting the above signals from others and give reasons such as 'It would be seen as weak', 'It would put me in a one down position', 'The other person wouldn't like it', i.e. I would lose positive approval, I would be a burden, I would be rejected, I don't trust others, They wouldn't understand me, It would give them too much control over me, etc. (Parry, 1988; and Brugha, chapter 14, this volume).

Investments and boosts to rank/status

Because, in humans, ranks are often linked with self-presentation signals, both sent and received, and the desire to be attractive to others and to elicit their voluntary bestowing of resources, there are many types of signal that can boost a person's sense of status and self-esteem. Basically these are signals that one is valued, approved of and that others are prepared to invest time, attention and resources (Gilbert, 1992a).

Investments are social rewards but also belong to what has been called *prosocial safety or reassurance signals* because of their general effects on psychobiological functioning and *social relations* (Gilbert, 1993). These signals convey to an individual that he or she can rely on others; that is, others are able and willing to invest in them (rather than challenge them, take things away or put them down). Bailey (1988; Bailey *et al.*, 1992) suggests that this is like treating others as though they were kin. Gilbert (1992a) suggests that this also involves sending signals that one supports the person as being a valued member of one's network of alliances and group. These signals have the effect of boosting the person's self-esteem and control, helping them to feel secure, content and happy (Price, 1988). They are likely to be especially effective if they have long-term implications.

Social investments from others can be seen as self-esteem 'boosting' signals. They include: *actual rewards*, such as acquiring control over resources, being awarded prizes, being helped to obtain a desired incentive, a voluntary bestowing of resources that is pleasurable for the receiver and giver; *social attention*, such as listening, valuing, empathising, taking interest in, approval, encouraging and acceptance; and *reassurance*, such as helping, offering support or sharing feelings, the positive exchange of facial signals (e.g. smiling), non-verbal behaviour (e.g. cuddling) and breaking down a sense of difference between people, etc. These rewarding and reassuring signals activate a sense of safeness (Gilbert, 1992a, 1993), encourage exploration and an openness of attention, trust and non-defensive behaviour.

In general the recipient of investment signals experiences two outcomes.

First, the social environment is experienced as beneficial, rather than harmful. Second, it boosts self-esteem and a sense of status and attractiveness to others, via the experience of being valued, approved of, desired, wanted, esteemed, helped, etc. Third, knowing that one is valued and accepted means that one does not involuntarily need to submit to others or be defensive. Rather one is free to make requests, put one's point of view, confide in others without risk of being put down, attacked or rejected. If one does not feel valued or is shame-prone (Kaufman, 1989) none of these things can be assumed.

Many therapies which provide interpersonal relationships where the therapist is empathic and listens in a friendly, reassuring way, are experienced as helpful and boosting (Frank, 1982; Bailey, 1988; Bailey *et al.*, 1992). Moreover, interpersonal therapists have noted that attention to both affiliative and status-enhancing messages is important (Horowitz & Vitkus, 1986; Bergner, 1988). Receiving social investments has positive effects on relationships and psychopathology. For example, supportive social interactions (e.g. befriending) have been shown to have positive effects on chronic, retarded psychiatric patients (Matson & Zeiss, 1979), while social support and access to a confidant have major effects on anxiety and depression (Brown *et al.*, 1986; Stokes & McKirnan, 1989; Brugha *et al.*, 1990) and other health indices (Argyle, 1987; Ornstein & Swencionis, 1990). Loss of esteem-supporting signals can have the reverse effect (Brown & Harris, 1978). Thus status modulations seem a salient dimension of how social support exerts its effects.

Affiliation, attachment and cooperation: the basis of belonging

A complication in understanding affiliative relationships is that they can be described as varying along a dimension of *intimate, personal, social* and *public* (Hall, 1979). Gilbert (1989) pointed out that there are important psychological differences between cooperation, caring-giving, care-eliciting, and status-enhancing behaviour which operate on this intimate–public dimension. Hence affiliation, love and trust/mistrust relate to the dimension of interpersonal spacing and not to cooperation, caring-giving, care-eliciting or status evaluations themselves. A few examples are offered below.

Caring/giving behaviour can be directed at other people, to oneself, to animals, to the environment or to inanimate objects such as a car or house (Fogel *et al.*, 1986). It involves a focus on another, evaluating their needs, and this may not be reciprocal. In its intimate forms it can involve love (as for a child, or even one's car) and attachment behaviour, but it need not. For example, charity work does not require close affiliations, attachments or love, nor desires to be with the targets of one's caring actions, nor expectations of repayment/reciprocation. Negatively, guilt may give rise to caring behaviour (one thinks one *ought* to help X), but there may be resentment for having to do it (Gilbert, 1992*a*). More positively one may experience pleasure for seeing others prosper from one's own caring behaviour. Indeed this pleasure is one reason that we care for each other in our multitude of ways, in addition to gaining status for it (Hill, 1984). Caring, unlike cooperation, does not require reciprocation or repayment.

Care/help eliciting is our primary mode of relating from the first days of life. We are born needing others to survive and mature. In the care-eliciting situation the self (or group, e.g. a nation asking for help with a famine) targets behaviours towards others who are seen to be capable of providing what is needed. In its pure form it does not involve reciprocation. Later in life, however, it may become difficult to elicit help without feeling a need to repay it, and thus turn it into a cooperative exchange (Buunk & Hoorens, 1992). There are many reasons for this, related to the fact that one has to signal need for help in some way. Some of these might include: (1) eliciting and receiving may invoke fears of being (seen as) inferior and shamed; (2) the 'what' of the need is seen as culturally unacceptable; (3) seeing others who are not so much in need as oneself invokes destructive envy, difficulties with gratitude and focuses the person on what they lack; (4) it may give too much control to others and smacks of dependency; (5) it can introduce concerns with obligations and feeling burdened and indebted ('If I don't want anything from them then they won't ask anything of me'). Again these may vary as to whether one is eliciting help for practical things or for more emotional–intimate needs.

Cooperative behaviour (in contrast to hostile individualistic competitiveness and possessiveness) in small close-knit communities was adaptive for early humans for very many reasons (e.g. protection against predators and other human groups, better utilisation of resources; Glantz & Pearce, 1989). It is focused on mutual gains, sharing, reciprocality, role enactments and growing/developing together. While cooperation may involve affiliation and closeness it does not always do so. An army can cooperate with rigid hierarchies but little affiliative behaviour up the ranks. Nations may form alliances for various reasons but still be mistrustful of each other. A person might be very good at giving social support that involves specific tasks (e.g. fixing things, specific actions/roles or lending money) but be very poor when it comes to intimate or emotional support-giving. Intimate cooperation, however, probably does involve affiliative emotions as well as marking the areas for what is shared. It probably also increases a desire for proximity and association.

Status enhancement is directed at boosting status/power and abilities of others. Teaching might be an example. It can recruit various aspects of caring behaviour and may or may not be affiliative. Psychotherapy, for example, can be seen primarily, as a status-enhancing interaction (Bergner, 1988) rather than a close cooperative relationship. This is because patients are not expected to get to know, help or support the therapist in any major way, and the problems of the therapist are kept out of the sessions; it is a mainly one-way transaction. What cooperation there is, is to help with the patient's difficulties only. Therapists are trained to send signals of valuing their patients (via empathy, positive regard, etc.) but also trained not to expect the patient to reciprocate these things. Indeed much training can be given to helping the therapist understand and deal with their own feelings when a patient is critical, disparaging or angry for perceived therapist failures. It is this aspect that raises difficult power issues. Moreover, therapists who have strong needs for their patients to like them, who stray too far into forming deep affiliative relations with their patients, or who sexualise them, can cause serious problems. It is these complications that make therapy such a paradoxical business.

Nevertheless, in everyday life, cooperative, caring and status-enhancing interactions often flow together. Being in a position to give support or help may also raise the status of the donor in the eyes of the receiver or onlookers (Hill, 1984). Successful efforts to help others (and at times the experience of their gratitude) may boost self-esteem.

An evolutionary perspective

The evolutionary perspective suggests that helping and support-giving are influenced by the relatedness of the participants (Trivers, 1985). The issue of relatedness, however, has two aspects. The first is direct genetic relatedness (kin altruism). Thus at the extreme someone who is affiliative with their own families can be extraordinarily vindictive to others. Some high-ranking Nazis, for example, could be affectionate to their own children only to walk out of the house to gas others. While we spend money on our own children (at Christmas and other times) we also know perfectly well that across the world many millions are starving. Although the evolutionary theorists argue that this is related to kin selection, xenophobia and other evolved traits, it is also the case that some individuals can take great risks to help others (Oliner & Oliner, 1988).

The second aspect of relatedness – via common/similar values, goals and personality type (Argyle, 1991) – arises from reciprocal altruism (Trivers, 1985) and forms the basis for ingroup–outgroup boundaries. It bears on what social psychologists have considered as equity theory (Brown, 1986; Buunk & Hoorens, 1992). With maturity the ability to form supportive relations outside the family become increasingly important. It allows helpful, supporting relations to form in the absence of known genetic relatedness but where an alliance would be of mutual gain. Thus human cooperation, which can lead to *companionable relating*, depends centrally on reciprocality, joint action and the type of attention being given and received. Heard & Lake (1986) capture this aspect well when they suggest that:

> The goal of companionable relating is reached whenever an individual construes from the emotive messages sent by companions, that they are taking interest in and showing appreciation of his contribution and the way he is making it; and at the same time, realises that the interest he is taking in the contribution of his companions is also appreciated.   (p. 431)

These aspects give us our sense of belonging, they root us in a social space, make the social environment predictable and offer an identity with which we can interact in the world. To lose a sense of belonging can lead to the experiences of being an outsider (Gilbert, 1992*a*).

Forms of affiliative–supportive relationships

Not surprisingly, then, research suggests there are many types of supportive and affiliative relationships. Hill (1984) found that people seek out others for various reasons and identified four major dimensions: (1) emotional support, (2) attention, (3) positive stimulation and (4) social comparison. Other researchers distinguish between gaining practical help, problem solving and emotional support. Weiss (1986) suggests six forms of what he calls 'social bonds': attachment, affiliation, collaboration, persisting alliances which are strongly associated with feelings of obligation to help the other, and help-obtaining which relates to relationships in which someone is perceived as a source of guidance.

Buunk & Hoorens (1992) also note that need for support (especially when others seem to be coping better than oneself) can be seen as status reducing and may lead to avoidance of acknowledging need (Fisher *et al.*, 1982). Also it may place burdens for subsequent repayment. Thus understanding the rank, social status/shame and reciprocal implications of help eliciting and receiving may help explain some of the negative (stress-increasing) effects of social support.

The breakdown of affiliative–supportive bonds

However we wish to describe affiliative and supportive bonds, when they break down they may be experienced as painful. Difficulty in forming, sustaining or losing long-term supportive relations are now known to be a marker for later psychopathology (Bowlby, 1980; Goodyer, 1990).

Biological effects of separation

A clue to this may be found in the effects of separation. There is now clear evidence that social separation, particularly disruptions of attachment bonds, causes major changes in many neurotransmitter systems (Reite & Field, 1985). Some of these early disruptions may have very long-term effects (Post, 1992). Animal work also suggests that previous experiences of separations affect later vulnerabilities to social disruptions (Reite & Field, 1985).

Coe *et al.* (1985) investigated the protective influence of social versus non-social familiar environments in primate infants separated from their mothers. The greatest protection was for infants in familiar cages with familiar others. Coe *et al.* conclude therefore:

> Thus, although overt care giving and solicitous behaviour does not appear to be a prerequisite for a beneficial effect to occur in the home environment, it does appear that social companionships are essential ... The social companions must be familiar to the infant in order for the beneficial effect to occur. (p. 174)

Alternative caregivers (aunts) and known peers appear to be of crucial importance in the capacity to cope with the distress of separation. Moreover, these social resources have protective influences on the activation of the HPAC system (Reite & Field, 1985). Although infant separation responses (both behavioural and biological) may be different from those of more mature animals, and we should be cautious about assuming otherwise, such work may still have important implications in psychological research on life events. Psychobiological research on the disruption of social bonds would seem the next logical step and would give more data on the value of social support whilst offering new psychobiological insights (especially if biological practitioners are going to take indices such as cortisol dysfunction as markers of a 'disease process' in the absence of concern with social relations). It would be very interesting to know whether those who have low social support demonstrate greater HPAC activity in the presence of exit life events (e.g. see Dolan *et al.*, 1985), and whether this is reversible with more advantageous changes in the social environment.

Conclusion

In this chapter we have explored an evolutionary view of social support. The propensities of our social behaviours arose from millions of years of evolving biosocial goals and stable strategies. So too did our need for supportive relations. Social relations serve many different purposes:

care-giving and care-eliciting, cooperation and status enhancement (rank). Changes in rank/status, attachment and cooperative opportunities appear to have many hormonal and neurotransmitter consequences. However, the need and use of social relationships change with development. The close attachments to caregivers are of primary importance in early life but with maturity there is a gradual movement to forming relations with non-kin, becoming a member of a peer group, seeking out peers for reciprocal, social support and status enhancement, and finding sexual partners, who may also become the sources of emotional support as well as cooperating in child rearing.

Family, cultural and economic values, such as gender scripts, acceptance of needs and vulnerabilities, tactics of face saving, and the avoidance of showing weakness and need, significantly interact with the preparedness, recognition and ability to both elicit and respond to self and others' particular needs (see Parry, this volume). Perhaps one reason why psychotherapies are so popular is that they provide very special types of relationship that are (supposed to be) affiliative, non-attacking, status-enhancing and allow communication of emotional needs.

As Parry (1988) and Buunk & Hoorens (1992) point out, to understand more fully the positive and negative effects of social support, greater consideration could be given to the psychological dimensions of social comparison and social exchange. Shame, for example, may help to explain why social support can have negative effects and why it is not sought out even if available. It has been argued that shame and fear of rejection in turn could be explored with an evolutionary perspective that sets social relationships in a bio-historical framework. This can act as a bridge between the psychosocial and physiological. As Hinde (1987, 1992) points out we need greater cross-disciplinary synthesis in our psychological theories, research endeavours and practice.

References

Abrams, D., Cochrane, S., Hogg, M. A. & Turner, J. C. (1990). Knowing what to think by knowing who you are: self categorization and the nature of norm formation, conformity and group polarization. *British Journal of Social Psychology*, **29**, 97–119.

Arana, G. W., Baldessarini, R. J. & Ornsteen, M. (1985). The dexamethasone suppression test for diagnosis of and prognosis in psychiatry. *Archives of General Psychiatry*, **42**, 1193–204.

Argyle, M. (1987). *The Psychology of Happiness*. London: Methuen.

Argyle, M. (1991). *Cooperation: The Basis of Sociability*. London: Routledge.

Bailey, K. G. (1987). *Human Paleopsychology Applications to Aggression and Pathological Processes*. Hillsdale, N. J.: Lawrence Erlbaum.

Bailey, K. G. (1988). Psychological kinship: implications for the helping professions. *Psychotherapy*, **25**, 132–41.

Bailey, K. G., Wood, H. & Nava, G. R. (1992). What do clients want? Role of psychological kinship in professional helping. *Journal of Psychotherapy Integration*, **2**, 125–47.

Barkow, J. H. (1975). Prestige and culture: a biosocial interpretation (plus peer review). *Current Anthropology*, **16**, 533–72.

Barkow, J. H. (1980). Prestige and self-esteem: a biosocial interpretation. In *Dominance Relations: An Ethological View of Social Conflict and Social Interaction*, ed. D. R. Omark, D. R. Strayer & J. Freedman. New York: Garland STPM Press.

Barkow, J. H. (1991). Precis of Darwin, sex and status: biological approaches to mind and culture (plus peer commentary). *Behavioral and Brain Sciences*, **14**, 295–334.

Barkow, J. H., Cosmides, L. & Tooby, J. (1992). *The Adapted Mind: Evolutionary Psychology and the Generation of Culture*. New York: Oxford University Press.

Baumeister, R. F. (1982). A self-presentational view of social phenomena. *Psychological Bulletin*, **91**, 3–26.

Baumeister, R. F. (1986). How the self became a problem: a psychological review of historical research. *Journal of Personality and Social Psychology*, **52**, 163–76.

Bergner, R. M. (1988). Status dynamic psychotherapy with depressed patients. *Psychotherapy*, **25**, 266–72.

Birtchnell, J. (1990. Interpersonal theory: criticism, modification and elaboration. *Human Relations*, **43**, 1183–201.

Bowlby, J. (1969). *Attachment and Loss*, vol. 1, *Attachment*. London: Hogarth Press.

Bowlby, J. (1973). *Attachment and Loss*, vol. 2, *Separation, Anxiety and Anger*. London: Hogarth Press.

Bowlby, J. (1980). *Attachment and Loss*, vol. 3, *Loss: Sadness and Depression*. London: Hogarth Press.

Bowlby, J. (1988). Developmental psychiatry comes of age. *American Journal of Psychiatry*, **145**, 1–10.

Brewin, C. R. & Furnham, A. (1986). Attributional and pre-attributional variables in self-esteem and depression: a comparison and test of learned helplessness theory. *Journal of Personality and Social Psychology*, **50**, 1013–20.

Broucek, F. J. (1991). *Shame and the Self*. New York: Guilford.

Brown, B. B. & Lohr, M. J. (1987). Peer-group affiliation and adolescent self-esteem: an integration of ego-identity and symbolic-interaction theories. *Journal of Personality and Social Psychology*, **52**, 47–55.

Brown, G. W. & Harris, T. (1978). *The Social Origins of Depression*. London: Tavistock.

Brown, G. W., Bifulco, A., Harris, T. O. & Bridge, L. (1986). Social support, self-esteem and depression. *Psychological Medicine*, **16**, 813–31.

Brown, R. (1986). *Social Psychology*, 2nd edn. New York: Macmillan.

Brugha, T. S., Bebbington, P. E., MacCarthy, B., Sturt, E., Wykes, E. & Potter, J. (1990). Gender, social support and recovery from depressive disorders: a prospective study. *Psychological Medicine*, **20**, 147–56.

Buss, D. M. (1991). Evolutionary personality psychology. *Annual Review of Psychology*, **42**, 459–91.

Buunk, B. P. & Hoorens, V. (1992). The role of social comparison and social exchange processes. *British Journal of Clinical Psychology*, **31**, 445–57.

Cacioppo, J. T. & Berntson, G. G. (1992). Social psychological contributions to the decade of the brain. *American Psychologist*, **47**, 1019–28.

Chamberlain, D. B. (1987). The cognitive newborn: a scientific update. *British Journal of Psychotherapy*, **4**, 30–71.

Chisholm, J. S. (1988). Toward a developmental evolutionary ecology of humans. In *Sociobiological Perspectives on Human Development*, ed. K. M. MacDonald, pp. 78–102. New York: Springer-Verlag.

Coe, C. L., Weiner, S. G., Rosenberg, L. T. & Levine, S. (1985). Endocrine and immune responses to separation and maternal loss in nonhuman primates. In *The Psychobiology of Attachment and Separation*, ed. M. Reite & T. Field. New York: Academic Press.

Cosmides, L. & Tooby, J. (1992). Cognitive adaptations for social exchange. In *The Adapted Mind: Evolutionary Psychology and the Generation of Culture* ed. J. H. Barkow, L. Cosmides & J. Tooby, pp. 163–228. New York: Oxford University Press.

Dolan, R. J., Calloway, S. P., Fonagy, F. W., De Souza, F. V. & Wakling, A. (1985). Life events, depression and hypothalamic-pituitary-adrenal axis function. *British Journal of Psychiatry*, **147**, 429–33.

Emmons, R. A. (1989). The personal striving approach to personality. In *Goal Concepts in Personality and Social Psychology*, ed. L. A. Pervin. Hillsdale, N. J.: Lawrence Erlbaum.

Fisher, J. D., Nadler, A. & Whitcher-Alagna, S. (1982). Recipient reactions to aid. *Psychological Bulletin*, **91**, 27–54.

Fogel, A., Melson, G. F. & Mistry, J. (1986). Conceptualising the determinants of nurturance: a reassessment of sex differences. In *Origins of Nurturance: Developmental, Biological and Cultural Perspectives on Caregiving*, ed. A. Fogel & G. F. Melson, pp. 53–67. Hillsdale, N. J.: Lawrence Erlbaum.

Frank, J. D. (1982). Therapeutic components shared by psychotherapies. In *Psychotherapy Research and Behavior Change*, vol. 1, ed. J. H. Harvey & M. M. Parkes, Washington, DC: American Psychological Association.

Gabbard, G. O. (1992). Psychodynamic psychiatry in the 'decade of the brain'. *American Journal of Psychiatry*, **149**, 991–8.

Gardner, R. (1988). Psychiatric infrastructures for intraspecific communication. In *Social Fabrics of the Mind*, ed. M. R. A. Chance, pp. 197–225. Hove: Lawrence Erlbaum.

Gilbert, P. (1984). *Depression: From Psychology to Brain State*. London: Lawrence Erlbaum.

Gilbert, P. (1989). *Human Nature and Suffering*. Hove: Lawrence Erlbaum.

Gilbert, P. (1990). Changes: rank, status and mood. In *On the Move: The Psychology of Change and Transition*, ed. S. Fisher & C. L. Cooper, pp. 33–52. Chichester: Wiley.

Gilbert, P. (1992a). *Depression: The Evolution of Powerlessness*. London/New York: Lawrence Erlbaum/Guilford.

Gilbert, P. (1992b). Defence, safe(ty) and biosocial goals in relation to the agonic and hedonic social modes. *World Futures, Journal of General Evolution*, **35**, 31–70.

Gilbert, P. (1993). Defence and safety: their function in social behaviour and psychopathology. *British Journal of Psychology*, **32**, 132–53.

Gilbert, P. (1994). Male violence: towards an integration. In *Male Violence*, ed. J. Archer. London: Routledge.

Glantz, K. & Pearce, J. K. (1989). *Exiles from Eden: Psychotherapy from an Evolutionary Perspective*. New York: W. W. Norton.

Goodyer, I. M. (1990). *Life Experiences, Development and Childhood Psychopathology*. Chichester: Wiley.

Hall, J. A. (1979). Proxemics. In *Nonverbal Communication*, 2nd edn, ed. S. Weitz. New York: Oxford University Press.

Harlow, H. F. & Mears, C. (1979). *The Human Model: Primate Perspectives*. New York: Winston.

Hartup, W. (1989). Social relationships and their developmental significance. *American Psychologist*, **44**, 120–6.

Heard, D. H. & Lake, B. (1986). The attachment dynamic in adult life. *British Journal of Psychiatry*, **149**, 430–8.

Henry, J. P. (1982). The relation of social to biological process in disease. *Social Science Medicine*, **16**, 369–80.

Henry, J. P. & Stephens, P. M. (1977). *Stress, Health and the Social Environment: A Sociobiologic Approach to Medicine*. New York: Springer-Verlag.

Hill, J. (1984). Human altruism and sociocultural fitness. *Journal of Social and Biological Structures*, **7**, 17–35.

Hinde, R. A. (1987). *Individuals, Relationships and Culture: Links Between Ethology and the Social Sciences*. Cambridge: Cambridge University Press.

Hinde, R. A. (1989). Relations between levels of complexity in behavioral sciences. *Journal of Nervous and Mental Disease*, **177**, 655–67.

Hinde, R. A. (1992). Developmental psychology in the context of other behavioral sciences. *Developmental Psychology*, **28**, 1018–29.

Hinde, R. A. & Groebel, J. (1991). Introduction. In *Cooperation and Prosocial Behaviour*, ed. R. A. Hinde & J. Groebel, pp. 1–8. Cambridge: Cambridge University Press.

Hooley, T. M. & Teasdale, J. D. (1989). Predictors of relapse in unipolar depressives: expressed emotion, marital distress and perceived criticism. *Journal of Abnormal Psychology*, **98**, 229–35.

Horowitz, L. M. & Vitkus, J. (1986). The interpersonal basis of psychiatric symptoms. *Clinical Psychology Review*, **6**, 443–70.

Howells, S. & Willis, R. (eds.) (1989). *Societies at Peace: An Anthropological Perspective*. London: Routledge.

Jenkins, J. H. & Karno, M. (1992). The meaning of expressed emotion: theoretical issues raised by cross-cultural research. *American Journal of Psychiatry*, **149**, 9–21.

Kaufman, G. (1989). *The Psychology of Shame. Theory and Treatment of Shame-Based Syndromes*. New York: Springer-Verlag.

Kemper, D. T. (1988). The two dimensions of sociality. In *Social Fabrics of the Mind*, ed. M. R. A. Chance, pp. 297–312. Hove: Lawrence Erlbaum.

Kemper, T. D. (1990). *Social Structure and Testosterone: Explorations of the Socio-Bio-Social Chain*. New Brunswick: Rutgers University Press.

Leary, T. (1957). *The Interpersonal Diagnosis of Personality*. New York: Ronald Press.

MacDonald, K. B. (1988). *Social and Personality Development: An Evolutionary Synthesis*. New York: Plenum Press.

MacLean, P. D. (1985). Brain evolution relating to family, play and the separation call. *Archives of General Psychiatry*, **42**, 405–17.

MacLean, P. D. (1990). *The Triune Brain in Evolution*. New York: Plenum Press.

McGuire, M. T. (1988). On the possibility of ethological explanations of psychiatric disorders. *Acta Psychiatrica Scandinavica*, (Supplement 341) **77**, 7–22.

Matson, S. T. & Zeiss, R. A. (1979). The buddy system: a method of generalised reduction of inappropriate interpersonal behaviour of retarded psychiatric patients. *British Journal of Social and Clinical Psychology*, **18**, 401–5.

Miedzian, M. (1992). *Boy Will Be Boys: Breaking the Link Between Masculinity and Violence*. New York: Virago.

Montagu, A. (1986). *Touching: The Human Significance of the Skin*, 3rd edn. New York: Harper and Row.

Nardi, P. M. (ed.) (1992). *Men's Friendships*. London: Saga.

Nesse, R. M. (1990). Evolutionary explanations of emotions. *Human Nature*, **1**, 261–89.

Oliner, S. P. & Oliner, P. M. (1988). *The Altruistic Personality: Rescuers of Jews in Nazi Europe*. New York: The Free Press.

Ornstein, R. & Swencionis, C. (1990). *The Healing Brain: A Scientific Reader*. New York: Guilford.

Parry, G. (1988). Mobilizing social support. In *New Developments in Clinical Psychology*, vol. 2, ed. F. N. Watts, pp. 83–104. Chichester: BPS Books/Wiley.

Post, R. M. (1992). Transduction of psychosocial stress into the neurobiology of recurrent affective disorders. *American Journal of Psychiatry*, **149**, 999–1010.

Power, M. (1992). *The Egalitarians: Human and Chimpanzee*. Cambridge: Cambridge University Press.

Price, J. S. (1988). Alternative channels for negotiating asymmetry in social relationships. In *Social Fabrics of the Mind*, ed. M. R. A. Chance, pp. 157–95. Hove: Lawrence Erlbaum.

Price, J. S. & Sloman, L. (1987). Depression as yielding behaviour: an animal model based on Schjelderup-Ebbe's pecking order. *Ethology and Sociobiology*, **8**, 85–98.

Price, V. A. (1982). *Type A Behaviour Pattern: A Model for Research and Practice*. New York: Academic Press.

Raleigh, M. J., McQuire, M. T., Brammer, G. L. & Yuwieler, A. (1984). Social and environmental influences on blood serotonin concentrations in monkeys. *Archives of General Psychiatry*, **41**, 405–10.

Raleigh, M. J., McQuire, M. T., Brammer, G. L., Pollack, D. B. & Yuwieler, A. (1991). Serotonergic mechanisms promote dominance acquisition in adult male vervet monkeys. *Brain Research*, **559**, 181–90.

Reite, M. & Field, T. (eds.) (1985). *The Psychobiology of Attachment and Separation*. New York: Academic Press.

Rippere, V. & Williams, R. (eds.) (1985). *Wounded Healers*. Chichester: Wiley.

Robson, P. J. (1988). Self-esteem: a psychiatrist's view. *British Journal of Psychiatry*, **153**, 6–15.

Sapolsky, R. M. (1989). Hypercortisolism among socially subordinate wild baboons originates at the CNS level. *Archives of General Psychiatry*, **46**, 1047–51.

Sapolsky, R. M. (1990*a*). Adrenocortical function, social rank and personality among wild baboons. *Biological Psychiatry*, **28**, 862–78.

Sapolsky, R. M. (1990*b*). Stress in the wild. *Scientific American*, [January], 106–13.

Scheff, T. J. (1988). Shame and conformity: the deference–emotion system. *American Review of Sociology*, **53**, 395–406.

Slavin, M. O. & Kriegman, D. (1992). *The Adaptive Design of the Human Psyche: Psychoanalysis, Evolutionary Biology, and the Therapeutic Process*. New York: Guilford.

Stokes, J. P. & McKirnan, D. J. (1989). Affect and the social environment: the role of social support in depression and anxiety. In *Anxiety and Depression: Distinctive and Overlapping Features*, ed. P. C. Kendal & D. Watson. New York: Academic Press.

Sullivan, H. S. (1953). *The Interpersonal Theory of Psychiatry*. New York: W. W. Norton.

Suls, S. & Wills, T. A. (eds.) (1991). *Social Comparison: Contemporary Theory and Research*. Hillsdale, N. J.: Lawrence Erlbaum.

Trivers, R. (1985). *Social Evolution*. California: Benjamin/Cummings.

Van Schaik, C. P. (1989). The ecology of social relationships amongst female primates. In *Comparative Socioecology: The Behavioural Ecology of Humans and Other Animals*, ed. V. Standen & R. A. Foley. Oxford: Blackwell.

Weiss, R. S. (1986). Continuities and transformation in social relationships from childhood to adulthood. In *Relationships and Development*, ed. W. W. Hartup & Z. Rubin, pp. 95–110. Hillsdale, N. J.: Lawrence Erlbaum.

Wenegrat, B. (1984). *Sociobiology and Mental Disorder: A New View*. California: Addison-Wesley.

Wiggins, J. S. &. Broughton, R. (1985). The interpersonal circle: a structural model for the integration of personality research. *Perspectives in Personality*, **1**, 1–47.

Wiggins, J. S. & Pincus, A. L. (1989). Conceptions of personality disorders and dimensions of personality: psychological assessment. *Journal of Consulting and Clinical Psychology*, **1**, 305–16.

Wilhelm, K. & Parker, G. (1988). The development of a measure of intimate bonds. *Psychological Medicine*, **18**, 225–34.

PART II

LESSONS FROM SELECTED OBSERVATIONAL STUDIES

6

Social support as a high-risk condition for depression in women

Hans O. F. Veiel

Introduction

Although the literature on social support and its influence on mental and physical health has grown exponentially over the last two decades, very few studies have compared the effects of support on mental health across basic sociodemographic categories such as defined by gender or marital status. This holds particularly for studies examining clinical samples. Many researchers seem to have implicitly assumed social support to be some kind of cultural constant, with comparable beneficial effect in all segments of the population. However, to expect social support to play the same or even similar roles for men and women, for the old and the young, and for the married and the single does not seem realistic: socialisation experiences, life conditions, and social roles and expectations differ enormously between these groups. The literature on gender-specific socialisation (e.g. Gilligan, 1982) and on the differentiation of support functions (e.g. Belle, 1982) suggests that men and women differ in their need for, and general approach to, social support. Indeed, two recent studies which have examined sociodemographic moderators of support effects on depression (Billings & Moos, 1985; Brugha *et al.*, 1990) have found such gender differences. These differences, however, were rather small and not as fundamental as the literature would lead one to expect. It is quite possible that distinguishing between sociodemographic categories on only one dimension at a time is not appropriate when the focus is on psychosocial conditions of mental health: the differences in the life conditions of, say, married and single women are perhaps as large as those between single women and single men, and comparing male and female samples containing both married and single individuals, or comparing single and married samples containing both men and women, may blur differences rather than reveal them

Social support and depression. There is now solid evidence regarding the protective role of social support in the aetiology of mental disorder, and particularly so for depression (e.g. Henderson, 1992; Monroe & Johnson,

1992). In contrast, negative, destructive social interactions and relationships and their role in the development of mental disorders have only comparatively recently received more than passing attention. Some studies have dealt with failed support attempts and their detrimental effects on health (e.g. Coyne *et al.*, 1988, 1990; Harris, 1992), others with effects of general aversive social interchanges in normal populations (reviewed by Rook, 1984, 1992). In clinical populations, it is primarily the concept of 'expressed emotion', referring to hostile and overbearing attitudes and behaviours of family members, which has been linked to relapses in schizophrenia (e.g. Vaughn & Leff, 1976) and, more recently, to depression as well (e.g. Hooley, *et al.*, 1986).

While these findings are concerned with patently disagreeable social interactions, genuine support, in contrast, is typically found to have a more or less beneficial effect on the recipient, to witness the vast literature on this topic. It is generally assumed that the term 'social support' refers to a class of behaviours and relationships which, even when not actually health-promoting, are at least neutral in this respect. Nonetheless, there have been several reports of detrimental effects on health of genuinely supportive relationships (e.g. Kobasa, 1979; Veiel & Kühner, 1990), warranting a closer look at this issue. Later in this volume, Kirke deals with a particular, indirect, example of this through the transmission of drug use among teenagers.

In the following, the results of two studies of depressed patients will be presented, which address the two issues touched upon above: the different role of social support in depression for men and women, and the issue of detrimental influences of support on recovery and relapse.

Method

Procedures

The two studies reported on here deal with the same sample of depressed inpatients. The first is a cross-sectional study, comparing patients who were recovered after discharge with those still severely depressed. The second study focuses prospectively on relapses of patients who were recovered at discharge.

The study population comprised all 18- to 60-year-old patients of the Psychiatric Clinic of the Central Institute of Mental Health in Mannheim, Germany, with prominent symptoms of depression who were admitted over a period of 3 years (1987–90). Patients were first approached by the psychiatrist in charge of their treatment and asked for their consent to be included in the study. They were then contacted by a psychologist or psychiatrist member of the research team (within 2 weeks of admission), who conducted a relatively brief screening interview and administered a depression questionnaire (see below). Patients were included in the study (*a*) if they had received a preliminary hospital diagnosis of primary unipolar depressive disorder (ICD-9 codes 290.0, 296.1, 300.4, 301.1, 309.1); or (*b*) if they had received a preliminary hospital diagnosis of other neurotic or personality disorders (ICD-9 codes 300–309), and if the screening assessment resulted in either a DSM-III research diagnosis of Major Depressive Episode or in self-reported levels of depression symptoms above a predefined cutoff (see the section on instruments below).

General exclusion criteria were indications of organic brain syndromes, illiteracy, mental retardation, bipolar disorder, obsessive–compulsive disorder, or schizophrenic or paranoid syndrome at any time during the study.

The primary baseline assessment (T1) was conducted 4 weeks after discharge when the patients had had time to readjust to their usual social environment but when relatively few changes in clinical status were thought to have taken place since discharge. This assessment consisted of an interview lasting, on average, about 3 hours, and included a variety of self-report and interview-based measures.

The follow-up (T2) assessment consisted of an interview of essentially the same format as used for T1, but it also included additional measures.

Sample characteristics

Three hundred and twenty-one patients were contacted at admission (T0), of whom about 10% refused to participate. Two hundred and twenty-one patients met the inclusion criteria, and 193 (84%) had complete baseline (T1) data. They constituted the sample for study 1 (cross-sectional examination of conditions of recovery). The sample included 125 (65%) women, which is typical for samples in treatment for depression, and its mean age was 41.6 years (SD 10.4 years). The mean level of depressive symptoms (mean IDD sum score = 38.2) at admission was comparable to figures reported for other acutely depressed samples (Zimmerman *et al.*, 1986). Seventy-two per cent had a partner, and 54% were employed at least half-time. Additional sample information is shown in Table 6.1.

Patients who dropped out between T0 and T1 included a significantly higher proportion of men (46% vs 36%) than the rest. Follow-up data (T2; 6 months after T1) were available for 105 patients, who were recovered at T1 and who constituted the sample for study 2 (longitudinal examination of conditions of relapse). Regarding the sociodemographic and clinical characteristics mentioned above, the samples were not significantly or appreciably different, with the following exception: dropouts between T1 and T2 were more likely to have been diagnosed as

Table 6.1. *Sociodemographic and clinical characteristics of the baseline sample*

Variables	All patients (n = 190)[a]	
	Mean/%	(SD)
Sociodemographic		
Age at admission (years)	41.7	(10.4)
Sex (% female)	65%	—
% with partner	72%	—
Education (% < 10 years)	58%	—
Occupational status (% employed)	54%	—
Clinical		
Symptoms at admission [b]	38.2	(12.6)
Length of index hospitalisation (weeks)	8.6	(5.2)
Duration of episode before admission (weeks)	23.1	(39.2)
Age at first MDE (years)	32.1	(14.3)
Previous chronicity (%) [c]	36%	—

Based on Veiel *et al.* (1992).
MDE, major depressive episode.
[a]Numbers vary slightly due to missing data.
[b]Symptom sum score (IDD).
[c]Presence of Dysthymic Disorder or full MDE syndrome during at least 2 years prior to admission.

having a Major Depressive Episode at T1 (46% vs 30%) and the size of their support network of friends was about one-third smaller than that of the T2 sample. No other differences (in age, sex, symptom scores, clinical history, or other support variables) was significant or sizeable. In particular, the means of the kin support variables were almost identical in the dropouts and the participants. Dropouts after T1 seem to have represented a more depressed and less sociable subgroup of patients.

Instruments and variables

Symptoms and clinical status

The Present State Examination (PSE, 9th revision: Wing *et al.*, 1974) was used as the major diagnostic instrument at T1 and T2. It had been expanded to yield DSM-IIIR diagnoses of Major Depressive Episode (MDE) and Dysthymic Disorder (cf. Maurer *et al.*, 1989). The PSE focuses on the 4 week period prior to the assessment date, which for the baseline assessment (T1) coincided with the time elapsed since discharge from hospital.

The Inventory to Diagnose Depression (IDD: Zimmerman *et al.*,

1986) was used for assessing self-rated symptoms at all assessment points (T0, T1, T2). It is designed to allow DSM-IIIR diagnoses of MDE in addition to yielding a sum score of depressive symptoms. An IDD-derived diagnosis of MDE or a sum score of 25 (about $1\frac{1}{2}$ standard deviations above the mean of a normal comparison sample examined concurrently) or higher at the screening assessment (T0) was used as the inclusion criterion for patients with primary hospital diagnoses other than depression (see above). The specificity of the IDD–MDE diagnoses with PSE diagnoses as a criterion is very high (95%; cf. Kühner & Veiel, 1992). This, together with the high cutoff for the IDD sum score as alternative inclusion criterion, ensured that only patients whose secondary depressions were severe were included in the sample. IDD sum scores were used to represent self-reported symptom levels at admission, baseline and follow-up (variables Symptoms at Admission, Symptoms T1, and Symptoms T2, respectively).

Patients were designated 'recovered' at T1 if they neither met the MDE criteria (based on the expanded PSE) nor scored 25 or higher on the IDD (the selection criterion at T0). The relatively stringent double criterion for recovery was selected because preliminary analyses indicated that patients meeting either criterion were more similar to those meeting both than to those meeting neither. For the purpose of study 2, patients were considered relapsed if they received a MDE diagnosis at T2.

Social support resources

The Mannheim Interview on Social Support (MISS: Veiel, 1990), a structured interview taking about 30–40 minutes to administer, was used to assess social support and social network parameters. It requires the subject to indicate for 12 prototypical support situations each actual (everyday situations) and/or potential (crisis situations) provider of support by name. For each situation, the subjects also indicate their satisfaction with the available support resources. In a second stage, the subjects describe each person mentioned on a number of factual and evaluative dimensions. The data are represented in a 'support matrix' of network members by support functions, from which a variety of indices can be derived, reflecting network categories, support categories, and specific supportive categories provided by specific segments of the social network. Although the MISS data reflect *perceptions* of available social support resources, the MISS's focus on specific situations and on single network members reduces the biasing influence of attitudes and mood on the subjects' responses, compared with more global assessments of aggregate support perceptions (relying on questions asking 'How many...' or 'How well...').

The following variables were derived from the MISS: satisfaction with available social support resources, averaged over the 12 different support functions (variable Satisfaction With Support); the size of the kin support network (variable Kin Network Size, representing all relatives who were named as providing crisis support functions, and/or who were named for everyday support functions *and* seen or spoken to at least once every 2 weeks); the size of the support network of friends and acquaintances (variable Non-kin Network Size); the number of kin and non-kin providers of at least one of three types psychological/emotional support in crises (variables Kin Psychological Crisis Support and Non-kin Psychological Crisis Support, respectively).

Moderator variables

To test for the hypothesised differences between male and female patients, those with and without partners, and between employed and unemployed patients, the corresponding variables Gender, Partnership Status (with/without a partner) and Employment Status (working less than half-time vs working more or being a full-time student or apprentice) were defined. The latter two were chosen as proxies for the patients' dependence on their families, which was thought to affect the reception as well as the provision of support, by family members as well as by friends and acquaintances.

Analyses

To examine the conditions of recovery at discharge (study 1), logistic regression with recovery status (recovered/non-recovered) as the dependent variable was used as the basic analytical framework. This approach was preferred over *t*-tests because it allowed direct comparisons between continuous and dichotomous variables as well as between zero-order and partial effects (see below). Also, logistic regression makes less stringent assumptions regarding the distribution of continuous variables than *t*-tests (Cleary & Angel, 1984). When appropriate, *t*-tests were also performed, but the results differed only marginally from those reported here.

Of the clinical and socioeconomic variables shown in Table 6.1, the patients' age and previous chronicity were the only ones significantly related to recovery status. In order to assess the spuriousness of apparent differences between recovered and non-recovered patients on account of these two variables, they were used as covariates in study 1, i.e. differences between recovered and non-recovered patients were evaluated with the effects of these two variables partialled out.

In study 1, the differences between recovered and non-recovered patients at T1 were examined on three levels: (1) zero-order effects were evaluated by entering the variables singly into the regression equations (comparable to performing straight *t*-tests); (2) the effects of covariates were partialled out by forcing them into the regression equations before the variables of interest; (3) interaction effects of Gender and Partnership Status were tested in two steps to keep the number of statistical tests to a minimum. In a first step, both two-way interactions were included simultaneously in the regression equations, and the improvement in overall predictive accuracy (or model fit) was tested (chi-squared with two degrees of freedom). If this was significant, the components of this chi-squared and the actual differences between subgroups were further examined.

For study 2, to examine relapses and increases in depressive symptoms between baseline (T1) and follow-up (T2), a multiple regression approach was also chosen as the principal analytical framework. Linear regression was used when Symptoms T2 was the dependent variable, and logistic regression when MDE T2 was predicted. Symptoms at Admission and Symptoms at T1 were always forced into the regression equations, as was the patient's gender. For making direct comparisons between the effects of a predictor variable in the linear regression analyses and its effects in the logistic regressions, partial correlations between the variable and the respective outcome were chosen to represent the strength of the associations in Table 6.2. For the linear regressions, partial product–moment correlations are used, and for the logistic regressions partial phi correlations were computed on the basis of the chi-squared associated with the respective effect. Product–moment and phi correlations are conceptually and numerically similar so that they can be compared directly (Guilford & Fruchter, 1978). As a more immediately interpretable (if less comparable) measure of association, unstandardised partial regression coefficients (for the continuous symptom score as dependent variable) and odds ratios (for the dichotomous MDE diagnoses as outcome) are also shown.

Results

Study 1: Correlates of recovery at discharge

At T1, i.e. 4 weeks after discharge from hospital, 61% of the patients had recovered from their depressive episode, i.e. they neither met the criteria for a MDE nor scored 25 or above on the IDD. (The proportions were about equal for men and women.)

Recovered and non-recovered patients differed significantly regarding Satisfaction With Support, but this difference was largely accounted for by the Chronicity and Age covariates, as the greatly reduced chi-squared in column 5 of Table 6.2 shows.

Neither the size of the kin support network, nor the number of kin available for psychological crisis support, differed substantially between recovered and non-recovered patients.

Table 6.2. *Differences in social support between recovered and non-recovered patients at baseline*

Variables	All patients (n = 190)[a]		Recovered (n = 115)[a]	Non-recovered (n = 75)[a]	p (diff) (χ^2, d.f. = 1)		Interactions sex and age (χ^2, d.f. =)[d]
	Mean	(SD)	Mean	Mean	b	c	d
Satisfaction With Support[e]	0.66	(0.27)	0.70	0.60	6.2*	2.2	0.7
Kin Support Network Size	4.0	(2.6)	4.1	3.7	1.1	0.4	1.2
Kin Psychological Crisis support[f]	2.3	(2.1)	2.4	2.1	1.2	0.2	0.8
Non-kin Support Network Size	6.0	(4.3)	6.2	5.5	1.4	3.4	7.5*
Non-kin Psychological Crisis Support[f]	2.7	(2.9)	2.8	2.6	0.2	0.9	13.7**

* $p < 0.15$; ** $p < 0.01$ (two-tailed).
[a] Numbers vary slightly due to missing data.
[b] Zero-order significance (two-tailed; based on logistic regression with recovery status as dependent variable).
[c] Significance after the effects of Age and Chronicity are partialled out.
[d] Significance of the compounded interactions with Partnership Status and Gender, after Age, Chronicity, and the respective main effects are partialled out.
[e] Range: 0–1.
[f] Number of network members named in response to at least one of three items targeting crisis support.

Table 6.3. *Non-kin Psychological Crisis Support, recovery, Gender and Partnership Status*

	Men		Women	
	With partner	Without partner	With partner	Without partner
Recovered	2.1	5.3	2.3	3.6
Non-recovered	1.1	2.4	3.6	2.0
Grand mean	2.7			
SD	2.9			

Reprinted from Veiel *et al.* (1992), with permission.
Figures represent mean numbers of friends providing support in psychological/emotional crises.
Variations of the association between Psychological Crisis Support and recovery across:
  Partnership Status: χ^2(d.f. = 1): 9.4 ($p = 0.003$)
  Gender: χ^2(d.f. = 1): 7.4 ($p = 0.007$)
(Effects represent interactions of Psychological Crisis Support with Gender and Partnership Status, respectively, in a logistic regression equation with recovery status [recovered/non-recovered] as the dependent variable.)

Although the overall association of the non-kin support variables with recovery status was very small, it varied significantly over different patient subgroups (cf. the last column of Table 6.2). Further analyses showed that the effect of Non-kin Network Size was completely accounted for by those network members who provided Psychological Crisis Support (who, of course, were included in the total support network). The following discussion will therefore focus on the crisis support variables. Table 6.3 presents the actual figures corresponding to its interaction effect.

It is evident that the interactions with both Gender and Partnership Status were due to women with partners, who showed a pattern of effects which was different from those of the other patient groups (men with and without partners, women without partners). Whereas among the latter, the recovered had about twice as many friends providing crisis support as the non-recovered, this proportion was reversed for women with partners.

Study 2: Prediction of relapse among recovered patients

In the subsample of recovered patients, Satisfaction with Support as well as the non-kin support variables measured at baseline (T1) showed small negative associations with Symptoms T2, which is in accordance with the expected beneficial effect of social support (Table 6.4).

In contrast, the T1 kin support variables showed significant positive

Table 6.4. *Baseline variables as predictors of relapse and of depressive symptoms at follow-up (recovered patients at baseline, n = 105)*

	Predicted variable at follow-up			
	Symptom sum score (linear regression)		Major Depressive Episode (log. regression)	
Predictors at baseline	r_0	r_p	phi_0	phi_p
Symptoms at admission	0.21*	—	0.022*	—
Symptoms T1	0.27**	—	0.03	—
Gender (M = 1; F = 2)	0.23*	—	0.15	—
Satisfaction with Support T1	−0.10	−0.08	−0.05	−0.06
Kin Support Network Size T1	0.34***	0.29**	0.23*	0.19
Kin Psychological Crisis Support	0.36***	0.31**	0.32**	0.33***
Non-kin Support Network Size	−0.13	−0.09	0.09	0.08
Non-kin Psychological Crisis Support	−0.07	−0.07	0.04	0.04

Based, in part, on Veiel (1993).
*$p < 0.05$; **$p < 0.01$; ***$p < 0.001$.
r_0, zero-order correlation with Symptoms T2; r_p, partial correlation with Symptoms T2, after Symptoms at Admission, Symptoms T1, and Gender are partialled out; phi_0, zero-order phi correlation with Symptoms T2; phi_p, partial phi correlation with Symptoms T2, after Symptoms at Admission, Symptoms T1, and Gender are partialled out.

correlations with T2 depression: a large number of supportive relatives was associated both with an increase in symptoms and with a higher probability of developing a MDE, with comparable zero-order and partial associations for Kin Psychological Crisis Support (phi = 0.32–0.33; r = 0.31–0.36).

This result seemed unusual, although a preliminary report (Veiel & Kühner, 1990) had suggested it. Further analyses showed that the detrimental effect of Kin Support Network Size was largely accounted for by the relatives mentioned as providers of psychological/emotional crisis support. The following discussion, therefore, will deal with the variable Kin Psychological Crisis Support as the more circumscribed and immediately meaningful variable.

The consistency of the detrimental effects of Kin Psychological Crisis Support, and of the lack of effects of non-kin support, was examined across the patient categories defined by Gender, Partnership Status, and Employment Status. Corresponding dummy variables were included in the regression analyses, and their interactions with the support variables were examined hierarchically. For Nonkin Psychological Crisis Support, none of the interactions approached significance. In contrast, very

Table 6.5. *Kin Psychological Crisis Support and symptoms at follow-up: effect sizes across subgroups of recovered patients defined by Gender and Employment Status*

	Predicted varaible			
	Symptoms T2 (linear regression)		MDE T2 (log. regression)	
Patient categories	β_p	r_p	OR	Phi_p
Men				
All ($n = 36$)	0.4[†]	0.12	—[a]	—
Working ($n = 31$)	0.8[†]	0.23	—	—
Not working ($n = 5$)[b]	—	—	—	—
Women				
All ($n = 69$)	2.5***	0.39	1.8**	0.38
Working ($n = 38$)	0.5[†]	0.07	1.7	0.27
Not working ($n = 31$)	4.1****	0.67	2.3**	0.52

Based, in part, on Veiel (1993).
*$p < 0.05$; **$p < 0.01$; ***$p < 0.001$; ****$p < 0.0001$; [†]$p > 0.20$.
Figures refer to effects of Kin Psychological Crisis Support in regression equations also containing Symptoms at Admission and Symptoms T1 as predictors.
β_p, unstandardised partial regression coefficient, indicating the mean net increase in Symptoms T2 for each additional supporter; r_p, partial correlation with follow-up symptoms after Symptoms at Admission and Symptoms T2 are partialled out; OR, odds ratio (increase in the odds of a MDE at T2 when the number of kin providing psychological crisis support is increased by 1, with all other predictors held constant); Phi_p, partial phi correlation with the criterion after Symptoms at Admission and Symptoms T2 are partialled out.
[a]Too few male patients (2) had relapses for analyses to be meaningful.
[b]n too small for meaningful analyses.

significant interactions with both Gender and Employment Status were revealed for Kin Psychological Crisis Support, when the continuous symptom score was the dependent variable (but not when they were tested by logistic regression analysis with relapse as the dependent variable). Thus, the detrimental effects of kin support differed significantly both between male and female and between working and non-working patients, at least with regard to self-reported symptoms.

The interactions involving Partnership Status were consistently small and non-significant.

For a closer examination of these interaction effects, the patients were separated into four groups representing the combinations of the Gender and Employment categories, and regression analyses were performed separately for each group. Table 6.5 represents the effects of Kin Psychological Crisis Support (T1) on T2 depression after the effects of Symptoms T0 and Symptoms T1 are partialled out.

Unfortunately, only five non-working men were recovered at T1, which precluded their separate examination. Also, only two recovered men had developed a MDE at T2, which ruled out logistic regressions with MDE T2 as dependent variable in the male subsample. The small cell sizes in the male subsample may have been partly responsible for the lack of interactions in the logistic regressions mentioned earlier.

It is apparent that the detrimental effects of kin support were restricted to the non-working women. In this subgroup, all other things being equal, each additional relative available for Kin Psychological Crisis Support increased the T2 symptom score by about 4 points ($\beta = 4.1$), which represents more than one-third of a standard deviation (cf. Table 6.1). This effect corresponds to a partial correlation of $r = 0.67$, and has a chance probability of less than 0.0001.

Each additional relative available for crisis support also more than doubled the odds of having a MDE at T2 for this subsample (odds ratio: 2.3). Although the odds ratio for the working women (1.7) was not significantly smaller, it must be kept in mind that only twelve women had relapsed, six each in the working and non-working subgroups. This greatly reduced the power to detect interaction effects, and the absence of significant interactions in the logistic regressions should therefore not be overinterpreted, considering the large absolute difference in the strength of the association (phi = 0.27 vs phi = 0.52) and the very significant interaction effects in the linear regression analysis.

When the analyses were repeated with a support score based only on relatives with whom the patients had indicated to have a satisfactory relationship, the results were only minimally different. In another supplementary analysis, a 'confidant' was defined as a person who was mentioned for three different psychological crisis support functions (confiding, consoling, and encouragement when depressed) and who was spontaneously named as 'particularly important' by the participant. The effect of having at least one such confidant, relative or friend, on symptoms T2 was also positively related to Symptoms T2 among recovered non-working women, although not significantly so (partial $r = 0.27$). This result makes it unlikely that one or two crisis supporters represented the support optimum, and that no supporters as well as too many were detrimental. It seems also safe to conclude that the detrimental effects of kin crisis supporters were not due to negative, destructive relationships.

Discussion

Beneficial effects of social support

The difference in Satisfaction With Support between recovered and non-recovered patients does not come as a surprise, confirming results of other studies (e.g. George *et al.*, 1989; Brugha *et al.*, 1990) that subjective measures of social support are negatively correlated with depression. It is, however, noteworthy that when the subjects' age and the chronicity of depression are taken into account, the association between recovery status at discharge/baseline and the patients' satisfaction with available support resources was reduced considerably. This, together with the latters' lack of prospective beneficial effects independent of baseline depression levels, suggests that it reflected, rather than influenced, the subjects' level of depression at the time of assessment. Without specific evidence to the contrary, therefore, negative appraisals of support should be regarded as concomitants of chronic depression rather than as a causal factor.

The overall size of the support network, whether of family or of friends, made little difference for recovery during inpatient treatment, pointing to a reduced importance of social contacts during hospitalisation. This is not surprising given the regulated hospital environment, which is bound to restrict the opportunity for individual needs and network structures to bear on actual social interactions.

The available crisis support from friends, however, was of critical importance for the hospitalised women without partners and for the men; here the non-recovered had far less support. It is quite conceivable that the prospect of returning to an accepting and supportive circle of friends – perhaps reinforced by their frequent visits to the hospital – boosts the recovery process by giving a patient something to look forward to no matter how difficult and stressful the rest of his or her life may be (provided they are in a position to make use of it: see below). Regardless of the specific processes involved, it would seem that in severe depressive states specific provisions of social support do indeed aid recovery, even when social contacts are generally restricted.

In contrast, it is noteworthy that supportive social networks did not reduce the probability of relapse after patients had returned to their normal social environment. This may reflect a process of continuing recovery or reconvalescence which cannot be substantially furthered by the social environment. Such an explanation makes intuitive sense: the patients' particular social environments had not prevented them from becoming depressed in the first place, and negative factors (such as stressful relationships, persistent economic or other difficulties) must have been present which outweighed whatever positive social influences existed. Thus, the very fact of the patients' depression suggests the ineffectiveness of their social support networks, large or small, good or bad. It is therefore not altogether surprising that they failed to prevent subsequent relapses. (In this context, it should be noted that possible 'stress buffering' effects of social support were not examined. However, preliminary analyses of patients with severe stressful life events after discharge did not indicate such buffer effects.)

Specific detrimental effects of support on women

Whereas the beneficial effect of non-kin crisis support on recovery is in line with the bulk of findings reported in the literature, the reverse pattern in women with partners was unexpected. One possibility was that the reliance on crisis support from friends represented a reaction to a largely unsupportive and even destructive relationship with the partner, which prevented recovery. However, 68% of the recovered and 59% of the non-recovered women with partners mentioned them as providing crisis support: the difference is non-significant and much too small to account for the differences regarding friends.

While social support networks did not have any beneficial effects on the probability of relapse after discharge, and only partly on recovery during hospitalisation, their influence was distinctly detrimental in some female patients. Although the deleterious effects on recovery and on relapse after discharge involved different segments of the support network, both these effects point to a specific vulnerability of women who are socially dependent. Before elaborating on this point, I will briefly discuss the apparent differences in the effects on recovery and on relapse.

While in hospital, the patients were cut off from their normal social environment. This, in most cases, meant a relatively greater reduction of contact with family members than with friends – the former are usually seen more frequently. Whatever influence, beneficial or otherwise, the kin support network usually had, the patients' physical removal from it must have reduced it considerably. In contrast, close friends (who may visit patients in the hospital) are likely to become relatively more important than in the patients' normal lives: in the hospital, there are usually few of the many everyday obligations which leave too little time to meet with friends and to appreciate their support and help. The situation is reversed after patients are discharged from hospital and the family again looms large in their lives, frequently eclipsing the actual and potential support from friends.

It is arguable that the relationship with one's partner is the one least affected by the hospitalisation: it is the partner, if anyone, who visits the patient and maintains regular contact – hence the importance of partners for the utilisation of non-kin support during hospitalisation, but not afterwards. On the other hand, a patient's regular occupation reflects little on his or her life in the hospital. Thus, being a homemaker, which made female patients vulnerable to detrimental effects of kin support after discharge, was of no consequence for effects on recovery in hospital.

As is set out in detail elsewhere (Veiel, 1990, 1993), a number of psychosocial and psychological mechanisms provide plausible explanations for the observed detrimental effects of support networks on relapse.

In particular, the reciprocity of supportive social structures seems to play a major role (see also, in particular, Gilbert, this volume). Good supportive relationships tend to be symmetrical, and a recovered patient returning into a supportive family environment without a visible need for support will probably be under the obligation to provide a fair amount of support, help, etc., him- or herself. In the long run, these demands may well be too much for the patient to handle, even if she or he does not realise it at first.

Such a situation is particularly likely to arise for non-working women. Women are part of someone else's support network more frequently than men (Buhrke & Fuqua, 1987; Veiel & Herrle, 1991; Veiel *et al.*, 1991). Female patients, therefore, are more likely than men to be faced with demands for support when they are recovered and return from hospital. If, in addition, they are not working, they have few opportunities to escape their families' explicit or implicit demands: the proportion of homemakers' social lives that is not shared by the rest of their families tends to be limited, and most of the time they are physically available to other family members.

In a similar vein, crisis support from friends may be helpful only for those women whose relational capacity is not already taken up by maintaining a relationship with a partner (cf. Brown *et al.*, 1986). When experiencing extreme levels of distress during an episode of clinical depression, a large number of supportive friends may represent an additional emotional burden rather than provide succour and relief. This burden may consist of vicarious experiences of stress as well as of outright demands for support (cf. Turner & Avison, 1989).

Since the present study is the only one of its kind which distinguishes between relapses and failures to recover, it has to remain open to what extent sample peculiarities have contributed to its results. Relatively permanent individual attributes, however, do not represent a sufficient explanation for the absence of social support effects. The sample examined consisted of non-selected patients of the major psychiatric inpatient facility in its catchment area, and the patients' sociodemographic characteristics were typical for clinically depressed samples. On the other hand, the particular stage of the depressive disorder, i.e. the first months after a recovery from a severe depressive episode, clearly distinguished the present sample from those examined in most similar studies. It is arguable that this period represented a phase of recovery and reconvalescence which cannot be much facilitated, but only hindered, by the social environment.

Regardless of the actual psychological and psychosocial mechanisms involved in the relative importance of families and friends during and after hospitalisation, it is significant that the detrimental effects of supportive social networks on both recovery and relapse involved women who were dependent on their families. Having a (male) partner and being a homemaker often implies that they are dependent, emotionally as well as economically, on their families. It is argued that this dependency on one's family alters the way social support is solicited, received and given, both within the family and without.

It would also follow that many aftercare strategies for depressed patients, which rely on the involvement of supportive family members, may have decidedly counterproductive consequences. The time after a woman's recovery from severe depression seems to represent a period of specific vulnerability to familial burdens and obligations. A therapeutic strategy that takes this into account could go a long way to decreasing the relapse rate for depressed women. Similarly, the effect of a partner on the utilisation of support from friends would deserve closer scrutiny, both in research and in clinical practice. (Differences in the way people need and use support are also the subject of the following chapter by Miller.)

Acknowledgement

The research reported in this paper was supported by the German Research Association (DFG; grant no. Ve97/2) and the German Federal Ministry of Research and Technology (grant no. 0701632/5). Some of the results presented here have been previously reported in Veiel et al. (1992) and Veiel (1993).

References

Belle, D. (1982). The stress of caring: women as providers of social support. In Handbook of Stress, ed. L. Goldberger & S. Breznitz, pp. 496–505. Free Press: New York.

Belsher, G. & Costello, C. G. (1988). Relapse after recovery from unipolar depression: a critical review. Psychological Bulletin, 104, 84–96.

Billings, A. G. & Moos, R. H. (1985). Psychosocial processes of remission in unipolar depression: comparing depressed patients with matched community controls. Journal of Consulting and Clinical Psychology, 53, 314–25.

Brown, G. W., Andrews, B., Harris, T. O., Adler, Z. & Bridge, L. (1986). Social support, self-esteem, and depression. Psychological Medicine, 16, 813–31.

Brugha, T. S., Bebbington, P. E., McCarthy, B., Sturt, E., Wykes, T. & Potter, J. (1990). Gender, social support and recovery from depressive disorders: a prospective clinical study. Psychological Medicine, 20, 147–56.

Buhrke, R. A. & Fuqua, D. R. (1987). Sex differences in same-and cross-sex supportive relationships. Sex Roles, 17, 339–52.

Cleary, P. D. & Angel, R. (1984). The analysis of relationships involving dichotomous dependent variables. Journal of Health and Social Behavior, 25, 334–48.

Coyne, J. C., Wortman, C. B. & Lehman, D. R. (1988). The other side of support. In *Marshaling Social Support*, ed. B. H. Gottlieb, pp. 305–30. Newbury Park: Sage Publications.

Coyne, J. C., Ellard, J. H. & Smith D. A. F. (1990). Social support, interdependence, and the dilemmas of helping. In *Social Support: An Interactional View*, ed. B. R. Sarason & I. G. Sarason, pp. 129–49. New York: Wiley.

George, L. K., Blazer, D. G., Hughes, D. C. & Fowler, N. (1989). Social support and the outcome of major depression. *British Journal of Psychiatry*, **154**, 478–85.

Gilligan, C. (1982). *In a Different Voice*. Cambridge, Mass.: Harvard University Press.

Guilford, J. P. & Fruchter, B. (1978). *Fundamental Statistics in Psychology and Education*. New York: McGraw-Hill.

Harris, T. (1992). Some reflections on the process of social support: the nature of unsupportive behaviors. In *The Meaning and Measurement of Social Support*, ed. H. O. F. Veiel & U. Baumann, pp. 171–92. New York: Hemisphere.

Henderson, A. S. (1992). Social support and depression. In *The Meaning and Measurement of Social Support*, ed. H. O. F. Veiel & U. Baumann, pp. 85–92. New York: Hemisphere.

Hooley, J. M., Orley, J. & Teasdale, J. D. (1986). Levels of expressed emotion and relapse in depressed patients. *British Journal of Psychiatry*, **148**, 642–7.

Kobasa, S. C. (1979). Stressful life events, personality, and helath: an inquiry into hardiness. *Journal or Personality and Social Psychology*, **37**, 1–11.

Kühner, C. & Veiel, H. O. F. (1992). Psychometrische und diagnostische Eigenschaften einer deutschsprachigen Version des Inventory to Diagnose Depression (IDD). *Diagnostika*, **39**, 299–321.

Maurer, K., Biehl, H., Kühner, C. & Löffler, W. (1989). On the way to expert systems: comparing DSM-III computer diagnoses with CATEGO (ICD) diagnoses in depressive and schizophrenic patients. *European Archives of Psychiatry and Neurological Sciences*, **239**, 127–32.

Monroe, S. M. & Johnson, S. L. (1992). Social support, depression, and other mental disorders: in retrospect and toward future prospects. *The Meaning and Measurement of Social Support*, ed. H. O. F. Veiel & U. Baumann. New York: Hemisphere.

Rook, K. S. (1984). The negative side of social interaction: impact on psychological well-being. *Journal of Personality and Social Psychology*, **46**, 1097–108.

Rook, K. S. (1992). Detrimental aspects of social relationships: taking stock of an emerging literature. In *The Meaning and Measurement of Social Support*, ed. H. O. F. Veiel & U. Baumann. New York: Hemisphere.

Turner, R. J. & Avison, W. R. (1989). Gender and depression: assessing exposure and vulnerability of life events in a chronically strained population. *Journal of Nervous and Mental Disease*, **77**, 443–55.

Vaughn, C. E. & Leff, J. P. (1976). The influence of family and social factors on the course of psychiatric illness. *British Journal of Psychiatry*, **129**, 125–37.

Veiel, H. O. F. (1990). The Mannheim Interview on Social Support:

reliability and validity data from three samples. *Social Psychiatry and Psychiatric Epidemiology*, **25**, 250–9.

Veiel, H. O. F. (1993). Detrimental effect of kin support networks on the course of depression. *Journal of Abnormal Psychology*, **102**, 419–29.

Veiel, H. O. F. & Kühner, C. (1990). Relatives and depressive relapse: the critical period after discharge from in-patient treatment. *Psychological Medicine*, **20**, 977–84.

Veiel, H. O. F. & Herrle, J. (1991). Geschlechtsspezifische Strukturen von Unterstützungsnetzwerken. *Zeitschrift für Soziologie*, **20**, 237–45.

Veiel, H. O. F., Crisand, M. & Stroszeck-Somschor, H. *et al.* (1991). Social support networks of chronically strained couples: similarity and overlap. *Journal of Personal and Social Relationships*, **8**, 279–92.

Veiel, H. O. F., Kühner, C., Brill, G. & Ihle, W. (1992). Psychosocial correlates of clinical depression after psychiatric in-patient treatment: methodological issues and baseline differences between recovered and non-recovered patients. *Psychological Medicine*, **22**, 415–27

Wing, J. K., Cooper, J. E. & Sartorius, N. (1974). *Measurement and Classification of Psychiatric Symptoms*. Cambridge University Press: Cambridge.

Zimmerman, M., Coryell, W., Corenthal, C. & Wilson, S. (1986). A self-report scale to diagnose major depressive disorder. *Archives of General Psychiatry*, **43**, 1076–81.

7

The importance of context: who needs and who does not need social support among college students?

Patrick McC. Miller

The extent to which people need or indeed are able to use personal relationships is found in the literature in various different forms. In the field of applied psychology an early distinction was made between person-oriented and task-oriented group leaders and a theory of group behaviour in the work situation was built around this (Fiedler, 1967). The work of Eysenck and others on extraversion–introversion is extremely well known (e.g. Eysenck & Eysenck, 1985). The tradition started by Murray (1938) and continued by McClelland and others (Atkinson, 1958) of describing peoples' needs and motives has led to work on the need for power and the need for intimacy (McAdams *et al.*, 1984). Finally, and perhaps most relevant, come the ideas of Beck and others on sociotropy and autonomy. Sociotropy or social dependency

> 'refers to the person's investment in positive interchange with other people. It includes passive–receptive wishes (acceptance, intimacy, understanding, support, guidance): narcissistic wishes (admiration, prestige, status) ... Individuality (autonomy) refers to the person's investment in preserving and increasing his independence, mobility and personal rights: freedom of choice, action and expression: protection of his domain ... and attaining meaningful goals'. (Beck, 1983)

Given that there may be individual differences (however described) in the need for social interaction and that social support on the whole seems to prevent symptoms, various questions arise: Do all types of people have an equal need for social support in time of trouble? Are there circumstances in which social support is not helpful? Are there circumstances in which it is helpful to some but not to others?

There appears to be very little evidence concerning the first question. However, two surveys of women were carried out by the Bedford College team on the Scottish Hebridean islands of Lewis and Norst Uist (Brown, *et al.*, 1977; Prudo, *et al.*, 1984). Women who were more integrated into the local community had lower rates of depression but *higher* rates of anxiety. Compared with women in Camberwell, London, the Hebridean

163

women tended to be more vulnerable to psychiatric disorder following personal loss (Prudo et al., 1981) and also had a greater tendency to show lack of self-confidence. While one must clearly be cautious in translating integration as social support and lack of self-esteem as lack of autonomy, to the extent that these interpretations can be made this suggests that social support might reduce depression but raise anxiety among sociotropic people.

O'Hara (1986) found that women who were depressed prepartum felt more able to turn to a confidante other than a spouse for emotional support. These women tended to rate their spouses as less supportive and their confidantes as more supportive than did non-depressed subjects. It seems possible that lack of support from the spouse may have first contributed to the depression and that the women then sought support elsewhere, thus producing the relationships seen. Goldstein (1980) found that, for female dental students at the start of their second semester, emotional support was associated with high anxiety, depression and physical symptoms and with low academic performance. However, the pattern for male students was, if anything, the opposite.

There seems to be somewhat more evidence regarding circumstances where social support appears to be unhelpful. Foorman & Lloyd (1986) found that, half way through their first year, medical students with high levels of support showed higher symptoms than other students. During a time of intense academic pressure, too much social support may have been perceived as detrimental to academic success and hence led to symptoms. Where there is conflict or upset in a relationship this may outweigh any helpful qualities (Fiore et al., 1983; Pagel et al., 1987). In fact, in these last two studies, upset was related to depression but there was little evidence that helpfulness was. Other examples are to be seen in the well-known work by Vaughn, Leff and others discussed later in this volume by Kuipers. Coyne & DeLongis (1986) suggest that 'an apparent deficit in supportive relationships may be the result of a deliberate effort to retreat from and avoid negative and overwhelming social involvements'.

To summarise, there seems to be very little work concerned directly with individual differences in the need for social support, but rather more concerning circumstances in which support might not be helpful. In the latter case it seems usually to be the nature of the support offered that is crucial rather than that there are particular situations where some kind of social support might not be beneficial. A further discussion relating to this issue with respect to discharged psychiatric inpatients is provided by Hans Veiel in the preceding chapter of this volume.

A study was carried out by the author and Camille Lloyd on medical students in two centres, either side of the Atlantic Ocean (see also Surtees & Miller, 1990; Miller & Lloyd, 1991; Miller & Surtees, 1991), to attempt to discover individual differences in the usefulness of social support. At the times of the study (1986–7 in Edinburgh, Scotland, and a year later in Houston, Texas) the first-year medical courses at both universities were highly demanding. There was little patient contact, a heavy academic workload and little time left over for other activities. Many students found this highly stressful, and this seemed particularly true at the start of the year and at Edinburgh, where 49.7% of students in the sample scored above the cutoff point suggesting possible psychiatric illness on Goldberg's (1978) 30-item General Health Questionnaire (GHQ). At Houston, where the students were 4 years older and had already gained a university degree, the corresponding figure was 25.2%. However, at both centres the academic workload and, later in the year, examination pressure were clearly sources of stress. This makes it appropriate to test whether, in the face of this, social support and personality would affect symptomatology, which is the subject of this chapter.

The relevant part of the study design required that information regarding personality variables would be collected at the start of the year and data on social support and symptoms later when examination pressure was high.

Eleven personality variables were initially chosen, all of which might relate to a person's ability to form and benefit from social relationships. Six of these were selected from the Personality Assessment Schedule (PAS) devised by Tyrer & Alexander (1985). The PAS scales 24 personality traits using an interview method, which involves asking a number of standard key questions about each trait and then probing the responses given. Due to shortage of resources, this procedure was modified to use just some of the key questions rendered into a Likert scale format. The Traits chosen and the key questions we used were as follows:

Introspection. Do you think a great deal about how you feel and what you do? Do you prefer being on your own than being with other people?

Shyness. Are you normally a shy person? Do you get to know people quickly or do you take a long time before feeling at ease with them?

Aloofness. Are you a person who likes to stay apart from other people or do you like to have close relationships? Do you need people in any way or can you do without them?

Sensitivity. Are you a sensitive person or does it take a lot to upset you?

Vulnerability. Do you find that when things go wrong in your life it disturbs you a great deal?

Suspicousness. Do you normally trust other people or do you mistrust them at least at first?

In the Edinburgh subsample the full procedure was also given and the correlations between the two methods of administration ranged from

0.45 to 0.65. In addition to these six traits, the Rosenberg Self-Esteem scale (Rosenberg, 1965) and the four Parental Bonding measures, i.e. Paternal Caring, Maternal Caring, Paternal Overprotection and Maternal Overprotection, developed by Parker *et al.*, (1979) were included.

On factor analysing the data from both centres, it seemed prudent to reduce these 11 traits to six. Sensitivity and Vulnerability were closely related and were summed to give a scale which we termed Reactivity. Likewise Aloofness and Introspection were combined into Reserve. Only one factor could be extracted from the four Parental Bonding scales and accordingly these were also coalesced into one measure defined as Parental Bonding = Maternal Caring + Paternal Caring − Maternal Overprotection − Paternal Overprotection.

At the time of second testing, i.e. when examination pressure was high, measures of social support, symptoms and life stress which had occurred during the year were collected. There were five measures of social support:

1 *Romantic Relationship.* The students were classified as those who: (*a*) had a steady partner throughout the study period, (*b*) gained a boy/girlfriend during the period, (*c*) lost a boy/girlfriend during the period, (*d*) had no boy/girlfriend during the period.
2 *Local Friend.* Presence/absence of a close friend in Edinburgh/Houston.
3 *Relative.* Presence/absence of a relative in whom to confide.
4 *Classmates.* Number of classmates regularly talked to, coded 0–10, 11–20, 20+.
5 *Confidants.* Total number of people seen as confidants, coded 0, 1–3, 4+.

Symptoms were measured by the GHQ, and by analogue line ratings of depression and anxiety during the past month used in previous studies (e.g. Miller & Ingham, 1979). In this measurement method five anchor statements, representing increasing symptom severity, are placed along a 10 cm line at 0, 2, 4, 6, and 8 cm. For anxiety the anchor statements are 'I never worried about anything', 'I got a bit worried occasionally', 'I often got worried about things', 'I tended to worry a great deal' and 'I was always in a terrible state of worry and anxiety'. For depression they are 'I never felt unhappy', 'I sometimes felt a bit unhappy', 'I was quite often in low spirits', 'I frequently felt very miserable' and 'I always felt very miserable and depressed'. The subject places a mark anywhere on the line to indicate how he or she personally felt over the past month and the distance from the no-symptom end of the line to this mark is measured to the nearest half centimetre, yielding a 20-point scale.

Life stresses during the year were assessed by a questionnaire covering academic work, personal and family relationships, money, health and personal injury, housing, deaths, legal problems, emergencies and stresses that happened to close relatives and friends of the subject. In Edinburgh, this initial questionnaire was followed by in-depth interviewing along the lines of the Life Events and Difficulties Scales (e.g. Brown & Harris, 1978), and various measures, including long-term threat, loss and impaired relationship stress, were derived.

It was expected that, in general, high levels of support would be associated with low levels of symptoms. On the whole, this was true, although the types of support that were most relevant turned out to be centre-specific. In Edinburgh, high levels of classmate contact were significantly associated with lower levels of symptoms on all three symptom scales (GHQ, anxiety and depression). Good support from a relative went with lower GHQ and anxiety scores. In Houston a high number of confidants was significantly related to lower anxiety and depression. However, the first result against the usual trend was seen on examination of the romantic relationship variable. When the Houston and Edinburgh samples are combined, it emerges that those students who did not have a boy/girlfriend during this first year were significantly *less* anxious then the rest. Those who had lost a boy/girlfriend were the *most* anxious, and the other two groups (those who gained one and those who had one throughout) were intermediate. Similar trends just failed to reach significance on the GHQ and on depression. An explanation in terms of the conflicting demands inherent in having a close romantic relationship while struggling with an extremely exacting academic course would fit these data. Some of the comments of the students at Edinburgh, which were obtained during the life event interviews, support this view. Here is a selection:

> I didn't realise how much time and effort medicine takes.
> Very boring – particularly anatomy. It is soul destroying to master. I am stuffing it in. It was a novelty at first, but now just a chore.
> Overload of work makes me feel like reconsidering my career.
> I feel I am missing out on what university has to offer – just sitting up here all the time.
> My girlfriend doesn't get upset if I have to work. She works in an office.
> Nearly all my friends have problems keeping up with former boyfriends at home and making new ones at university.
> I only go out on Friday and Saturday nights. Otherwise I don't have enough time. There is no time for clubs and societies.
> Almost everyone failed Physiology because there was no time to study it.
> Because of the pressure, I am getting irritated by the people around. I can't relax.

The main effects of the six personality variables in predicting symptoms were much as expected. They are fully set out in a table available on request from the author. In summary, reactivity, self-esteem, parental bonding and suspiciousness are significantly related to symptoms in Edinburgh, and the relationships are largely in the same direction but non-significant in Houston. Reactivity, by definition is likely to be related to symptoms. Likewise the associations between Self-esteem, Parental Bonding and symptoms have been seen before (e.g. Brown *et al.*, 1986; Ingham *et al.*, 1987; Richman & Flaherty, 1987) and there has been debate on whether self-esteem should sometimes be regarded as a symptom rather than a personality trait. In Houston the lack of significant relationships may well be due to the smaller numbers of subjects. However, some correlations, particularly those for parental bonding, do look numerically lower and this could be due to the greater maturity of the Houston students (on average 4 years older than those in Edinburgh).

The main interest of the study was not, however, in the effects of social support and personality taken separately but in their interaction. Do there exist types of people for whom social support in the face of (mainly) academic stress would not be beneficial and could even be harmful? To examine this question the interactions between the six personality traits and the five types of support were formed and tested in both universities, using fairly stringent significance criteria as there are so many tests (see Miller & Lloyd, 1991, for details). A number of significant interactions did emerge and several of these suggested that reserved students and students high in suspiciousness might not always benefit from social support. Here we will concentrate on two of these interactions: Classmate Support × Suspiciousness and Romantic Relationship × Reserve.

Classmate Contact × Suspiciousness improves prediction of both anxiety and depression in the combined samples (after the main effects of classmate contact and suspiciousness have been controlled). Table 7.1 sets out the effects. On all three symptoms there is a tendency for low suspiciousness subjects to have lower symptom scores when well supported. For the high suspiciousness subjects (those who mistrust other people for a long time after first meeting), this does not hold. For anxiety and the GHQ the tendency is the other way. Miller & Lloyd (1991) suggested two possible explanations. Firstly, the high suspiciousness students with support might want this support; however, in showing mistrust, they might alienate those giving it, thus increasing their own unhappiness. Secondly, suspicious students might only seek support as a last resort, after they are already anxious and depressed.

Here these two alternatives will be probed further, using other information contained within the study. If the first possibility is true, a greater number of rows and arguments with others might be manifest among the suspicious students who are well supported. If it is the latter, the suspicious students might turn out to be shy, reserved and reactive but with no greater tendency towards strained interpersonal relationships.

Table 7.1 *Symptom scores broken down by suspicious personality and classmate support*

	Low support	High support
Anxiety		
Low suspiciousness	0.12[a] (*n* = 77)	−0.24 (*n* = 130)
High suspiciousness	0.42 (*n* = 13)	0.57 (*n* = 29)
Depression		
Low suspiciousness	0.18	−0.27
High suspiciousness	0.58	0.49
GHQ		
Low suspiciousness	0.15	−0.24
High suspiciousness	0.21	0.60

[a]Since the mean symptom scores differed between the two universities they were converted to Z-scores within each separately. These Z-scores are shown here.

The students in the combined samples were first classified into four groups: high and low on suspiciousness and support. Discriminant function analysis was then used to see whether shyness, reserve, reactivity, personal and family relationship stress and some other variables could distinguish these groups.

Five variables discriminated significantly after being entered in stepwise fashion. There were two dimensions along which discrimination could be made and overall 51.8% of cases could be correctly classified. Mean values of the groups on the five discriminating variables are set out in a second table available on request from the author.

The findings with respect to the various groups may be summarised as follows:

Group 1: low suspiciousness–low support. This relatively large (*n* = 77) group of students have good self-esteem, are not aloof and introverted but are somewhat shy. They are also somewhat sensitive and vulnerable and have some tendency to have rows with those around them.

Group 2: low suspiciousness–high support. The majority of students (*n* = 130) belong to this group. They are *not* shy, *not* aloof and introverted, *not* sensitive and vulnerable, have high self-esteem and have few rows with those around them.

Groups 3: high suspiciousness–low support. This is the smallest group – only 13 students. They are shy, introverted and aloof, with poor self-esteem and a tendency to have rows with those around them. They are *not* sensitive and vulnerable.

Group 4: high suspiciousness–high support. These 29 students have poor

Table 7.2. *Depression scores[a] broken down by reserved personality (aloof and introspective) and romantic relationship*

	Low reserve	High reserve
Steady relationship throughout university	0.13 $(n = 49)$	−0.09 $(n = 28)$
Gain of boy/girlfriend since coming to university	−0.20 $(n = 23)$	0.46 $(n = 14)$
No boy/girlfriend while at university	0.05 $(n = 56)$	−0.37 $(n = 43)$
Loss of boy/girlfriend since coming to university	0.13 $(n = 26)$	0.44 $(n = 10)$

[a] Z-scores of line ratings of depression normalised within each university separately.

self-esteem, are aloof and introverted and have rows with others. They are distinguished from group 3 by being less shy but more sensitive and vulnerable.

While these results are not very conclusive, on the whole they seem in favour of the contention that suspicious students with support have symptoms because they are poor at handling the relationships with those giving the support, rather than that they seek the support only as a last resort. These students seem to be somewhat ambivalent about personal relationships. Shyness is the main correlate of classmate support and these students are not shy. However, they *are* aloof and introverted. They are also suspicious, sensitive, vulnerable and tend to have rows with others. One is not surprised that they have high symptoms.

Suspicious students without support look as though they may tend to have withdrawn from personal relationships, perhaps because they find them too difficult to handle or feel they do not need them. These students still tend to have rows with those around them but say they are not sensitive and vulnerable. They are shy, introverted and aloof. Both groups of suspicious students pay a high price in symptoms compared with other students who are low suspiciousness–high support (see Table 7.1).

Turning to the romantic relationship × reserve interaction, Table 7.2 sets out the findings. This interaction was significant only for depression, although it came close to holding for anxiety also (see Miller & Lloyd, 1991). The main conclusions to be drawn are that:

1 Gain of a romantic relationship is associated with high depression in reserved students and with low depression in non-reserved students.
2 Reserved students who never had a boy/girlfriend are particularly low scorers.
3 Loss of a boy/girlfriend is particularly associated with high depression in reserved students.

Following the strategy used above, a discriminant analysis was run to see whether further characteristics of the eight groups in the table could be found, which could explain these results. Three such variables were found, namely shyness, personal and family relationship stress and self-esteem. Three dimensions were significant in the analysis, each characterised by one of the three variables. The means of the groups on the variables are given in a third table, obtainable on request.

Among those who gained a romantic relationship, highly reserved students exhibited higher levels of interpersonal stress and were more shy than low reserved students. Surprisingly, both groups who gained a romantic relationship were on the low side in self-esteem. Students who were high on reserve and had no romantic relationship showed the lowest levels of all on interpersonal stress and were second highest on shyness. Their self-esteem was in the middle range. None of the three predictors variables distinguished high and low reserved students among those who lost a romantic relationship.

Thus, once more, the somewhat strange finding that reserved students who gained a boy/girlfriend show higher depression levels than those who did not seems explicable in terms of the difficulties these students have in handling personal relationships, particularly when academic stress levels are high.

Conclusions

The main conclusion to be drawn from these results and from the literature seems to be that there is little evidence of the existence of a truly hardy personality – a person who remains asymptomatic under stress, does not need the help and support of other people and genuinely does as well or better without it. There are indeed people who find personal relationships difficult and may only add to their stress levels when they seek support, but they are not asymptomatic when under stress and the impression is that they could still benefit from the right kind of support. The introverted and aloof person, the shy person, the suspicious person, the autonomous person, the person who lacks the need for intimacy may all get along very well most of the time while stresses are few. When real trouble comes, they all need the help of those around them. To be sure, better studies are needed to establish the point conclusively. It would be desirable, for instance, to follow groups of high suspiciousness and low suspiciousness people much more closely through a particular crisis in their lives and observe carefully what support they seek and actually obtain with that crisis. Older people and people in positions of leadership might also repay study, and, finally, very close attention should be paid to the precise nature of the support offered.

References

Atkinson, J. W. (1958). *Motives in Fantasy, Action and Society.* Princeton, N.J.: Van Nostrand.

Beck, A. T. (1983). Cognitive therapy of depression: new perspectives. In *Treatment of Depression: Old Controversies and New Approaches*, ed. P. J. Clayton & J. E. Barrett, pp. 265–90. New York: Raven Press.

Brown, G. W. & Harris, T. (1978). *Social Origins of Depression: A Study of Psychiatric Disorders in Women.* London: Tavistock.

Brown, G. W., Davidson, S., Harris, T., Maclean, U., Pollock, S. & Prudo, R. (1977). Psychiatric disorder in London and North Uist. *Social Science and Medicine*, 11, 367–77.

Brown, G. W., Bifulco, A., Harris, T. & Bridge, L. (1986). Life stress, subclinical symptoms and vulnerability to clinical depression. *Journal of Affective Disorders*, 11, 1–19.

Coyne, J. C. & DeLongis, A. (1986). Going beyond social support: the role of social relationships in adaptation. *Journal of Consulting and Clinical Psychology*, 54, 1–7.

Eysenck, H. J. & Eysenck, M. (1985). *Personality and Individual Differences.* New York: Plenum Press.

Fiedler, F. E. (1967). *A Theory of Leadership Effectiveness.* New York: McGraw-Hill.

Fiore, J., Becker, J. & Coppel, C. (1983). Social network interactions: a buffer or a stress? *American Journal of Community Psychology*, 11, 423–39.

Foorman, S. & Lloyd, C. (1986). The relationship between social support and psychiatric symptomatology in medical students. *Journal of Nervous and Mental Disease*, 174, 229–39.

Goldberg, D. (1978). *Manual of the General Health Questionnaire.* Windsor: National Foundation for Educational Research.

Goldstein, M. B. (1980). Interpersonal support and coping among first year dental students. *Journal of Dental Education*, 44, 203–5.

Ingham, J. G., Kreitman, N. B., Miller, P. McC., Sashidharan, S. P. & Surtees, P. G. (1987). Self-appraisal, anxiety and depression in women: a prospective enquiry. *British Journal of Psychiatry*, 151, 643–51.

McAdams, D. P., Healy, S. & Krause, S. (1984). Social motives and patterns of friendship. *Journal of Personality and Social Psychology*, 47, 828–38.

Miller, P. McC. & Ingham, J. G. (1979). Reflections on the life-events-to-illness link with some preliminary findings. In *Stress and Anxiety*, vol. 6, ed. I G. Sarason & C. G. Spielberger, pp. 313–36. Washington, D.C.: Hemisphere.

Miller, P. McC. & Lloyd, C. (1991). Social support and its interactions with personality and childhood background as predictors of psychiatric symptoms in Scottish and American medical students. *Social Psychiatry and Psychiatric Epidemiology*, 26, 171–7.

Miller, P. McC. & Surtees, P. G. (1991). Psychological symptoms and their course in first-year medical students as assessed by the Interval General Health Questionnaire (I-GHQ). *British Journal of Psychiatry*, 159, 199–207.

Murray, H. A. (1938). *Explorations in Personality.* New York: Oxford University Press.

O'Hara, M. W. (1986). Social support, life events and depression during pregnancy and the puerperium. *Archives of General Psychiatry*, **43**, 569–73.

Pagel, M. D., Erdly, W. W. & Becker, J. (1987). Social networks: we get by with (and in spite of) a little help from our friends. *Journal of Personality and Social Psychology*, **53**, 793–804.

Parker, G., Tupling, H. & Brown, L. B. (1979). A parental bonding instrument. *British Journal of Medical Psychology*, **52**, 1–10.

Prudo, R., Brown, G. W., Harris, T. & Dowland, J. (1981). Psychiatric disorder in a rural and an urban population. II. Sensitivity to loss. *Psychological Medicine*, **11**, 601–6.

Prudo, R., Harris, T. & Brown, G. W (1984). Psychiatric disorder in a rural and an urban population. III. Social integration and the morphology of affective disorder. *Psychological Medicine*, **14**, 327–45.

Richman, J. A. & Flaherty, J. A. (1987). Adult psychosocial assets and depressive mood over time: effects of internalised childhood attachments. *Journal of Nervous and Mental Disease*, **175**, 703–12.

Rosenberg, M. (1965). *The Measurement of Self-Esteem: Society and the Adolescent Image*. Princeton: Princeton University Press.

Surtees, P. G. & Miller, P. McC. (1990). The interval general health questionnaire. *British Journal of Psychiatry*, **157**, 679–86.

Tyrer, P. & Alexander, J. (1985). *Revised Classification of Personality using the Personality Assessment Schedule*. Nottingham: Mapperley Hospital.

8

Teenage peer networks in the community as sources of social problems: a sociological perspective

DEIRDRE KIRKE

In previous chapters the potential for harm to mental health through social processes and social relationships was discussed. This chapter discusses how teenagers' peer networks which develop within their community are the source of their drug use. The peer relationships that teenagers form, develop and change over time providing the teenagers with continually changing peer networks. Drug use is introduced to those peer networks when one member takes drugs. It is diffused throughout the peer network when that individual gives the drug and social support for its use to other members of the network or when the individual provides social support to others members of the network for the use of drugs which they have procured elsewhere. Changes in peer relationships over time facilitate the continued diffusion of drugs within the peer networks and between peer networks. Social support in this context contributes to the initiation and continuation of a deviant behaviour and could, therefore, be considered to have a negative effect. The social support of their teenage peers plays an important part, however, in the normal psychosocial development of teenagers (see also Champion, this volume). It would seem important that clinicians take account of the importance of teenagers' peer networks in dealing with the source and treatment of their individual psychosocial and social crises. This could most usefully be done by examining the teenagers' peer networks in the concrete way in which they are examined in this chapter, rather than dealing with the abstract concepts of peers, peer group and peer influence as has traditionally occurred.

Drug abuse has been recognised as a major social problem in many European countries and in the United States of America since the 1970s. A primary focus of research during this time has been on the causes of drug abuse. Researchers have been interested in trying to understand and explain the factors associated with the initiation into and continuation of drug abuse. Inevitably this research has centred on teenagers because it is during the early teenage years that young people are most likely to start using drugs.

One particular finding has superseded all others in much of this research. Numerous studies have confirmed that the predominant influence on teenagers becoming drug users is peer influence (Akers *et al.*, 1979, p. 644; Kandel, 1978*a*, p. 24; Kandel, 1980, p. 269; Dembo *et al.*, 1982, p. 376; Brook *et al.*, 1983, p. 276; Jessor & Jessor, 1978, p. 69). It has been demonstrated that when the teenagers' peers are drug users, or are perceived by the teenagers to be drug users, the teenagers are likely to become drug users too. One author suggested that the strength of this influence was so great that, if the teenagers were not similar in their drug behaviour, they would either change their drug behaviour or their friend in order to maximise similarity (Kandel, 1978*b*, pp. 433, 435). Gilbert (this volume) clearly sets out the importance of relationships with similar others, who are of the same social rank. The process of influence was identified by Kandel (1978*a*, p. 24) as one of both imitation, through which adolescents imitate or model their drug behaviour on the actual or perceived drug use of their peers, and social reinforcement, through which teenagers who perceive that their peers' attitudes are tolerant of drug use, are likely to use drugs. While there is no direct evidence in these studies that particular peers influenced particular teenagers into taking drugs, the evidence from longitudinal research confirmed that teenagers whose peers took drugs were likely subsequently to take drugs. On the basis of these findings the assumption was that if peers' drug use preceded (in time) the teenagers' drug use and the teenagers subsequently took drugs, the peers influenced the teenagers' drug use. From this evidence there seemed little doubt that the primary source of the social problem of drug use among teenagers was the teenagers' own peers.

The research methods used in these studies were longitudinal and covered large numbers of teenagers. Some of the most important examples are the study by Kandel (1973, p. 1067), which was longitudinal and collected data from 8206 adolescents, and the work of Jessor & Jessor (1978, pp. 46, 47), which was longitudinal and covered 432 high school students and 205 college students. These studies traced the changes in teenagers' drug use over time and confirmed that peer influence was the main influence in teenagers' drug use. Methodological advances which have occurred since the time these studies were done suggest some important shortcomings in their methodologies. In particular, the availability of social network analytic techniques highlights the inadequacy of using individual-level data to explore the concept of peer influence when peer relationship data are more appropriate. Kandel (1973) had analysed dyadic relationships between adolescents and their best friends. No study has been found, however, which analysed peer relationships beyond the dyad. The question that arises, therefore, is whether data based on peer relationships beyond the dyad would support the evidence based on individual-level data or on dyadic data of the importance of peer influence in spreading drug use.

A second difficulty was that most of the studies relied on 'perceived peer data'. Teenage respondents were asked to report on their peers' attitudes to drugs *and their peers' use of drugs*. The difficulty is that perceived peer data have been noted to exaggerate peer effects (Kandel, 1980, pp. 269, 270). Again one exception is Kandel's (1973) study in which she obtained self-reported data from teenagers and their best friends. No study was found in which self-reported data were obtained from peers other than the best friend. The question that arises from these findings, therefore, is whether there is evidence of peer influence when self-reported peer data are available from best friends and other peers.

In an attempt to overcome the shortcomings of earlier research and to examine the concept of peer influence in a more stringent manner, the author designed a study that would collect peer relationship data at a number of levels of analysis (details in Kirke, 1990) and would cover peer relationships at various levels of closeness from best friend to pal. The interviews would also collect all drug-related data *directly* from each teenager and from each peer. Interviewers did *not* ask respondents about the drug use of *others* in their peer network, thus avoiding the bias inherent in 'perceived peer data'. The research methods are described below.

Research methods

A cross-sectional study of the total population of teenagers living in one working-class electoral area in Dublin, Ireland, was carried out. This area had a total population of about 2500 residents living in approximately 500 houses. (Exact details are not given to protect the anonymity of the area.) It was known from census data (Central Statistics Office, 1981, 1986) that a large proportion of the population was below 25 years of age. It was expected, therefore, that a study of this area would provide a sufficient number of teenagers who were drug users and would also provide controls, i.e. people who were living in exactly the same social environment as the drug using teenagers but who had not taken drugs.

Survey research data on individuals: sources of the data

Total coverage of every 14- to 18-year-old teenager ($n = 298$) living in this electoral area was attempted. This strategy ensured that self-reported drug data and self-reported peer data were collected directly from the teenagers and directly from their peers who resided in this area. The response rate was 91%. Data were also collected from a 'snowball sample' of some of the teenagers' friends and pals, i.e. peers, outside the population ($n = 106$). The response rate to the snowball sample survey was 92%.

Methods of data collection

Personal interviews using structured questionnaires were conducted with the teenagers. A team of six interviewers, trained and supervised by the author, completed the interviews. A census of every house in the selected electoral area was conducted first to locate the teenagers aged 14–18 years who were living there. The interviewers sought the permission of the parents to speak to their children who were aged 14–18 years and then requested the teenagers to do the interview. All interviews were completed between October and December 1987. The questionnaire included questions on the respondents and their families, their associations with peers, the identity of those peers, and the respondents' smoking, drinking and drug behaviour. Questions relevant to this chapter are given in the Appendix. For example, the indicator of providing 'social support for the teenager's drug use' was that that person had been in the company of the teenager during their first drug use (see Q142 and Q146 in Appendix).

Social network data

Peer relationship data collected in the survey of the total population of teenagers were the source of the social network data. During the interviews teenagers were asked to identify by name, and later by address, all of their best friends, boyfriends, girlfriends, good friends, friends and pals (i.e. people with whom they spent free time but were not as close as friends). The relationships identified were the teenagers' peer ties. These peer ties were strong peer ties. Other less close ties could be described as the teenagers' weak peer ties. These would, for example, be people with whom the teenagers were acquainted or to whom they spoke on the street but with whom they did not spend any free time. The peer relationship data were then prepared for social network analysis and were analysed using the social network analysis programme, Gradap (Sprenger & Stokman, 1989).

Due to the fact that peer data had been collected from a total population of teenagers, peer data in this study were produced on a complete network. A complete network is covered when all relationships existing between all actors within a particular population are identified (Knoke & Kuklinski, 1982, p. 17). The advantages of using a complete network for this study were that an accurate estimate of the peer structure existing in the complete network could be obtained and, through this, the naturally existing peer networks could be identified. Thus, the peer relationships and peer networks existing between all of the teenagers ($n = 298$) in one community ($n = 2500$) were identified. This made it possible to analyse the peer relationship data at the level of the dyad (i.e. peer ties), partial network (i.e. peer network/peer group) and complete network (i.e. the peer ties existing within the population of teenagers). Another advantage was that data on the structures (i.e. the peer networks) and the units that formed those structures (i.e. teenagers and peers) could be identified simultaneously and the relative impact of units on structures and structures on units could be assessed (Wellman, 1988, p. 26). The findings are given in the next section, beginning with a description of drug diffusion throughout the population of teenagers, followed by a detailed case study of one network.

Findings

Findings are presented on the peer networks identified in this community, drug use among members of these peer networks and how the formation and development of the peer network is the source of the teenagers' drug use. The peer networks were identified by using the social network analysis programme, Gradap, to identify the weak components. Weak components include all of those who are directly or indirectly connected to one another by a relationship (Sprenger & Stokman, 1989, pp. 261–3). The weak components in this study included all the teenagers directly or indirectly (i.e. through another teenager) connected to one another through a peer relationship. The weak components identified were the teenagers' peer networks. No one in any one of these networks was connected through a peer tie, either directly or indirectly, with any person in any other peer network. A total of 35 discrete peer networks of varying size were identified in the population of teenagers. These peer networks are presented in Fig. 8.1 in proportion to the number of teenagers they contain. The peer networks are numbered 1 to 35 and the number of teenagers in each network is given alongside it. Ninety-eight teenagers had no peer ties with any other teenager in the population. These 98 teenagers appear as isolates and are represented by small squares in the centre of the diagram. (All but two of these teenagers had friends or pals outside the population, many of whom were interviewed in the snowball sample.)

In order to understand the relevance of these data to the diffusion of drug use throughout a population of teenagers it is necessary to examine them in the context of other findings from this study. These findings (based on individual-level, self-reported data) confirmed that there was an association between the teenagers' self-reported ever use of drugs and

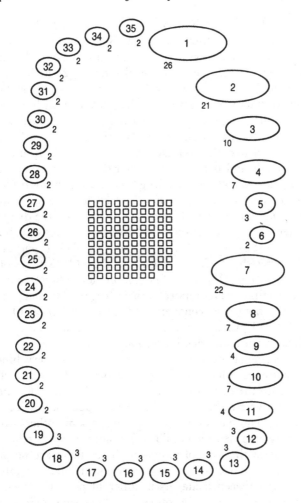

Figure 8.1. Peer networks in population study.

their peers' self-reported ever use of drugs ($\chi^2 = 22.44$; 1 d.f.; $p < 0.0001$). The association was relatively weak (phi = 0.36). Just 16.9% (45) of the teenagers interviewed (267) in the population study had ever used drugs. Their peers had influenced the drug use of 88.9% (40) of these teenagers. Drugs diffused to these 40 teenagers by their friends and pals were either marijuana (25 teenagers), inhalants (10 teenagers), both marijuana and inhalants (3 teenagers), stimulants (1 teenager) or tranquillisers (1 teenager). Sixty per cent (27) of the teenagers had been supplied with the drug and social support for its use by their friends and pals. If the teenagers had been in the company of friends during their first drug use, those friends were assumed to have provided social support for their drug use. A further 28.9% (13) had either been given the drug or social support for its use by their friends and pals. Thus, only 11.1% (5) of the teenagers who had taken drugs had not been influenced by their peers in doing so. Three of the five had got the drug (2 other opiates, 1 tranquillisers) in their own home and had taken it while alone. One had got the drug (inhalants) at home and had taken it with a sibling (a brother). The other teenager had been given the drug (marijuana) and social support for its use by a friend's sibling (the friend's brother). These findings confirmed that the teenagers were more likely to use drugs if their peers (friends and pals) also reported that they were doing so.

The teenagers who got their first drug from friends or pals usually took their first drug with friends or pals (27 of 28 teenagers). (The other teenager who had got his first drug from a friend took the drug alone.) Most of the teenagers who got their first drug some other way, however, also took their first drug with friends or pals (12 of 17 teenagers). (The other 5 teenagers either took the drug while alone (3), with a sibling (1) or with a friend's sibling (1)). These findings provide indirect confirmation of the suggestion that social support for their drug use was being provided by those with whom the teenagers took their first drug. Otherwise, teenagers who had procured the drug some other way need not have taken the drug with their friends and pals.

If teenagers wished to use drugs, therefore, it would be very difficult for them to do so unless they had drug-using peers who were willing to supply them with the drug and to provide social support for their first drug use, or who were willing to provide social support for their first drug use to teenagers who had procured the drug in some other way.

The peer networks identified in Fig. 8.1 indicate the peer relationships of the teenagers at the time of interview. Since there are no peer ties between teenagers across the peer networks, peer influence into drugs could not occur between teenagers in different peer networks. (Links across the peer networks may, of course, exist between people other than the 14- to 18-year-olds and links may be formed when teenagers change their friends or make new friends. For the moment these are not relevant.) Fig. 8.2 indicates the peer networks that had drug-using members and those which had not at the time of interview in 1987. Those that had drug-using members are highlighted with stippling. The number of drug users in each peer network is given alongside the network. Sixteen (45.7%) of the 35 peer networks had drug-using members. Only in these networks were there drug-using peers who could influence other teenagers into drug use. It is only in these peer networks, therefore, that drug diffusion was likely to take place at the time the teenagers were interviewed.

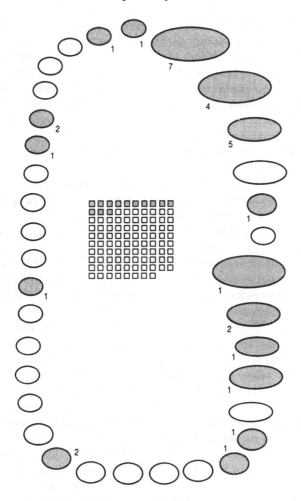

Figure 8.2. Peer networks with drug users (stippled).

A case study of one peer network

Ideally longitudinal data are needed to demonstrate the process of peer tie formation and change and its connection with the diffusion of drug use through peer ties. Such data are not available in this study; nor, indeed, are they available in the drug literature. Retrospective data are, however, available in this study which demonstrate this process. When interviews were conducted in this study, teenagers were asked to state when (i.e. month and year) they had formed each of the peer ties they had at the time of interview and when they had first taken drugs. From these data it was possible to trace the formation and development of the peer networks from their inception, when the first peer tie was formed, to their structural composition in 1987, when the data were collected. Individual-level data relating to the timing of the teenagers' first drug use and the process through which drug influence had occurred were superimposed on these structural data. Selective findings for *one* peer network, in which drug use had occurred and had apparently diffused to other members, is presented below as a detailed case study in order to demonstrate how the peer network of the teenagers is the source of their drug use. The overall findings are summarised and discussed later, beginning on page 188.

The network on which the detailed case study is performed is Peer Network No. 3. In this case study, the peer ties with people in the snowball sample are also included. The peer network includes 10 teenage males who were interviewed in the population study, and 6 teenage males who were interviewed in the snowball sample. A six-digit identification number is used for the respondents. The first two digits indicate the road on which the person lives. These roads were numbered 00 to 09 in the population study. In order to indicate that a person was interviewed in the snowball sample, 11 was entered in the space for the road number. The next three digits are the family's identification number. These are numbered consecutively along each road and indicate, therefore, how near families live to each other. The final digit indicates how many teenagers in the family are interviewed.

All 16 members of the network were teenagers of 15–19 years when interviewed in 1987. The 19-year-old was in the snowball sample and did not, therefore, have to be between 14 and 18 years. Each teenager's age is given in the diagram beside the identification number (M15 means male of 15 years). Six of the 16 members (37.5%) had taken drugs. Three (033851, 033961 and 043771) were current drug users; the other three (033971, 034191 and 115761) were previous drug users. The data presented trace the formation and development of this network over time and indicate when and how drugs were introduced to its members.

Possible weaknesses of the data should be borne in mind. The first is that, while the analysis traces the historical formation and continuation of the peer ties that still existed in 1987, it does not trace all the ties formed in each specific year which were subsequently broken. The second is that the respondents who had taken drugs were not asked to name those who had given or sold the drugs to them; nor were they asked to name the people with whom they had taken drugs. They were, however, asked to state the relationship they had with these people and whether they were male or female. It is these data on relationship and gender, combined with the structural formation of the network at a particular time, which provide clues as to who influenced whom into using drugs. This second 'weakness' of the data may have resulted in loss

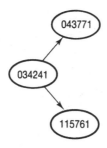

Figure 8.3. Peer relationship in 1970. Key to Figs. 8.3–8.7: D, drug user; [year], person started using drugs in that year and stopped using drugs in the same year; [year–year], person started using drugs in the first year mentioned and stopped using drugs in second year mentioned; [year–, person started using drugs in the year mentioned and was still using drugs when interviewed in 1987; ——→, person at head of arrow was mentioned as a friend or pal by person at the tail of the arrow (unreciprocated tie); ←—→, each person mentioned the other as a friend or pal (reciprocated tie); M number, male age in years (e.g. M15, male 15 years old).

of data on the social context of drug diffusion behaviour, but it retained the 'strengths' of reducing the likely bias in 'perceived peer data' and retained the trust and rapport developed with the respondents, thus ensuring the successful completion of the interviews in the community.

Data on the formation and development of the network and on the timing of the drug use of members are presented graphically in five figures. In the interests of brevity and clarity this detailed material is kept to a minimum. The first connections in this network formed in 1970 when 034241 became friends with 043771 and 115761 (Fig. 8.3). Note that these are unreciprocated ties as neither 043771 nor 115761 said that 034241 was their friend in 1970. New peer ties continued to be formed and some ties were reciprocated over the years, so that by 1982 this network had 12 members (Fig. 8.4). In 1982 a member of the network (034191), who had joined in 1979, took drugs for the first time. The drugs, inhalants, had been given to him by members of his peer network. He had been given the drugs by his male friends, had taken the drugs with his male friends and said that he had taken them because his friends in the neighbourhood were taking them. These friends do not appear in this network in 1982 because 034191 had since ceased being friends with them. From 1982, when this member took drugs, the possibility of peer influence into drugs existed for the other members of the network, in particular for anyone directly connected to the drug user.

During 1983 and 1984 new direct ties were formed between those previously indirectly connected (e.g. 033961 and 033971) and previously

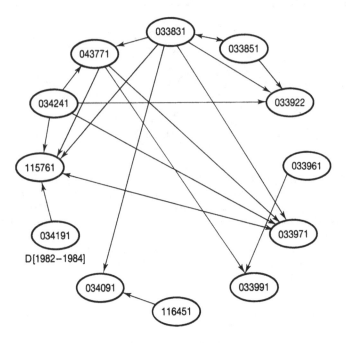

Figure 8.4. Peer relationships in 1982. (For key see legend to Figure 8.3.)

unreciprocated ties were reciprocated (e.g. 043771 and 033971). The result of these changes was that this network was becoming increasingly more densely connected. Density in social network analysis refers to the ratio of the actual number of ties in the network to the number which would be present if all individuals were connected to all others (Scott, 1988, p. 114). The importance of the density of the network to drug diffusion within it is that drug use is more easily spread to others when the network is more densely connected.

In 1984 three members (033971, 115761 and 033851) took drugs for the first time (Fig. 8.5). Their own replies indicate how they started to use drugs. Number 033971 said that he had taken drugs because 'me friend had some'. That male friend had given him the drug, inhalants, and he had taken the drug in the company of that friend and other male friends. He was no longer friends with the person who had given him the drug. Number 115761 had bought the drug, marijuana, from a drug dealer who was not a friend then or later. He had taken the drug, however, in the company of his male friends. Number 033851 said that he started taking drugs 'through friends'. It was not a friend, however, who had given him the drug, i.e. marijuana. He had been given the drug by his 'friend's big brother' and had taken the drug with that person. Although apparently different, there are similarities in the circumstances

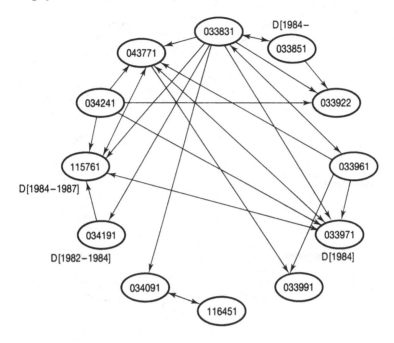

Figure 8.5. Peer relationships in 1984. (For key see legend to Figure 8.3.)

surrounding the initiation into drugs of the three boys. The source of their drug use was their peer network. With four members of the network using drugs in 1984 the possibility of drug diffusion within this network had increased because most drug-free members of the network were at the time directly connected to drug users. These connections may be traced in Fig. 8.5.

Two members of the network stopped taking drugs in 1984. Number 033971 started and stopped taking drugs during Easter 1984. On his second use of inhalants he had taken a bad trip and had not used any drug since that time. Number 034191 stopped taking drugs in December, 1984 when he said he realised it was 'stupid'. Their peer ties, it should be noted, were unaffected by their changed drug status. Both continued to be members of the network.

In 1985 043771 took drugs for the first time (Fig. 8.6). His first drug was marijuana. He took it because his 'friends were taking it, I wanted to try it'. One of his male friends gave him the drug and he took it with a number of male friends. He was still friends in 1987 with the person who gave him the drug and, since all of the friends he mentioned in 1987 were interviewed, the person who gave him the drug was one of the members of this peer network interviewed in 1987.

In 1986 four new peer ties were formed by 033851. All were male.

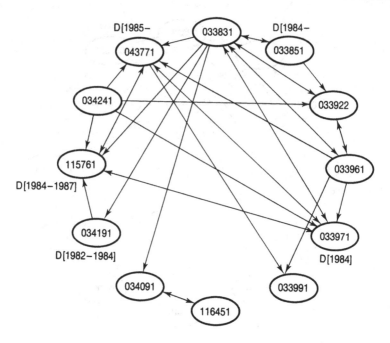

Figure 8.6. Peer relationships in 1985. (For key see legend to Figure 8.3.)

None was a drug user. No member of the network was initiated to drugs in 1986. In 1987, however, 033961 took drugs for the first time (Fig. 8.7). He started drugs because he was fed up and 'needed something to do'. He was given the drugs, marijuana and inhalants, by a male friend and had taken the drugs with his male friends. Since he took drugs for the first time in 1987 and the interview was conducted in that year, it can be assumed that his friendships had remained the same between the time he first took drugs in February 1987 and the time he was interviewed in November 1987. Six of his seven male friends had been interviewed and were in this peer network. This information suggests that the male friends with whom he had first taken drugs were in the peer network. Since one of the seven friends was not interviewed, the person who had given him the drug may or may not have been in the network in 1987. Since, however, three of his friends (033851, 043771 and 115761) who were in the network were current drug users at the time he was initiated, it seems quite likely that one of them may have given him the drug. His peer network had, therefore, been the source of his drug use by giving him the drug and the social support for its use.

One drug user stopped taking drugs in 1987. Number 115761, who had started taking drugs during 1984 (he did not state the month), stopped in May 1987. His reason for stopping taking drugs was related to

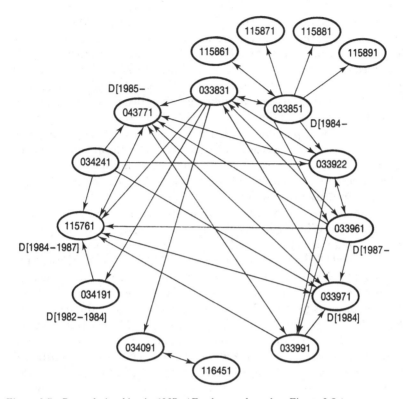

Figure 8.7. Peer relationships in 1987. (For key see legend to Figure 8.3.)

a bad drug experience as a result of which he 'ended up in hospital'.

To *summarise* the data on the initiation into drugs of the six drug users in this peer network, the findings presented confirm that their peer network had been the source of the drug use for five of them (034191, 033971, 043771, 033961 and 115761). His peer structure had indirectly influenced the drug use of the sixth person (033851), whose friend's brother had initiated him into drugs. The findings also confirm, however, that other teenagers in this network had not ever taken drugs although their peers had been drug users.

These peer network data provide a number of insights into the process of peer influence which were not available in previous drug research that relied on individual-level, dyadic or perceived peer data. They demonstrate that peer influence is not a one-way process with drug-using peers influencing non-drug-using teenagers to use drugs. The teenagers studied are peers to each other. Thus, while the teenagers' peers (i.e. friends and pals) may influence their behaviour by facilitating their drug use, those teenagers are peers to others and may facilitate those friends and pals in taking drugs. The relationships between the teenagers do not seem to be based on a power base, in which one influences the other, but on mutual trust, respect and tolerance of difference. The slowness of the drug diffusion process in this network (as well as in all other networks examined in this study) suggests that there was no overt effort on the part of the drug users to influence others to use drugs. The findings suggested that if the teenagers wished to use drugs their drug-using peers would facilitate the process; if the teenagers wished to discontinue using drugs the peer relationship did not stop. The work of Kandel (1978*b*, pp. 433, 435) had suggested otherwise. Also, in contrast with other studies, the peer network data demonstrated that when information is available on a range of peer ties and not simply on best friend dyads, the likelihood of similarity in drug use is weaker.

Teenagers were not asked any questions relating to their friends' or pals' drug use. When the relationship ties were constructed using social network analysis and the individual-level data on drug use were superimposed on them, it became clear which peers were drug users and which peers were not. Such data are superior to perceived peer drug data because perceived data are known to exaggerate the behaviour and attitudes of peers to make them seem more like those of the respondent (Kandel, 1980, pp. 269, 270; Laumann, 1973, p. 39). The peer network data presented above demonstrated an apparent tolerance of difference in the drug use of teenagers linked by peer ties. They also demonstrated that these differences persisted over a number of years in some peer relationships without apparently damaging the relationship. The level of difference and tolerance of difference in the drug use of peers over time would not have been anticipated from earlier research which had all been based on individual-level perceived peer data or on dyadic self-reported data.

Only one case study has been included in this chapter. All of the peer networks of seven or more members, which had at least two drug users, have, however, also been examined. The results confirm those presented in the case study (Kirke, 1990).

Discussion and conclusion

The findings presented in this chapter have demonstrated that peers influence the drug use of other teenagers. They have also demonstrated how that influence occurs. It is more likely to occur when drug-using peers provide the drug and social support for its use to the teenagers or when the peers provide social support for the teenager's initiation into drugs with drugs the teenager has procured elsewhere.

While teenagers who got their first drug from friends or pals usually took their first drug in the company of their friends or pals (27 of 28 teenagers), teenagers who got their first drug some other way also took their first drug in the company of their friends or pals (12 of 17 teenagers). These findings suggest that social support was being provided by their friends and pals for the teenagers' initiation into drugs.

The drug literature supports the idea that the use of many of the drugs of abuse, in particular marijuana, is a shared activity and that those with whom the activity is shared are usually close associates (Becker, 1973; Rubin & Comitas, 1975; Willis, 1978). When the drug activity is shared, information is given about the correct mode of ingestion to be used and the effects which are expected from the use of the drug. The actual effects experienced are also shared and enjoyed with those present. In this way social support is provided by those present for each other's drug use. In the author's study the use of marijuana and inhalants were shared activities. All 38 teenagers who had taken marijuana or inhalants as their first drug had taken the drug in the company of their friends or pals.

The findings of the author's study confirm that some peer networks are the source of drug use and that the community in which these peer networks are formed is the source of the drug use of the individual teenagers. If the peer networks which are formed between teenagers in a community include drug users, drug use is likely to diffuse within that community. The diffusion will not, however, be random. Only teenagers who, at a particular time, are friends or pals (i.e. peers) of other individuals, who are drug users, are likely to be influenced.

The diffusion of drugs occurs, therefore, within peer networks. When diffusion is complete within particular peer networks it can only continue when changes in peer relationships occur which link new friends or pals to the peer network or when new peer ties are formed which link formerly separate peer networks. This occurs when a friendship is formed between an individual in one network and an individual in another.

Implications for prevention and treatment

These findings suggest that a most useful strategy for the prevention of drug use among teenagers would be to focus on peer relationships and peer networks rather than on individuals. The peer networks in which teenagers are located at any particular time are crucial to whether or not they are likely to become drug users. Whether the teenagers become drug users at a later time depends on changes which occur in those relationships over time and on whether any of the individuals with whom they have peer relationships are drug users.

Preventive programmes should take account of these findings.

Preventive programmes are generally aimed at teenagers advising them to resist peer influence to take drugs. For example the National Institute on Drug Abuse drug prevention literature 'Just Say No' is designed to help teenagers to resist the pressure to take drugs when faced with peer influence to take them (Department of Health and Human Services, 1983). Such prevention programmes remove responsibility for drug diffusion from the teenager and place it firmly on their peers. They do not take account of the fact that teenagers will only take drugs if and when they choose to even when their peers are drug users and that teenagers are peers to other individuals. As well as directing teenagers to resist peer influence, therefore, they should request teenagers not to initiate new users. Teenagers then have the responsibility of modifying their own influence on others as well as resisting the influence of others on them.

The findings presented in this chapter may also have implications for the work of clinicians such as psychiatrists, psychologists, psychotherapists, counsellors and social workers who deal with teenagers who are experiencing psychosocial or social problems. While family members are often included in treatment plans, the teenagers' peer networks are unlikely to be included. Consideration of peer networks as sources of teenagers' problems could be valuable. It would enable the clinician to consider the individual teenager's problem in the social context in which it may have arisen. Clinicians should also keep in mind, however, that the social support teenagers give each other in their peer networks is crucial to their normal psychosocial development (see Champion, this volume). Resources that the teenagers' peer networks provide could be very valuable in dealing with teenagers' psychosocial problems such as drug abuse, drug addiction, problem drinking and depression that may be triggered by adversity (Lloyd, this volume). Peer networks could, therefore, be valuable as an aid to recovery. They could provide the much-needed social support to teenagers in dealing with particular crises.

Before applying such techniques in a clinical setting there seems to be a need for research on the value of such an approach and an evaluation of applications in pilot projects. Such research should ideally be interdisciplinary, with clinical practitioners, who deal with individual cases, and sociological researchers, who deal with the broader social dimension of relationships and social structures, working cooperatively together. Such research would require a complex methodology. It would require research methods that can be used to produce individual-level and social network data, to examine the interaction of the individual and the structural, and to examine changes in both and in their interaction over time. Recent advances in social network analysis make it possible to begin conducting such complex research.

Appendix

PEER RELATIONSHIP QUESTIONS

This brings us to questions about your friendships and
relationships with people of your own age.
Could you tell me first about your friends - starting with
your best friend - then boyfriend or girlfriend - then
other good friends - and then anyone else who is a friend
of yours?
Put names across top of sheet

Will you also tell me the other people of around your age
that you pal around with (e.g. in school or at discos) but
who are not as close as friends? This list should cover
all the people of your own age that you spend any free time
with.
Put names across top of sheet

Note whether person is BF (best friend), BOYF
(boyfriend), GIRLF (girlfriend), GF (good friend), F
(friend) or PAL

Q62 Name_____

Q63 Age_____
Q64 Gender: Male_____
             Female_____
Q67 Since when have you been best friend, friend, etc.?
     Month Year:_____

DRUG QUESTIONS

Q132 Have you ever used/or even tried any of these drugs?
Use show card

                                                  Yes No

Marijuana (Cannabis, Pot, Hash,
  Grass, etc.,_____
Inhalants (Glue, Tippex, Petrol,
  Lighter fluid, Solvents, Gas, etc.)_____

Hallucinogens (LSD, Acid,
  Psilocybin-Magic Mushrooms, PCP,
  Angel Dust, etc.)_____
Cocaine_____
Heroin_____

Q133 Drugs on this list are usually prescribed by a doctor. I want to ask you if you have used any of them at a time when they were not prescribed for you by a doctor.
Use show card

                                                    Yes No

Other opiates (Codeine, Cough Syrup,
  Painkillers, Morphine, etc.)_____
Stimulants (Amphetamines, Speed,
  Uppers, Ups, Pep Pills, etc.)_____
Sedatives (Barbiturates, Downs, etc.)_____
Tranquillisers (Valium, Librium, etc.)_____

Q134 Have you used any other drug that is not on these lists?
Yes Name of drug:_____
No

Ask all who have taken a drug
Q140   Age when first used?   When was that?

                                                Month   Year

Marijuana_____
Inhalants_____
Hallucinogens_____
Cocaine_____
Heroin_____
Other opiates_____
Stimulants_____
Sedatives_____
Tranquillisers_____
Other_____

Q142 When taking/using your first drug were you: On your own?_____

or with others?_____
No names-relationship then-male or female
Q146 Did you get it (i.e. first drug) from a friend_____
or some other person?_____
No names-relationship then-male or female

References

Akers, R. L., Krohn, M. D., Lanza-Kaduce, L. & Radosevich, M. (1979). Social learning and deviant behavior: a specific test of a general theory. *American Sociological Review*, **44**, 635–55.
Becker, H. S. (1973). *Outsiders: Studies in the Sociology of Deviance*, enlarged edn. New York: Free Press.
Brook, J. S., Whiteman, M. & Gordon, A. S. (1983). Qualitative and quantitative aspects of adolescent drug use: interplay of personality, family and peer correlates. *Psychological Reports*, **51**, 1151–63.
Central Statistics Office (1981, 1986). Census of population. Dublin: Central Statistics Office.
Dembo, R., Schmeidler, J. & Burgos, W. (1982). Processes of early drug involvement in three inner-city neighborhood settings. *Deviant Behavior*, **3**, 359–83.
Department of Health and Human Services (1983). Publication no. (ADM) 83-1271. Washington, DC.
Jessor, R. & Jessor, S. L. (1978). Theory testing in longitudinal research on marijuana use. In *Longitudinal Research on Drug Use: Empirical Findings and Methodological Issues*, ed. D. B. Kandel, pp. 41–71. New York: Hemisphere Publishing/Halsted Press.
Kandel, D. B. (1973). Adolescent marijuana use: role of parents and peers. *Science*, **181**, 1067–70.
Kandel, D. B. (1978a). Convergences in prospective longitudinal surveys of drug use in normal populations. In *Longitudinal Research on Drug Use: Empirical Findings and Methodological Issues*, ed. D. B. Kandel, pp. 3–38. New York: Hemisphere Publishing/Halsted Press.
Kandel, D. B. (1978b). Homophily, selection, and socialization in adolescent friendships. *American Journal of Sociology*, **84**, 427–36.
Kandel, D. B. (ed.) (1978c). *Longitudinal Research on Drug Use: Empirical Findings and Methodological Issues*. New York: Hemisphere Publishing/Halsted Press.
Kandel, D. B. (1980). Drug and drinking behavior among youth. *Annual Review of Sociology*, **6**, 235–85.
Kirke, D. M. (1990). Teenage drug abuse: an individualistic and structural analysis. Unpublished PhD thesis, University College Dublin.
Knoke, D. & Kuklinski, J. H. (1982). *Network Analysis*. Sage University Paper Series on Quantitative Applications in the Social Sciences, series no. 07-028. Beverly Hills and London: Sage Publications.
Laumann, E. O. (1973). *Bonds of Pluralism: The Form and Substance of Urban Social Networks*. New York: Wiley.

Rubin, V. & Comitas, L. (1975). *Ganja in Jamaica: A Medical Anthropological Study of Chronic Marijuana Use*. The Hague: Mouton.
Scott, J. (1988). Trend report social network analysis. *Sociology*, **22**, 1, 109–27.
Sprenger, C. J. A. & Stokman, F. N. (eds.) (1989). *Gradap: Graph Definition and Analysis Package*. Groningen: ProGamma.
Wellman, B. (1988). Structural analysis: from method and metaphor to theory and substance. In *Social Structures: A Network Approach*, ed. B. Wellman & S. D. Berkowitz, pp. 19–61. Cambridge: Cambridge University Press.
Willis, P. E. (1978). *Profane Culture*. London: Routledge and Kegan Paul.

PART III

LESSONS FROM
INTERVENTION STUDIES

9

Social network and mental health: an intervention study

Odd Steffen Dalgard, Trine Anstorp, Kirsten Benum
and Tom Sørensen

Introduction

The first two chapters in Part III have been included to provide readers
with a deeper understanding of the benefits of and the challenges posed
by conducting experimental intervention studies. In this chapter we
describe a preventive programme aimed at improving mental health by
improving social networks, which was carried out in a recently established
working-class/middle-class neighbourhood with mainly high-rise houses
on the outskirts of Oslo, Norway ('satellite town'). The target group was
middle-aged women with poor social networks, low quality of life and a
high load of stress symptoms, identified by a survey of a representative
sample of middle-aged women in the neighbourhood.

As shown in a previous study from Oslo (Dalgard, 1986), having a
qualitatively poor social network increases the risk of mental disorder,
especially when living in a new and poorly integrated neighbourhood.
Being a woman, especially when middle-aged, adds to this risk (Dalgard,
1980). However, it can not be decided, on the basis of such a
cross-sectional study, to what extent a poor social network contributes to
the development of mental disorder, possibly as a vulnerability factor, or
rather is a consequence of poor mental health. Longitudinal studies and
intervention studies are necessary to shed more light on this question.
The present chapter describes an intervention project, designed on the
basis of the epidemiological study referred to above.

In brief, the study group was randomly split in two, resulting in an
experimental group ($n = 26$) and a control group ($n = 29$). Both groups
were interviewed four times: at the beginning of the intervention
programme, after the programme was terminated, 2 years later, and 6
years later, allowing for a comparison with respect to social network,
quality of life and mental health. The intervention programme lasted for
1 year and consisted of weekly group meetings with between five and
seven of the women participating in each group. The groups were led by
two psychologists. The group aims were the stimulation of social

interaction and the enlargement of the women's social networks. Some of the groups were combined with physical training and practical activity (porcelain painting).

The intervention project

The project was an attempt to prevent the development of mental disorder by influencing the social network in a positive way, i.e. by social network stimulation. By this systematic manipulation of the social network, and by recording any effects on mental health, one is not only evaluating an intervention programme, but as the same time studying the aetiological effect of the social network.

Other studies with the same aim are described in the literature (Levander, 1985; and elsewhere in this volume), and there are numerous reports about the positive effect of strengthening the social network of psychiatric patients and people in emotional crisis. However, when this study was being planned there were, to our knowledge, no other studies of its kind, i.e. community-based social network programmes with a preventive purpose which had been subjected to systematic evaluation, including the use of a control group.

Selection of target group

In order to be able to demonstrate the preventive effect of social network stimulation on mental health, we had to select a population group in which the high risk of mental disorder was associated with poor social networks, and then expose this group to the programme.

On the basis of findings from the epidemiological study referred to above, we decided that our target group should be middle-aged women living in a new and poorly integrated urban neighbourhood and having a poor social network. To these criteria we added poor quality of life and symptoms of stress, but without requiring the women to be current psychiatric patients. By including a high score of stress symptoms among our criteria, we deviated from dealing strictly with a programme of primary prevention. Thus the study encompassed, rather, a mixture of primary and secondary prevention components, with the aim of preventing symptoms of stress from developing into manifest psychiatric disorder, as well as preventing existing mental disorder from developing into a more chronic form of mental disorder.

Poor quality of life was also included among the criteria because this variable is closely related to mental disorder, especially anxiety and depression, and probably acts as an intervening factor between life problems and mental health.

To select the target group as defined above, a new community survey had to be carried out. This was the only way to identify a group representative of the defined high-risk population, allowing for generalisations applicable to the community. From a practical point of view this procedure was, of course, very awkward, but from a methodological point of view it was indispensable.

The community survey covered, according to our high-risk criteria, a representative sample of women in the age group 45–54 years living in a new and poorly integrated neighbourhood similar to that described in the first epidemiological study. This sample was drawn from the population register of Oslo, and consisted of 318 women out of 645 possible women in the selected age group, in a neighbourhood fulfilling our criteria of social disintegration.

To identify those of the 318 women with a qualitatively poor social network, poor quality of life and symptoms of stress, the women were interviewed with respect to these characteristics. The quality of each social network was measured in the same way as in the first epidemiological study (Dalgard, 1986), using questions about feelings of closeness, cohesiveness and reliability in relation to family and friends (Appendix A). Information was also gathered about frequency of contacts with network members.

Quality of life was measured by several subscales, referring to the state of affect as well as feeling of self-realisation, combined with more general questions about life satisfaction and happiness. Among the questions relating to quality of life, was one concerning how content the respondent was with herself as a person. This was supposed to give an indication of self-esteem (Appendix B).

To measure symptoms of stress, two different scales were used: GHQ, 20 items (Goldberg, 1972) and SCL-90 (Derogatis, 1977). As the SCL-90 was judged to be more suitable for measuring change over time, only this scale will be referred to as the outcome measure in this account of our study.

To select the target group (middle-aged women in a poorly integrated neighbourhood who also had a poor social network, poor quality of life and a high level of stress symptoms) the following procedure was followed: Those belonging to the poorest third with respect to quality of social network, as well as with respect to quality of life and symptom score, were selected. This provided a group of 100 women, of whom 57% were 'psychiatric cases' according to the GHQ-20 (cutoff between 3 and 4). Twenty-eight per cent had consulted a psychiatrist at some time during their life, but none were under psychiatric treatment when the programme started. As mentioned earlier, this means that the aim and scope of the project embraced both primary and secondary prevention, with some of the participants already having developed mental disorder whilst the remainder had at least a number of stress symptoms.

Design of the intervention study

To compare the development of the group exposed to our programme, i.e. the experimental group, with a comparable control group, the 100 high-risk women referred to above were randomly allocated to two groups of equal size. Both these groups then became somewhat reduced, due to a move away from the area or lack of time or interest on the part of the subjects. This left 26 women in the experimental group and 29 in the control group. There were no significant differences between groups with respect to any of the variables included. With respect to the SCL-90 symptom score, the averages were 81.2 for the experimental group and 79.1 for the control group.

Both groups were interviewed again at the start of the intervention programme, at the end of the programme and 2 and 5 years after this. The experimental group was also interviewed in the middle of the programme. At all these time points core questions were repeated, covering social network, quality of life and mental health (Appendixes A and B). For the experimental group data were also gathered about their behaviour in the programme. This was based on the observations of the group leaders, and qualitative interviews about the participants' attitudes, expectations and reactions to the group and its activities. In order to describe each women's relationship to her social network members at different points in time, possibly including other members of the experimental group, a so-called network circle questionnaire was used. Very simply, the respondent was asked to plot her network members in a first, second or third circle from the centre (herself), according to the closeness of the relationship.

The design of the study is summarised in Fig. 9.1.

The intervention programme

To achieve the objective of social network stimulation, it was necessary to decide whether the programme should aim either at strengthening the participants' existing networks or at developing new social relationships. We decided to focus upon the latter. We invited the women to take part in various group activities together with women randomly picked from the target group, led by two research psychologists. By choosing the group approach we accorded with the views of Kurt Lewin who argued that: 'It is generally easier to induce social change by involving groups

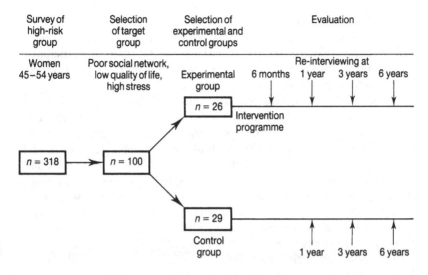

Figure 9.1. Design of the intervention study.

rather than through individuals directly' (Lewin, 1944). Through the group intervention the intention was not to change symptoms directly, but to increase the women's power or competence to do something themselves with their life situation.

The concrete organisation of the groups was centred around activities that the women themselves had chosen. (The importance of choice is discussed by Brugha in the final chapter of this volume). A total of six groups were established: two for physical training, two for porcelain painting and two social activity groups. Some women participated in more than one group, each consisting of between five and seven participants. The social activity groups were led by two research psychologists, whereas the two other types of groups were led by professional instructors in addition to the psychologists. All groups were organised in the neighbourhood, and were free of charge. In general the group meetings took place once a week, and the programme lasted for 1 year.

Even among women who had initially expressed interest in the group activities, much work had to be devoted to *motivating* them actually to come to the meetings. Physical health problems and problematic life events were often put forward as excuses for not coming to the meetings, whereas psychiatric symptoms as such were not mentioned so often. The consequence of this resistance against joining the meetings was that it took about half a year before the programme was fully operational.

To a certain extent, *methods of social network stimulation* had to be developed during the programme, taking into consideration the perceived needs and interests expressed by the participants themselves. To offer the women a given model, previously developed in another type of social setting, could easily have led to many more refusing to participate. Ideally, these are issues that could be resolved as part of a pilot project before such an experiment is begun.

The aim of the programme was, as mentioned before, to initiate among the women a process of being acquainted, and even to make friends. The process was supposed to continue after the intervention programme was finished, hence leading to the establishment of self-sustaining social networks. At the *individual level* the programme consisted of four main elements: to develop/strengthen self-esteem; to learn to give and receive social support; to learn to function as a member of a group; and lastly to strengthen the person's motivation to make and deepen social relationships. On the *group level* the key elements were to create a safe atmosphere, to develop group cohesion and to talk about and solve conflicts.

In the following section the different elements will be explained in more detail, in the light of experience gained with the participants.

Key elements of the programme

To develop/strengthen self-esteem

In our original survey, low self-esteem turned out to be one important negative factor preventing contact at an *individual level* (see also Brewin, Lloyd and Gilbert, this volume). In the group sessions the women would either talk extremely negatively about themselves or their families, or would be completely silent. The group leaders spent some time trying to model how to present oneself in a more adequate way.

To get to know other people one has to present oneself, and in some way give information about oneself that will make other people interested in getting in contact. Accordingly the group leaders concentrated on positive qualities, made comments on positive experiences the women had had in life, gave compliments and paid much attention to each individual. In this way the leaders wanted to model, or reinforce, positive attempts to communicate. The programme also included some elements of assertiveness training, such as how to give and take criticism, how to present demands to others, and so forth.

The learning of certain skills in the porcelain painting group and the physical training group was, of itself, important for raising the women's self-esteem.

To give and receive social support

Initially the married women participating in the programme complained about lack of support from their husbands. They did not seem to have compensated for this situation by developing close relations with friends or other family members.

Our eventual intention was to show the women how to give and receive social support from people outside their family network. We also wanted to demonstrate that belonging to a group might be an alternative to having only close family relations. To influence this process, little by little we requested more initiative from the women themselves. They were asked to contact each other between the group sessions, make phone calls, and so on. Every tendency of tolerance and approval among the women was systematically reinforced by the group leaders. The problem seemed to be how to maintain and develop deeper engagement when contact was established. In Parry (this volume) there is a further discussion of methods for recognising and making use of support offered by others in existing relationships.

To function as a member of a group

These women were not accustomed to belonging to organisations. They were typical 'non-participants' in society. If they had any experience from groups outside the family, it was from more informal girlfriend groups or 'chatty groups'. These groups were perceived as negative: 'There is too much gossip, where the strongest people decide everything, I can never say a word', or 'I don't like to talk about meaningless things'. These informal groups are characterised by having no leader to structure the rules and to pay attention to the communication. Consequently the leaders spent much time teaching the women how to listen to each other rather than all speaking at the same time.

Making the women commit themselves to group participation in general had to be one of the main tasks. Because of caretaking obligations in the family, or fear of involving themselves too much in the programme, the women would reject obligations. The group leaders tried to delegate some responsibility to each of the women, such as making coffee in the group sessions. Some of the women became informal group leaders in the different groups, but no one wanted to take any formal responsibility.

To strengthen motivation

It is not enough to have the skill or ability to act if the motivation is not present. Our experience was that many of the women came to a point where they had to choose between either being isolated and safe, as before, or taking the initiative and being tense. Their previous contacts having been close and intimate, we learned that some of the women thought of all social relations as either intimate or very distant (e.g. professional). They would get disappointed easily if their initiative in starting a friendship was rejected by the other. This of course affected negatively any further motivation to deepen a relationship.

The group leaders tried to stress the fact that belonging to a group might be a way to have social contact in itself. This was a new experience to many of the women.

At the *group level*, the following elements were considered to be especially important:

To create a safe atmosphere

The methods applied to influence the group atmosphere positively were: to initiate talk about familiar topics, to use humour, to serve coffee and cakes, to arrange the chairs in order to sit relatively close together, and to reinforce positive feelings towards each other. Commenting upon the atmosphere seemed to reduce tension.

To develop group cohesion

In creating group cohesion the group leaders used well-known methods such as introducing common tasks in order to create a common history and common goals in the groups. In the activity groups this seemed to be easy. The common task was how to learn porcelain painting or do physical exercise. The social group made food, visited the theatre and took trips into town. Talking about the aims of the project also stimulated group cohesion.

To talk about and to solve conflicts

Tendencies to hide conflicts, or gossiping behind others' backs, were obvious in all groups at the beginning. Irritation towards dominant participants was shown indirectly. Rules about group norms had to be outlined. The problem for the group leaders was not to intervene too much, as they did not have any contract that involved changing individual behaviour explicitly. The purpose was to keep the discussion at a group level and not to individualise it too much.

One important topic of discussion was whether the groups should allow talk about personal problems, or whether the group should be a pleasant place to meet, drink coffee, paint porcelain and chat. The women were all engaged in this question, and they made a decision to try to be open about their own situation. This decision contributed to a more consolidated and safe atmosphere. At the same time the group leaders tried to redefine problems and symptoms in a more positive way. The aim was not to minimise but to generalise problems, and to focus upon common concerns such as self-image, myths about the menopause, women's role in general, children leaving home, and so on. Another aspect was to invite the women to criticise the group leaders or the programme, in order to legalise criticism.

Evaluation of the intervention programme

The programme was evaluated with respect to *effectiveness* by comparing various *outcome* variables in the experimental and control groups, as well as with respect to *process*. Evaluation of effectiveness alone would not say anything about how the programme worked. Process evaluation alone would not reveal whether the same results would have been obtained without any programme at all, or with another programme.

Process evaluation

As mentioned earlier, it took about 6 months to establish a working relationship with all the women who expressed an interest in participating in the programme. From then on the groups developed through the following three phases:

Initial phase. This phase, which was characterised by considerable uncertainty and social insecurity on the part of the participants, lasted for about 6 months. The group leaders spent much time trying to promote an atmosphere of trust and caring, and played an active role in structuring the groups and deciding the nature of the activities.

Consolidation phase. During the next 4–5 months the interpersonal activity in the groups increased, and contacts between the women outside the meetings started to develop. At the same time the expectations towards the leaders as friends/or problem-solvers increased. The leaders worked on developing group norms and group identity, and at the same time encouraged extra-group contacts between the participants.

Independence phase. During the last couple of months the group leaders worked on transferring responsibility for the groups to the participants themselves, preparing leadership withdrawal from the programme. In this phase the groups started to develop their own life with closer contacts among the women.

In an attempt to describe the qualitative aspects of group participation, the women were classified along four dimensions: active/passive, personal/not personal, establishing contact/not establishing contact, and interest/no interest in continuing the groups after withdrawal of the leaders. As would be expected, there was a strong positive association between the number of meetings attended and the qualitative participation of the women. Half of the 26 women participated in all meetings in their group, and at the same time showed maximum qualitative participation in terms of personal involvement. However, there were also women who in spite of being present at all, or almost all meetings, showed very little personal involvement and, conversely, strongly involved women who participated in only a few meetings.

To what extent the women established new friendships in the groups may to a certain degree be reflected in the network circle questionnnaire referred to above. Whereas only 7 women indicated group members in their circles after 6 months of the programme, this number was increased to 15 by the end of the programme.

Outcome evaluation

In the following the results are shown in terms of percentage improvement of the various variables. With respect to the SCL-90, a difference of more than 5 points is required to be regarded as a change.

Of the experimental group ($n = 26$), 21 were interviewed again 2 years after the programme had terminated; the number interviewed again from the control group ($n = 29$) was 20. The reasons for this drop-out were partly moving away from the area, partly lack of time, and partly lack of interest; in no case was drop-out caused by mental health problems.

Table 9.1 gives the results 3 years after the programme had started (i.e. 2 years after its termination). For most of the variables there is a tendency for the higher percentage improvement to occur in the experimental group. Taken separately, this difference is statistically significant for only one variable: self-esteem ($p = 0.02$). The overall distribution of the variables is, however, statistically significant ($p = 0.05$).

There is a trend towards least improvement in the experimental group with respect to quality of family relationships (Table 9.1, Appendix A). This may simply be a consequence of the small and unstable numbers, but may also indicate that the participation of the women in activities outside the family had led to problems at home.

To achieve more conclusive results from the point of view of statistical power the sample would have had to be about twice as large. With the given distribution, to achieve a power of 80% with an α risk of 5% and a reached effect quantified by a relative risk of 2.0, the sample size needed for most of the variables would have been 36 in both the experimental group and the control group.

Process and outcome

Those who were most active in the groups and most successful in making new friends, were also those who made the most improvement in their mental health (table available from authors). There was a trend for most variables indicating that those who had been relatively active in the

Table 9.1. *Outcome after 3 years for the experimental group and control group*

	Percentage improved	
	Experimental ($n = 21$)	Control ($n = 20$)
Social network		
Frequency of seeing friends	43	19
Quality of relationship: friends	43	43
Quality of relationship: family	40	55
Satisfaction with family/friends	33	20
Quality of life		
Life useless/worthwhile	38	24
Life meaningless/meaningful	50	35
Life disappointing/rewarding	45	25
Feel free/tied down	30	14
Feel able/unable to use own potential	45	33
Feel life is full/dull	40	35
General satisfaction with life	24	19
Self-esteem	71	30*
Health		
Satisfaction with health	52	24
SCL-90	67	50

Chi-square for the overall distribution: $p = 0.05$.
*$p = 0.02$.

group meetings improved more than did passive participants. With respect to change in symptoms, the passive members were the same as the controls, with 50% improving (and 50% getting worse or showing no change). In contrast, the active participants showed improvement in 75% of cases. When we examined the symptom score at the beginning of the study there was no association between this, the activity in groups and improvement.

As expected, there was a relationship between activity in the group meetings and keeping in contact with other group members after the programme was terminated, and between keeping in contact and improvement with respect to mental health. Of those who had been relatively active in the group meetings, 83% had been in touch with one or more of the group members during the last year of the follow up when interviewed 2 years after the end of the study, whereas the corresponding figure for the passive members was 44% (table of further results available from authors). There is a trend, especially with respect to mental health and general satisfaction with health (Appendix B), for those who have kept up social contact with other group members to have improved more often than the rest. For the other variables the pattern is less clear.

The findings have not as yet been fully analysed with respect to the follow-up 5 years after the termination of the programme. There seems, however, to have been a general trend towards a reduction in the differences between the two groups during the last 3 years (Lilljeqvist, 1993).

Conclusion

Our impression is that the programme worked, and more or less in the way we expected. At follow-up the outcome appeared to be more positive in the experimental group than in the control group with respect to social network and quality of life, as well as mental health. The group meetings stimulated social interactions and network formation, and this was associated with a positive development of quality of life, self-esteem and mental health. Even so, the programme did not seem to be very successful in promoting lasting relationships between the women, which was the intention. The positive effect of the programme seemed to be related as much to the stimulation of existing social networks as to the creation of new ones. In accordance with this, most of the friends identified in the outcome variables involved references to old friendships and not to new ones that had been established in the programme. Thus, the group meetings may have functioned as a social learning process, making the participants more open about social interaction in general, rather than as an arena for obtaining new friends.

The programme seems to have been more clearly successful in strengthening the self-esteem of the participants – also one of its main goals. Others have found also that self-esteem acts as a major explanatory variable between the social environment and mental health (Brown & Harris, 1978; and elsewhere in this volume).

The criteria used for selecting the participants in our programme identified a group of women with generally low social and interpersonal competence. This made it particularly difficult to motivate the women to join the programme and, for some, to stay in it. Hence we would advise, when selecting self-help group participants, the inclusion of some with more individual resources and social skills who might stimulate the group process and probably develop into group leaders.

When motivating people to join a programme it is important to listen to what the subjects themselves are interested in doing. It seems important that the group programme includes practical activities: doing things together tends to reduce anxiety and may act as a means for the development of group cohesion.

To develop the group into a self-help group it has to be made clear from the very beginning that the professionals will participate only for a limited period.

Discussion: disease prevention or health promotion?

According to the common definition of *disease prevention*, such projects address themselves to high-risk groups and the intervention is quite specific. This project could be characterised as a mixture of primary and secondary prevention, all the participants having developed at least some symptoms of stress although only a certain proportion were actually identified as patients with psychiatric disorders.

Was it necessary to employ psychologists to run the groups? It is quite expensive to engage professionals to run such programmes. By choosing professionals there is less inducement for lay people and the non-professional community to develop supporting social structures. Could the local community have met the need for social contact and stimulation of these women equally well and more cheaply? We do not think so. These particular women had too many problems to be likely participants in ordinary community groups – though a better-organised neighbour-hood, with various possibilities for contact and social interaction, might have met the needs of such people. Hence any effort to make such socially poorly integrated neighbourhoods into a better place to live may also be important from a health point of view. Such work would be an example of *health promotion*.

Could *both* psychiatric prevention and mental health promotion benefit the community? By producing general improvements in commu-nity organisation, it may be easier for professionals to motivate and refer high-risk individuals to existing groups and activities. Similarly, people working in health promotion could profit from the insights of mental health workers with respect to the basic psychosocial needs of the population.

Finally, we wish to emphasise the importance of the planning of new neighbourhoods as a tool for mental health promotion. Risk-producing factors could have been better managed in the planning process (Dalgard, 1986), particularly when large numbers of people move into a new neighbourhood at the same time. Among the most important negative factors are the lack of suitable opportunities for social contact and recreation, lack of various public and private services, the relatively high rent of the housing and possibly also the skewed age distribution, with almost all of the people aged less than 40 years. In this respect it is a step forward that the psychosocial aspects of the planning of new neighbourhoods have come to be emphasised in the statements and plans of the central housing and health authorities in Norway.

Appendixes

Appendix A. Questions about quality of the social network

<u>Family</u>
Do you find it difficult to know the points of view and
opinions of your close family?
    Often   1
    Sometimes   2
    Never   3

By and large do you feel that you can be yourself in
relation to your close family?
    Always   1
    Usually   2
    Seldom or never 3

Do you feel that your <u>close</u> family gives reasonable
emphasis to your opinions?
    Always   1
    Usually   2
    Seldom or never 3

<u>Friends</u>
Do you feel closely attached to your friends?
    Always   1
    Usually   2
    Seldom or never 3

Do you feel that your friends give reasonable emphasis to
our opinions?
    Always   1
    Usually   2
    Seldom or never 3

Do you feel apart, even among friends?
    Often   1
    Sometimes   2
    Never   3

<u>Question about frequency of contact with friends</u>
How often do you see your friends?
    Have none   0
    Daily   1
    Each week, but not daily   2
    Each month, but not each week   3
    Several times a year, but not each month   4

About once a year   5
Seldom or never   6

Appendix B. Questions about quality of life

Taken overall, how satisfied would you say you are with
your life nowadays? Would you say that you are:

Extremely satisfied   1
Very satisfied   2
Quite satisfied   3
Not sure   4
Quite unsatisfied   5
Very unsatisfied   6
Extremely unsatisfied   7

Take your time to go through the pairs of words and put a
circle around the number which best describe how your
life is nowadays.

My life is:

Worthless	1 2 3 4 5 6 7	Useful
Meaningless	1 2 3 4 5 6 7	Meaningful
Disappointing	1 2 3 4 5 6 7	Rewarding
I feel free and can decide about my own life	1 2 3 4 5 6 7	I feel trapped and tied up
I feel that I can use own skills and potentials	1 2 3 4 5 6 7	I feel that I cannot use my skills and potentials
I feel that life is providing deep and intense experiences	1 2 3 4 5 6 7	I feel that life is grey and monotonous

To what extent are you satisfied with the following
aspects/parts of your life?

Your health and physical condition   1 2 3 4 5 6 7
The time spent with family and friends   1 2 3 4 5 6 7

(Other aspects of life were also included in the
questionnaire, but they were less relevant to the study.)

References

Brown, G. W. & Harris, T. (1978). *Social Origins of Depression.* New York: Free Press.

Dalgard, O. S. (1980). *Bomiljø og psykisk helse.* Oslo: Universitetsforlaget.

Dalgard, O. S. (1986). Living conditions, social network and mental health. In *Social Support: Health and Disease,* ed. S. O. Isacsson & L. Janzon, pp. 71–84. Stockholm: Almquist & Wiksell.

Derogatis, L. R. (1977). SCL-90: administration, scoring and procedures manual 1 for the R version. Baltimore: Derogatis.

Goldberg, D. P. (1972). *The Detection of Psychiatric Illness by Questionnaire.* Oxford: Oxford University Press.

Levander, S. (1985). Community work as part of the psychiatric services of Nacka. In *Preventive Psychiatry: Methods and Experiences,* ed. O. S. Dalgard. *Acta Psychiatria Scandinavica Supplementum 337,* 21–9.

Lewin, K. (1944). Field theory and experiment in social psychology: conceptual methods. *American Journal of Sociology,* **44**, 868–96.

Lilljeqvist, A. -C. (1993). Sosialt nettverk, livskvalitet og psykisk helse Thesis, University of Trondheim.

10

A test of the social support hypothesis

Bryanne Barnett and Gordon Parker

Background to the social support study

The study we undertook was part of a larger programme of research on childhood antecedents of adult psychosocial difficulties and psychiatric disorders (some of which has been discussed by Champion and by Brewin in this volume). We were particularly interested in the behaviour and attitudes of parents towards their children and the consequences of this for the children. It is, therefore, relevant to outline the prior stages of the research programme as well as describing the models which guided our thinking. Accordingly, the general question of social networks and social support; the measurement of these; attachment theory and related research, which are discussed in earlier chapters, will be mentioned briefly first, followed by the findings which prompted our intervention study, the study itself and the results.

Social networks and social support

Social network

What is a 'social network' and who should be included in any measurement of it? How are the positive and negative aspects of the various relationships to be weighted, and how do these relate to the concept of 'social support' and to the question of morbidity? In spite of intensive research and theoretical speculation these questions remain difficult to answer.

The social network of any individual may be held to comprise those with whom the person has regular face-to-face interaction and some degree of commitment (Broom & Selznick, 1973). From this group, the individual is thought to obtain certain basic supplies defined by Weiss (1974), including attachment, as discussed earlier. Three levels or circles of relationships are required: (1) confiding, intimate relationships; (2) reasonably close friendships; and (3) a wider circle of more casual acquaintances.

How do these concepts of social provision relate to families? Is this pattern interrupted, for longer or shorter periods, in late pregnancy and while the woman has small children at home to care for? The changes may include benefits such as not having to travel to and from work, but also entail: loss of financial independence, loss of adult company for at least part of the day, and in general a loss of the spontaneous quality in day-to-day decisions and activities. There may also be the move to a new neighbourhood. These changes may be experienced as a major loss.

Some women may quickly and successfully negotiate a new network, for example, appropriately including other women with children, while others do not. Some have a mother and perhaps extended family to fill the gaps; other do not. In Australia, with a high proportion of the population consisting of immigrants, a large network of relatives and all the cultural supports of ritual and custom are likely to be missing for many young couples.

Social support

Social support may be seen simply as the provision of help and advice by other people. The description offered by researchers such as Sarason is that such support implies the perception that others are available in times of need and satisfaction with the adequacy of that available support (Sarason *et al.*, 1983). This seems very close to Bowlby's notion of secure attachment (see below).

The association between lack of social support and an increase in physical or psychological morbidity has been the subject of considerable speculation and research interest (e.g. Henderson *et al.*, 1981; Greenblatt *et al.*, 1982; Brugha *et al.*, 1982, 1990; Broadhead *et al.*, 1983; Heller, 1986). Henderson has listed three separate hypotheses about the effects of social support and suggests there may be others (Henderson, 1988). First, 'that it has a direct and independent effect in its own right on mental and/or physical health, whether or not adversity is also present'; second, 'that it provides a buffer or cushioning effect against stress, but has no independent effect in its absence'; or third, 'that in persons who have already developed affective or neurotic symptoms, it has a therapeutic effect shortening the episode and reducing symptoms'. Henderson *et al.* (1981) in their extensive study concluded 'under adversity, it is those who construe their social relationships as inadequate who are more likely to develop symptoms'. Other workers (Maddison & Walker, 1967; Maddison & Viola, 1968) seem to invoke both possibilities – perceived and actual social network – as operative.

The question of the importance of close relationships was particularly relevant to our study. Marital satisfaction affects adaptation (Paykel *et al.*, 1980; Crnic *et al.*, 1983). Wandersman *et al.* (1980) reported that support from the spouse bore a positive relation to parental skills, although not to parenting attitudes, and that network support was not related to parental competence. Crnic *et al.* (1983) similarly reported that spousal support was positively and directly related to more effective mothering, while network support was associated with a more positive attitude towards the mothering role. Intimate relationships were related to satisfaction with life in general and with parenting. Brown *et al.* (1975) found marital satisfaction buffered stress, but these workers concluded that spouse support was essential to well-being and no other individual could fill the gap if such support were lacking (Brown & Harris, 1978). Others have, however, reported that support from other persons in the network is also of importance (Andrews *et al.*, 1978).

Measurement of the social network/social support

Many research groups have attempted to devise a reliable and valid instrument for measurement of social network (McCallister & Fisher, 1978; Winefield, 1979; O'Connor & Brown, 1984). But the one which best fitted our view of the function of attachment and social support at this developmental stage, i.e. becoming a parent, was the Interview Schedule for Social Interaction (ISSI: Henderson *et al.*, 1980), which was referred to by Brugha in the opening chapter of this volume. The ISSI is based, in part, on the notion of social provisions described by Weiss (1974) and introduced by Brugha. Henderson gave the highest priority to attachment, which he considered 'to deserve the greatest representation, on the grounds that attachment theory leads one to predict that it will have the strongest association with the development of psychiatric symptoms'.

The ISSI is a measure of the perceived availability and adequacy of support from intimates and the wider social network. The structured interview contains 52 questions which assess, at three levels (i.e. close and confiding, friendship and acquaintanceship) the social relationships which the respondent reports to be currently available to her, and also assess how adequate she feels they are in meeting her needs. The four main scale scores derived from the ISSI are availability and adequacy of attachment (AVAT, ADAT) and availability and adequacy of social integration (AVSI, ADSI). The questionnaire also enquires about unpleasant interaction with intimates and acquaintances.

Attachment

Clinical work with patients in both child and adult psychiatry is a constant reminder of how the interactions between parents and children influence – for better and for worse – psychosocial development in the children. The work of John Bowlby and his followers (e.g. Mary Ainsworth and Mary Main) on attachment and its significance throughout the life cycle, is, of course, central to any discussion on this topic (Parkes & Stevenson-Hinde, 1982) already explored in the chapters by Champion, Brewin and Gilbert in this volume. Methods are now available for measuring not only infants' and children's models of the relationship with their parents, but of parents' models for specific children and of the adult's 'current state of mind with respect to attachment' (Ainsworth *et al.*, 1978; Bretherton *et al.*, 1989; Main & Goldwyn, 1990).

Research on attachment offers an understanding not only of how patterns are constructed and carried internally, but also how they are transmitted from generation to generation. Very specific primary preventive intervention then becomes a possibility. If the adult's internal model is used as a guide or filter in the relationship with her or his own children, perhaps the model can be modified or a new one constructed, for example through the medium of a therapeutic relationship.

Attachment theory predicts that when individuals are stressed they are more likely to manifest attachment behaviours. Their attachment figures are expected to *provide* a feeling of security (i.e. 'support'). When a couple is making the important transition from dyad into family, these issues might be expected to achieve high salience.

The Sydney Research Programme

The Parental Bonding Instrument

An important corollary of attachment research is that simple observation of parental behaviours is regarded as grossly inadequate for making any judgements regarding the parent–child relationship as it 'does not capture the meaning of the behaviours for a given dyad' (Zeanah & Barton, 1989). It is the subjective experience of each party which is important: 'what is communicated and experienced within that pattern about the caregiving relationship, the self, and the other' (Zeanah & Barton, 1989).

Early in the course of the research programme, a scale known as the Parental Bonding Instrument (PBI) was developed (Parker *et al.*, 1979). This is a 25-item, self-report measure of the respondent's perceptions, or subjective experience, of two important dimensions of parental behaviour, namely care and protection, as the respondent experienced them up to the age of 16 years.

The care dimension measures a range of qualities from empathy and affection at the positive end to coldness, neglect and hostility at the negative end. The protection (i.e. control or limit-setting) dimension reflects a spectrum from a positive pole of appropriate encouragement of independence through to a negative pole of overprotection, control, intrusiveness and infantilisation. The instrument has been shown to be reliable and valid, as a measure both of perceived and of actual parental style (Parker, 1983), and has gained wide acceptance (Parker, 1992).

Applied research using the PBI has led to the conclusion that insufficient parental care and/or overprotection are associated with neurotic anxiety and depressive disorders in both clinical and non-clinical populations (Parker, 1983).

Influences on maternal protectiveness

Another study (Parker & Lipscombe, 1981) considered possible determinants of maternal overprotection. In particular, the question was asked as to what produced the behaviour which the child interpreted as both uncaring and overly protective (i.e. affectionless control) and which appeared to be the style most clearly linked with neurotic symptoms in adulthood.

A non-clinical group of 75 postgraduate trainee teachers completed the PBI and gave permission for their own mothers to be contacted for interview. The index child's developmental history and the mother's responses to and involvement with that child were explored. Two subgroups of mothers were formed: 15 who were rated as 1 SD above the mean on the PBI protection scale by the index child, nominated the 'overprotective mothers', and the remaining mothers ($n = 60$) who were rated at 22 or less on that protection scale.

Index children of the overprotective mothers rated them as significantly less caring. Overprotective mothers had a significantly lower level of education and women of Mediterranean birth were overrepresented in this group. The overprotective mothers scored their own mothers on the PBI as having behaved in a significantly more controlling and less caring way towards them. When asked to complete the PBI as they believed they had related to the index child, the overprotective mothers scored themselves significantly higher on the protection scale, but did not differ in rating themselves on the care scale. High anxiety, several subscales of the Fear Survey Schedule (Marks & Mathews, 1979), Type A characteristics, obsessionality and external locus of control also differentiated the two groups significantly. Regression analyses established that maternal trait anxiety was a highly significant predictor of how her child rated that mother on the PBI protection scale.

The social support intervention study

As anxiety in the mother appeared to be associated with an overprotective style of parenting, we next wished to examine this connection prospectively. In addition, if mothers with high trait anxiety found the maternal role difficult, could we reduce their anxiety and thus assist both mother and child?

The aims of our applied research were, therefore, (1) to examine the effects of maternal anxiety on the mother–infant relationship, (2) to assess whether interventions successfully reduced anxiety in a high trait anxious mother, and (3) to discern whether such anxiety reduction altered the mother–child relationship (specifically, the attachment pattern) and the hypothesised tendency to pathological psychosocial development in the child.

A randomised intervention design was incorporated into a naturalistic cohort study. It was designed to assess the longitudinal adaptation, specifically during the first year of their infant's life, of primiparous mothers who differed in terms of having, by self-report, high, moderate or low levels of trait anxiety. The two interventions comprised (a) allocation of the subject to an experienced mother who had volunteered to be readily available for 'support' (i.e. commonsense advice and practical help), such as might be offered by a good neighbour; (b) allocation to a social worker who would make contact and provide 'support' according to her usual professional strategies, and so aim to promote the self-esteem and confidence of the new mother while monitoring the mother–infant and marital relationships. Contact in both interventions was to be maintained for 12 months.

The study is reported elsewhere (Barnett & Parker, 1985), but will be described briefly at this point. A series of 630 consecutive primiparous women was recruited on the third or fourth day post-partum from two major obstetric hospitals. Subjects were required to have adequate command of English to give informed consent and to complete the questionnaire in that language, to be married or living in a stable *de facto* relationship, to have had a healthy, singleton baby and to be living in an accessible geographical area (approximately within 30 kilometres of the centre of Sydney). They were asked to complete state and trait anxiety scales (Spielberger *et al.*, 1970). Three women refused. Subjects were then randomly assigned to one of three groups on the basis of their trait anxiety score: 40 or above was designated as reflecting 'high anxiety'; 25 or less 'low anxiety'; and intermediate scores 'moderate anxiety'. Additional high anxiety subjects were recruited as interventions were to be offered to two groups of these, while the third comprised the control group. After the initial interview, 89 subjects remained in the high anxiety groups and 29 in each of the others. Eleven subjects had refused and three did not complete the initial interview.

Of the 89 high anxiety subjects, 30 were allocated to the 'lay intervention' group and 31 to the 'professional intervention' group (see below). The high anxiety control group ($n = 28$) received no intervention over the course of the year.

Rationale and details of the interventions

If pregnancy and the postnatal period are viewed as a transitional stage – a developmental crisis – (Benedek, 1959; Pines, 1972; Raphael-Leff, 1980), there exists the potential for the individual to mature, but also a possibility of losing psychological ground, becoming emotionally disturbed or even psychiatrically ill, for example in the postpartum period (e.g. Kendell *et al.*, 1976; Kumar & Robson, 1984; O'Hara *et al.*, 1984). Since deficiencies in social support had been reported to be a risk factor for neurotic disorders in times of adversity (Henderson *et al.*, 1981), we hypothesised that ensuring availability of social support for the highly anxious mothers might prove beneficial. Intervention was, therefore, based on the notion of providing 'support' in various ways for the woman in her transition to a new role.

Groups 1 and 2 of the high trait anxious mothers were offered lay (contact with a 'support mother') or professional (contact with a social worker) support, respectively. The two groups of assistants were collectively referred to as support workers.

The helpers for group 1 were drawn from a panel of 35 volunteers who already had one or more children of their own, owned a car and lived within 10 minutes' driving time from the allocated subject. It was intended that each should have two subjects as far as was geographically possible, in order to minimise overinvolvement. Seven volunteers were allocated two subjects each, while 18 were allocated one, as it quickly became evident that one was all they could be expected to manage. Because some of the subjects as well as some support mothers moved house during the year, not all subjects had the same person attached to them throughout the 12 months (three study mothers were prematurely separated from any support because of moving interstate or overseas).

A panel of six (one reserve for illness and holidays) female social workers was recruited for the professional support group. Four were employed as preschool social workers, while the other two worked in both hospital (including the maternity wards) and community in the field of infants, children and families. A total of six subjects was allocated to each of the five social workers, but, because of employment problems at one hospital, one of the sets of six mothers was attached to five different workers over the course of the year.

The support workers were aged between 25 and 40 years. Written guidelines for the strategies to be employed were drawn up after discussion with the volunteers themselves; each was given a copy (see Appendixes A and B). All were told to use their own discretion if the guidelines were unclear in any particular situation. The basic schedule of contact was organised so that telephone calls and home visiting were more frequent in the early weeks and months, but maintained over the whole year. It was suggested that contacts should be reduced in the second half of the year, in order that the subject did not become dependent and then suddenly find herself cut off from a supportive figure.

All support personnel were asked to keep a diary of contacts with their study subject(s). A pre-printed form was provided for this purpose, and termed 'Bonding Study Diary'. The main aims of this were to ascertain whether the workers kept their part of the contract; whether their estimates of the interaction and its content tallied with those of the subject; and whether the subjects ever spontaneously contacted their support person.

Support workers were given written information regarding the office and home telephone numbers of one of the investigators (B.B.), and knew they could make contact at any time. Meetings were held regularly with small groups of support mothers to ensure mutual support and encouragement, and to discuss any concerns they had or strategies they wished to try. There was a meeting with the professional workers on a social basis (a group dinner) on five occasions over the year – primarily to ensure that their interest in the study was maintained, as they were adamant that they must be given a free hand and that this was their area of expertise. They were encouraged to use their own judgement regarding the intervention, although keeping the guidelines (which they themselves had suggested) in mind.

A token payment, to cover petrol and telephone expenses only, was made to each support mother and social worker at the end of her commitment to the research. More details and qualitative information on the intervention process are given later in this chapter.

Procedures

All study subjects were visited at home by the same rater (B.B.) within 3 weeks of leaving the maternity hospital. A prior telephone call to the women reminded them that the researchers were interested in the difficulties mothers face with new babies, especially the first, and that the initial visit was to discuss this further.

A semi-structured, pre-coded interview was administered to collect sociodemographic data and information about the pregnancy and delivery, the mother's developmental history, her physical and mental health, and the relationship with her family and partner. Several questionnaires were completed, including the Costello–Comrey (1967) trait anxiety and trait depression scales (since these had been used in the earlier studies); the Beck Depression Inventory (Beck et al., 1961); the Eysenck Personality Inventory (Eysenck & Eysenck, 1964); the Hereford Parent Attitude Scale (Hereford, 1963); a life event scale devised specifically for women in the pregnant and postnatal stages (Barnett et *al.*, 1983); and the Interview Schedule for Social Interaction (ISSI; Henderson *et al.*, 1981).

The ISSI was administered at the beginning of the interview to avoid contamination. To obtain the maximum information on how pregnancy and mothering affected the social network, how women perceived this new situation, and what might be helpful to others in similar circumstances, the ISSI was completed on two occasions: around the time of the baby's birth and when the infant was 12 months old.

The interviewer remained unaware of each subject's group allocation until the interview and questionnaires were completed, when an envelope containing the result of the previous allocation was opened. High anxiety subjects had been randomly allocated to lay or professional intervention or control (i.e. no intervention) groups.

Subjects were asked to complete and return questionnaires at 3, 6 and 9 months, and to attend a 1-year follow-up interview, with trait and state anxiety scores being measured on each occasion. At 6 months the mothers were sent an infant temperament questionnaire to complete (Persson-Blennow & McNeil, 1979), and at 12 months, the PBI (Parker *et al.*, 1979). At the second interview at 12 months, many of the questionnaires were repeated, including the ISSI.

A standardised laboratory procedure, the Strange Situation Procedure (SSP: Ainsworth *et al.*, 1978; and described by Champion, this volume), was used at 12 months to assess three main categories of infant–mother attachment pattern: category B, described as 'secure'; category A, 'anxious-avoidant'; and category C, 'anxious-resistant'. Infants classified as 'secure' are likely to be distressed when separated from the mother, but are effectively comforted by her upon reunion and confidently return to exploration of the environment. Infants with the attachment pattern known as 'anxious-avoidant' (category A) are held to have learned to be independent and self-sufficient. They do not show distress when separated from mother and do not try to obtain comfort from her when reunited. In category C, i.e. 'anxious-resistant', infants who are reunited with their mother after a separation make it clear that they are angry with her, demanding comfort but also rejecting it; their ambivalence is obvious.

Results

Anxiety

Data analysis was undertaken on the 147 of 152 subjects who completed all the scales. Compliance with the study requirements and with the interventions was very high on the part of the subjects; somewhat less so on the part of the helpers.

As hypothesised, high levels of anxiety in the mother were associated with a number of problems in the transition to parenthood, such as an increased incidence of prenatal complications, lower maternal self-confidence, more life events and greater distress experienced with these, more depression and greater dissatisfaction with various aspects of their social network. The infant was more likely to be dysmature and slow to suckle, and the mother had more concerns regarding the baby, her marriage and herself (Barnett & Parker, 1986).

Over the first year of the study (i.e. the active intervention period), minimal changes in anxiety levels were observed in subjects not receiving intervention, while there was a considerable lessening of state and trait anxiety in both non-professional (group 1) and professional intervention (group 2) subjects. Mothers in group 1 showed a rapid fall in anxiety levels over the first 3 months compared with group 2. Their levels remained more or less steady thereafter. Their trait anxiety score decreased over the year by 11% compared with 7% for the high anxiety control group (group 3). Group 2 subjects showed a reduction in trait anxiety scores of 13%. There was a 12% reduction in state anxiety levels for mothers in group 1, a 19% reduction for those in group 2 and a 3% reduction in group 3.

Although these results reached significance on the t-test analyses, when planned contrast analysis was applied, examining for linear and quadratic trends, it seemed that only the professional intervention had had a significant effect, successfully lowering state anxiety to a mean of 33.9 – a level within our designated 'moderately anxious' range (Barnett & Parker, 1985).

Social support

The social support hypothesis was tested by examining first for improvement in social support scores for those receiving active intervention, and, second, for a reduction in anxiety scores in those receiving an active intervention (Parker & Barnett, 1987).

ISSI results are limited to the 139 subjects who were able to attend the 12-month interview and thus complete the social interaction schedule a second time. The test–retest coefficients varied across the groups, with the coefficients for the total sample being 0.55 (AVAT), 0.57 (ADAT), 0.72 (AVSI) and 0.63 (ADSI).

The high anxiety subjects (i.e. those in groups 1, 2 and 3 and therefore irrespective of treatment status) differed both at baseline and at follow-up from the mothers with moderate anxiety (group 4) or low anxiety (group 5). At baseline, they reported significantly less adequacy of attachment (ADAT) and significantly less availability of social integration (AVSI). At follow-up, the high anxiety subjects differed significantly from the remainder on all four ISSI measures, in the direction of reduced availability and less adequacy in their attachments.

Anxious subjects thus returned ISSI scores suggesting certain deficiencies in social support, before and after our intervention.

At baseline and at the end of the year there were no significant differences in ISSI scores between those receiving an intervention and the high anxiety controls who received no intervention. On both occasions the professional intervention group reported greater adequacy of attachment (ADAT) than the other two high anxiety groups, but this difference was not significant.

In a more rigorous examination, planned contrast analyses assessed changes in ISSI scores over the 12 months. Such analyses were important to control for group differences at baseline and to avoid the risks of multiple inference associated with the large number of tests used in the initial analyses. In undertaking the analyses of variance with repeated measures, the technique accepted the distinction between two types of factors, namely, independent groups (i.e. treatment and control) and repeated measurement (i.e. baseline and follow-up scores). The Bonferroni procedure was used to control the Type 1 error rate for each family of contrasts at 0.05, and a critical F ratio of 8.53 was set to establish significant differences between groups and for interactions of groups with repeat measurements.

Examination for group differences on ISSI scale scores averaged over time showed significant differences for ADAT ($F = 13.46$) and AVSI ($F = 11.84$), but not for ADSI ($F = 4.46$) or AVAT ($F = 3.10$), when high anxiety subjects (groups $1 + 2 + 3$) were contrasted with the remainder (groups $4 + 5$). No differences were found on any scale when groups 1 and 3, or groups 2 and 3, were contrasted on scores averaged over time.

Interaction contrasts examined for changes between groups over time. When combined high anxiety subjects were contrasted with the remainder, there were no significant differences in change regarding availability or adequacy of either attachment or social integration. When groups 1 and 3 were contrasted, no significant differences in improvement were found over time for any of the four scales (AVAT, ADAT, AVSI or ADSI). Nor were significant differences found when groups 2 and 3 were contrasted.

In sum, at the end of the first postnatal year for these primiparae, anxiety was decreased in those high anxiety subjects receiving intervention (especially professional intervention) in comparison with the controls. Nevertheless, this improvement was not associated with any change in the four ISSI measures of their close and diffuse social relationships.

Attachment

The mother–infant attachment relationship was investigated at 12 months using Ainsworth's SSP (Barnett *et al.*, 1987). Of the 134 mother–infant pairs available for assessment, 70% were rated as category B (securely attached), 16% as category A (anxious-avoidant) and 14% as category C (anxious-resistant). Interestingly, the level of maternal trait anxiety was not associated with the infant's SSP category. When subjects whose state anxiety had decreased by 10% or more over the year were compared with those whose state anxiety had increased by a similar amount, no significant difference in SSP classification of their infants was found. There was also no significant difference in SSP rating between anxious mothers who had or had not received an intervention.

Variables which correlated significantly with the SSP category were: the mother's own maternal care score and her rating of one or both parents as both overprotective and uncaring on the PBI; availability of attachment (AVAT) at baseline, and her report at 12 months that she had had problems with people other than her husband during the year. For each of these variables, it was the mothers of category C infants who differed from the rest. When categories C and A infants were combined into a single 'insecure' group, again it was the mothers of insecure infants who perceived their situation more negatively; their mother as less caring; attachment figures as less available; and other people as more of a problem.

Our hypothesis that high trait anxiety mothers would have anxiously attached infants was not upheld and, possibly as a consequence, our hypothesis that lowering maternal anxiety would result in more secure infant–mother attachment, was also jeopardised.

The maternal anxiety study follow-up

Subjects were contacted and re-interviewed 5 years later to determine whether differences could be discerned at that stage among the anxiety groups in maternal or child adaptation, and whether any evidence of continuing advantage from the intervention in the first post-partum year could be found (Barnett et al., 1991).

High trait anxiety in general continued to be related to problematic maternal adaptation. Psychosocial difficulties, as measured by teacher and parent reports on the Child Behavior Checklist (CBCL: Achenbach & Edelbrock, 1981, 1983), were also evident in the children of such mothers.

At follow-up, subjects from the original group 2, who were offered professional support, were more confident in their maternal role, reported fewer psychological and financial problems, and were more likely to be involved in paid employment. Neither intervention group differed from the high anxiety controls (group 3) on any measure of anxiety at 5 years. In this context, however, it should be noted that the highest drop-out rate was recorded in group 3. Numbers remaining at 5 years in the other four groups varied from 20 subjects in group 2, to 23 in group 1, whereas only 14 were still available from the high anxiety control group.

Mothers with high trait anxiety scores in the first week post-partum continued to report more social and psychological problems, more depressive symptoms and episodes, less confidence in their own mothering capacity, fewer outside interests and to occupy a lower social stratum. They reported less adequacy of attachment, and less adequacy and availability of their wider social network. They described their children as having more behavioural problems and lower social competence – assessments with which their partners agreed.

Maternal psychopathology at 5 years was best predicted by the baseline measure of trait anxiety (Costello & Comrey, 1967) and by the 1-year neuroticism score (Eysenck & Eysenck, 1964). Inadequate social support was the other predictor of continuing and possibly increasing psychopathology.

The child's adaptation at follow-up (as measured by the CBCL) was best predicted by maternal variables of state and trait anxiety, depression, social network, and reported overprotection by the subjects' own fathers. Child factors also contributed to prediction through variables such as sex and aspects of temperament. The infant variables that best predicted behaviour problems or social competence on the CBCL at 5 years were four of the nine temperament variables measured (maternal ratings; Persson-Blennow & McNeil, 1979) at age 6 months, and the sex of the infant. The temperament items were: attention-persistence, approach, adaptability, and mood. Male sex predicted a greater likelihood of high externalising scores.

Anxious (category A or C) or secure (category B) attachment ratings from Ainsworth's SSP for the mother–infant pairs at 12 months again showed no clear association with maternal anxiety scores, i.e. the scores at 5 years. Girls assessed as category B (secure) rather than A or C at 12 months had fewer behavioural problems at 5 years.

Thus anxious attachment in 1-year-old infants was not simply linked with high anxiety in their mothers in an intergenerational way. This may be a reality (i.e. that anxiety is not intergenerational) or reflect methodological limitations, but, whatever the interpretation, it limited our capacity to demonstrate that reduction of high maternal anxiety would be of secondary benefit to the children in later years.

Discussion

Having ascertained from earlier studies that high trait anxiety in the mother might predispose her offspring to problems with anxiety and depression, we embarked upon a prospective study of such women. A non-clinical sample of women was recruited within 4 days of the birth of their first child. Subjects were assigned in a random, stratified fashion to subgroups designated 'high', 'moderate' and 'low' anxiety on the basis of their trait anxiety scores. The 'high anxiety' group were noted at baseline to evince other psychopathology – e.g. higher neuroticism and depression (state and trait) scores and more simple phobias, as well as high state and trait anxiety. They also reported less confidence in their own mothering capacity and coping ability, more likelihood of experiencing postnatal blues for more than 24 hours, more life events and higher levels of distress associated with those life events. They were more worried about themselves, the baby and their marriage compared with less anxious subjects. In view of this degree of psychosocial morbidity, attempts to intervene were justified.

Social support intervention

Overview

In designing our interventions we hoped to avoid some of the pitfalls reported in the literature by, for example, Gray & Wandersman (1980). These authors state that the changes the intervention hopes to procure should:

1 be compatible with the goals and aspirations of the subjects and their culture rather than with those of the interveners;
2 be realistically achievable;
3 have no undesirable side-effects, such as (in this research) increasing the burden on the mother, creating dependency on the therapist rather than promoting the confidence of the mother in her own coping skills, or undermining the marital relationship;
4 pay attention to the wider social environment and how the mother–child dyad relates to this;
5 be measurable in the short and long term if possible.

These changes must also be made by appropriate interveners – selected by gender, age, social class, education, and so on. The question arises whether volunteers or professionals should be the helpers. Volunteers tend to be difficult to screen, middle-class, unreliable, and to have difficulty in comprehending the theoretical underpinnings of the intervention effort and in being flexible in application. They may need much training and supervision. Nevertheless, they are economical and not hard to find, so successful programmes using volunteers can often be more easily generalised. In addition, some studies have found professionals and paraprofessionals to be equally effective (cf. Madden, Levenstein &

Levenstein, 1976). Whether professional or lay helpers are used, it can still be difficult to separate treatment effects from personal characteristics of the therapist.

Inspection of the relevant literature provides no unequivocal guidance regarding optimal hours per week or longitudinal duration of contact/intervention. Also, the possible ethical issue of not providing 'assistance' to the control groups must be addressed. In this study, there appeared to be no *a priori* justification for assuming that either intervention would necessarily be therapeutic and have no adverse effects. Finally, the effect of virtually saying to the control subjects that they do not need special help or treatment is difficult to assess – any such effects would also be likely to vary among the three (different) anxiety control groups (high, moderate and low). Clinical experience might suggest that the high anxiety control subjects, for instance, would be ambivalent – partly relieved and partly disappointed.

Experience suggested that having other new mothers to talk to (a peer group; see also Dalgard *et al.*, this volume), and having someone readily available from whom they could ask advice, would be helpful, although it was not obvious whether advice would be more acceptable from someone who had experienced the same stressful events or from an 'expert'.

Corse *et al.* (1990), in a recent controlled study of abusive mothers, found that abuse was more common where mothers were isolated, and found a link between social support and parenting beliefs. They suggested that 'the presence of peers in the network is related to greater enjoyment of and openness in parenting'.

Elizabeth Bennett's careful documentation of the experience of 'coping in the puerperium' lends weight to these considerations. When new mothers were asked to rate the importance of things that are helpful in the early stages with a new baby, there was close agreement about what was needed. The item which headed the list of 16 was 'someone to go to for advice'. Also in the top six were: someone to look after the baby occasionally while the mother went out with her partner or by herself, shopping assistance, 'reassurance about breast feeding' and 'friendship with and support from new mothers (Bennett, 1981). In a recent comprehensive review of 'Social and Community Intervention', Heller comments that interventions must recognise such factors as social context, gender and life stage (Heller, 1990). In Sydney, over 90% of primiparous mothers attend their local Baby Health Centre, but it is often the anxious mothers who find it difficult to go to the Centre, to ask for help and to cope with the conflicting advice mothers tend to receive from all sides at this time (cf. Bennett, 1981).

We devised two interventions in an attempt to address various aspects of social support in different ways, including an effort to promote the marital relationship. Both were intended to lower the mother's anxiety. Anxiety level was certainly lowered considerably over the year by both lay and professional intervention, but no evidence of a more secure attachment for the infant was found.

Partners

This non-clinical sample of mothers were all required to have a 'stable' partnership at entry to the study. At baseline (i.e. post-partum), the discernible differences on our social network measure, the ISSI, were that high anxiety subjects reported less adequacy of attachment (ADAT) and less availability of social integration (AVSI). By the end of the first post-partum year the situation had evidently deteriorated further. The high anxiety subjects differed significantly from the rest on all four measures: AVAT, ADAT, AVSI and ADSI.

In this context, the findings of Brown *et al.* (1986), discussed by Brugha in the opening chapter of this volume, seem particularly relevant. These authors reported a high risk for those women who 'did not receive the support which they might have expected in terms of the first interview', i.e. they were 'let down'. A similar violation of expectations may have occurred in our more vulnerable study subjects.

Support workers

Measurement using the ISSI of social network at baseline and at the end of the 1-year intervention gave no indication that the support personnel had become in any way key figures in the subjects' closer circle of intimates or among wider social contacts (see also Dalgard *et al.*, this volume). More direct questioning of the subjects about the support workers elicited only positive comments, but subjects may have felt constrained to respond in this way by the demand characteristics of the research setting. Although it was evident that a few helpers and subjects had become firm friends and that this would continue after the 12 months, nevertheless, for the majority, the contract of arranged contacts ceasing at 1 year was met. Knowledge of the stipulations of the contract, quite apart from actual events, may thus have affected the subjects' responses to the ISSI questions concerning their social network.

It is possible that the therapists were effective as social support figures but that improved social support was not detected by the ISSI, or perhaps they were effective independent of any social support role. Henderson and his colleagues (1981) found a link between higher neuroticism scores and lower availability and adequacy scores on the ISSI. They suggested that neuroticism might influence the capacity to form and maintain social relationships, and cause the individual to view his or her relationships as inadequate. Reduction of anxiety levels in such subjects might be expected to result in a more positive view of their social network and improvement in their relationships. This did not seem to occur in our study.

Even if deficiencies in social support do induce psychosocial morbidity, it does not necessarily follow that the provision of social support will relieve that morbidity, for causal and reparative pathways are not necessarily linked (see also Brugha, Chapter 1, this volume). Nor does successful intervention offer proof of a causal link (Brugha *et al.*, 1982).

Observations regarding the interveners

The following comments are based on subjective observations of one of the investigators (B.B.), and are included with an heuristic purpose. Some of our comments may be of benefit to readers planning similar intervention.

Because of changes of domicile on the part of supporters as well as subjects, there were situations where a subject had more than one support person attached to her during the 12 months. Problems in filling the social work position at one hospital meant that there were several changes of helper for that cluster of subjects. Those subjects fared as well as the others. Only one subject refused outright to accept intervention.

Most of the non-professional helpers appeared to be very capable, but many were diffident and their interpersonal styles varied from the open and direct to the gentle and indirect. They all had a reasonable idea of what the new mothers were experiencing, so presumably had been through much the same themselves. The investigator had wondered whether some of the support mothers would require considerable telephone contact or other support, but this did not occur; they usually waited for regular meetings and if they did telephone it was invariably appropriate.

Although the support mother could not be shown to have been incorporated into the social network of the study subject (Parker & Barnett, 1987), for many pairs the subject certainly became part of the helper's social network. At meetings, the support mothers would speak of 'my mother', and everyone would acknowledge with amusement when this resulted in an ambiguous statement.

Observation at the meetings suggested that some supporters, despite initial enthusiasm, found contact with their subjects anxiety-provoking. It seemed to reawaken memories of a time when they themselves had been anxious, depressed or not coping. Two had certainly had untreated postnatal depression. One of these was clearly struggling with the assignment and a way had to be found of letting her drop out without losing face.

Several had difficulty making or maintaining contact with their subjects, withdrawing as soon as the mother suggested she did not really need help. The professional workers would have recognised that such statements were not necessarily to be taken at face value. All support mothers expressed surprise that their subjects so rarely contacted them; they had been worried about overwhelming demands – a process parallel to the investigator's own apprehensions, as noted above.

The majority of subjects in group 1 commented during the review discussion of their first postnatal year and in the relevant forms they completed that it was helpful to have someone to talk to and obtain advice from, especially in the first few weeks. It also seemed to the interviewer that the support mother's encouragement or possibly her company had enabled the subjects to leave the house and socialise more, although the subjects themselves did not recognise this. In comparison, group 3 (the high anxiety controls) indicated difficulties with organising themselves and the baby for shopping or other expeditions and many lacked the confidence to contact neighbours, the Nursing Mothers Association of Australia or a nearby playgroup or Health Centre for support.

In the second half of the year, signs of strain within the marital partnership were evident for many high anxiety subjects. (This is not uncommon and, perhaps not surprisingly, all the *de facto* relationships which did not proceed with a formal marriage during the year actually split up). The situation may be difficult to discuss with a friend, whereas this is possible with a professional, who may even broach the topic if she discerns signs.

As we did not know what a support person should provide for an individual mother, whether they should be matched or whether it was better that they should or should not be close neighbours, it seemed best to allow the situation to unfold naturally and observe events. Nor did it seem reasonable to impose a management plan on the professionals, who were all highly skilled and very familiar with postnatal problems. The social workers were apprehensive about the possibility of non-professional helpers proving more effective and stated subsequently that perhaps they should have done more for their subjects. At the end of the year the social workers said it had all been harder than expected. They had thought these mothers would be part of their usual case-load but most were an addition to the normal clientele.

Because of the heavy clinical load, study subjects in group 2 received a fairly minimal intervention and were certainly encouraged to see the social worker in her office whenever possible. Contact was unlikely to be made between social workers and the subjects more frequently than the minimum suggested in the guidelines; the social workers quickly 'networked' (as is their custom) the subjects with other neighbourhood mothers, and referred them to other appropriate resources such as parent groups, local Nursing Mothers' Association chapters, Family Care

Cottages and mothercraft facilities if they were in trouble. They were probably viewed as reliable from the point of view of most of the subjects, but were in no position to become over-involved or promote dependency. In most instances, contact was minimal in the last quarter of the year, again suggesting that the social worker would not have been seen as part of the social network at that point, even if she had been earlier.

The fact that the professional was a woman, usually a mother herself, and clearly working full-time outside the home is also likely to have made some impact on the subjects in group 2. Clinical experience suggests that this situation legitimises any wish to return to outside work on the part of the mother. Returning to paid employment may be very helpful, as the work of Brown's group has attested (Brown & Harris, 1978). Mothers in this group were noted at follow-up to be more involved in activities outside the home, including employment (Barnett *et al.*, 1991).

Early intervention studies

Others have described difficulty with programmes of assistance to new mothers. Siegel *et al* (1980) assessed the effects of early and extended mother–baby contact in hospital, as well as of home visits by a trained para-professional, in 321 low-income women. Maternal attachment was only slightly (though significantly) affected by early and extended contact and was not affected by home visits. Neither intervention was related to reports of child abuse and neglect, or to utilisation of health care facilities. Larson (1980) carried out a controlled evaluation of the efficacy of home visits (by psychologists) designed to promote child health and development in working-class families. He found, as he had predicted, that such an intervention was only effective if commenced pre-natally. Field *et al.* (1980) provided a parent-training intervention for pre-term infants of teenage black mothers. Improved maternal attitudes and behaviour, and more optimal growth for the child, were found in comparison with a control group. Minde *et al.* (1980) arranged support groups for parents of low birthweight infants and reported an improvement in maternal confidence and behaviour towards the baby. Fleming *et al.* (1992) evaluated the effects on maternal mood, attitude and behaviour of providing a 'social support' group post-partum. Their intervention increased mothers' attention to their infants, but did not relieve depression and may even have had an adverse effect on self-confidence in the depressed subjects. While Bromwich & Parmelee (1979) reported good results for mothers and infants from a 2-year intervention, most evaluations have considered brief interventions and suggested rather nebulous advantages when any positive effects have been found. In contrast to the non-clinical population in our intervention project, most documented interventions at the time of our study were for disadvantaged or disturbed subjects: low income, single parent, adolescent, depressed – i.e. clinical populations. We hoped to produce secondary prevention for the women and primary prevention for the children.

Conclusion

If, in fact, the lay therapists principally provided 'support', while the professionals additionally provided more specific therapeutic stratagems to reduce anxiety, then 'social support' appears to be insufficient in itself. We do not know, however, whether these women would have fared even worse without this assistance, since a considerable number of the high anxiety controls had dropped out by the 5-year follow-up. If the lay and professional interventions had been equally successful, then there would have been considerable cost-benefit advantages in recommending the use of lay volunteers. The superiority of professional intervention, especially when it appears to have been fairly low in direct personal involvement of the professional herself, suggests that it would be difficult to argue for such a lay intervention, although discussion with the subjects certainly left the impression that the support mothers had offered valuable assistance at a crucial time. If such an intervention is to continue for longer than 8–12 weeks, it may be preferable to screen, train and support the interveners in a more intensive fashion. It is quite possible too that the interventions would have had different effects in clinical or in socially disadvantaged groups. Nonetheless, neither intervention seemed to improve parenting behaviour and attitudes to the extent that a measurable effect resulted for the infants.

What has been learned from this intervention attempt? Much of what was found corroborates clinical experience. In general, women who are stressed feel the need to talk to others and be heard, they need practical assistance, and they benefit from contact with others who have shared a similar experience (provided such contacts have at least partially resolved their own problems). To make contact prior to delivery (i.e. screen for those at risk of decompensation by using an anxiety scale or Eysenck Personality Inventory) might be useful, but this has proved difficult to implement.

To produce significant personality change may, therefore, require greater skill, training and sustained performance over a period of time. Attachment theory might suggest that, to be effective, intervention would need to modify maternal internal working models of attachment.

Heller (1990) states that 'There is now a fair amount of evidence from prospective studies indicating that social support serves as a protective factor, enhancing physical health and psychological well-being'. He goes on, however, to note that 'the social support intervention literature is much less consistent'. We would agree with him that the fundamental problems continue to be that we do not know when, how or under what conditions natural or artificially-induced support is effective.

There remains a pressing need to define precise intervention strategies that may readily be incorporated into health care programmes, and to demonstrate the optimal timing and duration of those strategies, as well as the benefits that might be expected. The challenges ahead are fully acknowledged in further discussion in Part III of this volume. Our study, using seemingly appropriate interventions and support groups, suggests the advantages and limitations so frequently described in intervention studies: in essence, minor therapeutic effects, with continuing generalised improvement in adaptation not clearly evident – in this case either for the mothers or for their children.

Appendixes

Appendix A. Guidelines for intervention: Group 1/support mothers (SMs)

Aims and goals
1. Provide support, commonsense advice, practical help.
2. Help the new mother to enjoy her baby in a relaxed way instead of being tired and worried all the time.
3. Help her achieve a sense of competence and fulfilment as a mother.

Methods
1. Home visiting. First visit within 1 week of the mother's interview with researcher; second visit within 1 week; minimum of three visits within the first month; minimum of one visit by SM to mother or mother to SM each subsequent month until baby is 6 months old; contact thereafter by visit or telephone as appropriate, but at least once per month until baby is 12 months old.
2. Telephone contact. Telephone before your first visit and leave your number with the mother after the visit; contact thereafter as SM and mother feel appropriate and within the guidelines given in (1).
3. Referral. Should this prove necessary (SM is to use her discretion), encourage the mother to attend e.g. the Nursing Mothers Association, new mothers group, family doctor.

Administration
Attend meetings (approximately monthly) with researcher and other SMs.

Complete diary forms with details of contacts with your
  study mother. Write notes as close to the time of
  contact as possible and do not be tempted to change
  them later! Hand in the forms at the meeting.
Contact the researcher whenever you wish.
Each SM may be allocated two mothers for the year, but,
both will not arrive at once!

Appendix B. Guidelines for intervention: Group 2/social workers (SWs)

Goals
  Reduction of maternal overprotection.
  Promotion of maternal care.
  Optimal mother–child relationship.

Aims
  To change attitudes and behaviour.
  To lessen anxiety.
  To promote self-esteem generally, and feelings of
  competence in the maternal role in particular.
  To discourage maternal overinvolvement with the baby.
  To encourage paternal involvement with the baby.
  To promote and strengthen the marital dyad.

Administration
  Attend meetings with researcher when arranged.
  Complete the monthly diary forms.
  Expect 6 mothers per SW.
  Contact researcher whenever you wish.

Methods
1. Interpersonal support:
(a) Indicate availability. Give telephone number if
  appropriate and, in all cases, leave a written note
  of name, clinic address and telephone number at first
  visit.
(b) Visit within 1 week of researcher's interview with
  the mother; minimum of three visits within first
  month; minimum of one visit to mother or mother to SW
  each month until baby 6 months; contact thereafter by
  telephone or visit as appropriate until baby is 12
  months old.
(c) Refer for any other support as necessary.
2. Specific anti-anxiety measures (SW or refer), e.g.
  relaxation, other behavioural techniques,

psychotherapy, anxiolytic drugs, books to read,
tapes.
3. Promote self-esteem and competence, e.g. modelling,
positive reinforcement.
4. Lessen intensity of mother-child interaction by
encouraging attendance at mothers' groups, social
activities, return to work, etc.
5. Enhance (4) by promoting paternal involvement with
baby. SW to meet father within the first month.
Encourage (a) activities with baby - not just play but
sharing in routine care, (b) support of wife by
assisting with household tasks and turning a blind eye
to domestic chaos, etc.; outings for her with baby and
for the couple together. Maintain contact with father
to monitor and provide reinforcement.
6. Maintain a watching brief on the marital
relationship: discuss problems, provide treatment if
required, promote communication.

References

Achenbach, T. M. & Edelbrock, C. S. (1981). Behavioral problems and
competencies reported by parents of normal and disturbed children aged
four through sixteen. *Monographs of the Society for Research in Child
Development*, serial no. 188, 46, 1. Illinois: University of Chicago Press.
Achenbach, T. M. & Edelbrock, C. (1983). *Manual for the Teachers' Report
Form and Teacher Version of the Child Behavior Profile.* Burlington: University of
Vermont, Department of Psychiatry.
Ainsworth, M. D. S., Blehar, M. C., Waters, E. & Wall, S. (1978). *Patterns of
Attachment. A Psychological Study of the Strange Situation.* Hillsdale, N.J.:
Lawrence Erlbaum.
Andrews, G., Tennant, C., Hewson, D. & Vaillant, G. (1978). Life event
stress, social support, coping style, and risk of psychological impairment.
Journal of Nervous and Mental Disease, **166**, 307–16.
Barnett, B. & Parker, G. (1985). Professional and non-professional
intervention for highly anxious primiparous mothers. *British Journal of
Psychiatry*, **146**, 287–93.
Barnett, B. & Parker, G. (1986). Possible determinants, correlates and
consequences of high levels of anxiety in primiparous mothers. *Psychological
Medicine*, **16**, 177–85.
Barnett, B. E. W., Hanna, B. & Parker, G. (1983). Life event scales for
obstetric groups. *Journal of Psychosomatic Research*, **27**, 313–20.
Barnett, B., Blignault, I., Holmes, S., Payne, A. & Parker, G. (1987). Quality
of attachment in a sample of 1-year-old Australian children. *Journal of the
American Academy of Child and Adolescent Psychiatry*, **26**, 303–7.
Barnett, B., Schaafsma, M. F., Guzman, A.-M. & Parker, G. B. (1991).

Maternal anxiety: a 5-year review of an intervention study. *Journal of Child Psychology and Psychiatry*, **32**, 423–38.

Beck, A. T., Ward, C. H., Mendelson, M., Mock, J. & Erbaugh, J. (1961). An inventory for measuring depression. *Archives of General Psychiatry*, **4**, 561–71.

Benedek, T. (1959). Parenthood as a developmental phase: a contribution to the libido theory. *Journal of the American Psychoanalytic Association*, **7**, 389–417.

Bennett, E. A. (1981). Coping in the puerperium: the reported experience of new mothers. *Journal of Psychosomatic Research*, **25**, 13–21.

Bowen, M. (1976). An interview with Murray Bowen. In: *Family Therapy in Clinical Practice*, ed. M. Bowen. New York: Aronson.

Bretherton, I., Biringen, Z., Ridgeway, D., Masun, C. & Sherman, M. (1989). Attachment: the parental perspective. *Infant Mental Health Journal*, **10**, 203–21.

Broadhead, W. E., Kaplan, B. H., James, S. A., Wagner, E. H., Schoenbach, E. J., Grimson, R., Heyden, S., Tibblin, G. & Gehlback, S. H. (1983). The epidemiologic evidence for a relationship between social support and health. *American Journal of Epidemiology*, **117**, 521–37.

Bromwich, R. & Parmelee, A. (1979). An intervention program for pre-term infants. In *Infants Born at Risk*, ed. T. Field, A. Sostek, S. Goldberg & H. H. Shuman. New York: Spectrum.

Broom, L. & Selznick, P. (1973). *Sociology*. New York: Harper & Row.

Brown, G. W. & Harris, T. (1978). *The Social Origins of Depression*. London: Tavistock.

Brown, G. W., Bhrolchain, M. N. & Harris, T. (1975). Social class and psychiatric disturbances among women in an urban population. *Sociology*, **9**, 225–54.

Brown, G. W., Andrews, B., Harris, T., Adler, Z. & Bridge, L. (1986). Social support, self-esteem and depression. *Psychological Medicine*, **16**, 813–31.

Brugha, T., Conroy, R., Walsh, W., Delaney, J., O'Hanlon, E., Dondero, L., Hickey, N. & Bourke, G. (1982). Social networks, attachment and support in minor affective disorders: a replication. *British Journal of Psychiatry*, **141**, 149–255.

Brugha, T. S., Bebbington, P. E., MacCarthy, B., Sturt, E., Wykes, T. & Potter, J. (1990). Gender, social support and recovery from depressive disorders: a prospective clinical study. *Psychological Medicine*, **20**, 147–56.

Corse, S. J., Schmid, K. & Trickett, P. K. (1990). Social network characteristics of mothers in abusing and nonabusing families and their relationships to parenting beliefs. *Journal of Community Psychology*, **18**, 44–59.

Costello, C. G. & Comrey, A. L. (1967). Scales for measuring depression and anxiety. *Journal of Psychology*, **66**, 303–13.

Crnic, K. A.., Greenberg, M. T., Ragozin, A. S., Robinson, N. M. & Basham, R. B. (1983). Effects of stress and social support on mothers of premature and full-term infants. *Child Development*, **54**, 209–17.

Eysenck, H. J. & Eysenck, S. B. G. (1964). *Manual of the Eysenck Personality Inventory*. London: University of London Press.

Field, T. M., Widmayer, S. M. & Stringer, S. (1980). Teenage, lower-class, black mothers and their pre-term infants: an intervention and developmental follow-up. *Child Development*, **51**, 426–36.

Fleming, A. S., Klein, E. & Corter, C. (1992). The effects of a social support group on depression, maternal attitudes and behavior in new mothers. *Journal of Child Psychology and Psychiatry*, **33**, 685–8.

Gray, S. W. & Wandersman, L. P. (1980). The methodology of home-based intervention studies: problems and promising strategies. *Child Development*, **51**, 993–1009.

Greenblatt, M., Becerra, R. M. & Serafetinides, E. A. (1982). Social networks and mental health: an overview. *American Journal of Psychiatry*, **139**, 977–84.

Heller, K. (ed.) (1986). Special series: disaggregating the process of social support. *Journal of Consulting and Clinical Psychology*, **54**, 415–70.

Heller, K. (1990). Social and community intervention. *Annual Review of Psychology*, **41**, 141–68.

Henderson, A. S. (1988). *An Introduction to Social Psychiatry*. New York: Oxford University Press.

Henderson, S., Duncan-Jones, P., Byrne, D. G. & Scott, R. (1980). Measuring social relationships: The Interview Schedule for Social Interaction. *Psychological Medicine*, **10**, 723–34.

Henderson, S. with Byrne, D. G. & Duncan-Jones, P. (1981). *Neurosis and the Social Environment*. Sydney: Academic Press.

Hereford, C. F. (1963). *Changing Parental Attitudes through Group Discussion*. Austin: University of Texas Press.

Kendell, R. E., Wainwright, S., Hailey, A. & Shannon, B. (1976). The influence of childbirth on psychiatric morbidity. *Psychological Medicine*, **6**, 297–302.

Kumar, R. & Robson, K. M. (1984). A prospective study of emotional disorders in childbearing women. *British Journal of Psychiatry*, **44**, 35–47.

Larson, C. P. (1980). Efficacy of prenatal and postpartum home visits on child health and development. *Pediatrics*, **66**, 191–7.

Madden, J., Levenstein, P. & Levenstein, S. (1976). Longitudinal I.Q. outcomes of the mother–child home program. *Child Development*, **46**, 1015–25.

Maddison, D. C. & Viola, A. (1968). The health of widows in the year following bereavement. *Journal of Psychosomatic Research*, **12**, 297–306.

Maddison, D. C. & Walker, W. L. (1967). Factors affecting the outcome of conjugal bereavement. *British Journal of Psychiatry*, **113**, 1057–67.

Main, M. & Goldwyn, R. (1990). Adult attachment rating and classification system. In *A Typology of Human Attachment Organization Assessed in Discourse, Drawings and Interviews*, ed. M. Main. New York: Cambridge University Press.

Marks, I. & Mathews, A. (1979). Brief standard self-rating for phobic patients. *Behaviour Research and Therapy*, **17**, 263–7.

McCallister, L. & Fischer, C. S. (1978). A procedure for surveying personal networks. *Sociological Methods and Research*, **7**, 131–48.

Minde, K., Shosenberg, N., Marton, P., Thompson, J., Ripley, J. & Burns, S. (1980). Self-help groups in a premature nursery: a controlled evaluation. *Journal of Paediatrics*, **96**, 933–40.

O'Connor, P. & Brown, G. W. (1984). Supportive relationships: fact or fancy? *Journal of Social and Personal Relationships*, **1**, 159–95.

O'Hara, M. W., Neunaber, D. J. & Zekoski, E. M. (1984). A prospective study of postpartum depression: prevalence, course, and predictive factors. *Journal of Abnormal Psychology*, **93**, 158–71.

Parker, G. (1983). *Parental Overprotection: A Risk Factor in Psychosocial Development*. New York: Grune & Stratton.

Parker, G. (1992). Citation classic. A parental bonding instrument. *Current Contents*, **24**, 14.

Parker, G. & Barnett, B. (1987). A test of the social support hypothesis. *British Journal of Psychiatry*, **150**, 72–7.

Parker, G. & Lipscombe, P. (1981). Influences on maternal overprotection. *British Journal of Psychiatry*, **138**, 303–11.

Parker, G., Tupling, H. & Brown, L. B. (1979). A parental bonding instrument. *British Journal of Medical Psychology*, **52**, 1–10.

Parkes, C. M. & Stevenson-Hinde, J. (eds.) (1982). *The Place of Attachment in Human Behavior*. London: Tavistock.

Paykel, E. S., Emms, E. M., Fletcher, J. & Rassaby, E. S. (1980). Life events and social support in puerperal depression. *British Journal of Psychiatry*, **136**, 339–46.

Persson-Blennow, I. & McNeil, T. F. (1979). Questionnaire for measurement of temperament in six-month-old infants: development and standardization. *Journal of Child Psychology and Psychiatry*, **20**, 1–13.

Pines, D. (1972). Pregnancy and motherhood: interaction between fantasy and reality. *British Journal of Medical Psychology*, **45**, 333–43.

Raphael-Leff, J. (1980). Psychotherapy with pregnant women. In *Psychological Aspects of Pregnancy, Birthing and Bonding*, ed. B. L. Blum. New York: Human Sciences Press.

Sarason, I. G., Levine, H. M., Basham, R. B. & Sarason, B. R. (1983). Assessing social support: the social support questionnaire. *Journal of Personality and Social Psychology*, **44**, 127–39.

Siegel, E., Bauman, K. E., Schaefer, E. S., Saunders, M. M. & Ingram, D. D. (1980). Hospital and home support during infancy: impact on maternal attachment, child abuse and neglect and health care utilization. *Pediatrics*, **66**, 183–90.

Spielberger, C. D., Gorsuch, R. L. & Lushene, R. E. (1970). *Manual for the State-Trait Anxiety Inventory (Self-evaluation Questionnaire)*. Palo Alto, California: Consulting Psychologists Press.

Wandersman, L. P., Wandersman, A. & Kahn, S. (1980). Social support in the transition to parenthood. *Journal of Community Psychology*, **8**, 332–42.

Weiss, R. S. (1974). The provisions of social relationships. In *Doing Unto Others*, ed. Z. Rubin. Englewood Cliffs, NJ: Prentice-Hall.

Weiss, R. S. (1981). Attachment in adult life. In *The Place of Attachment in Human Behavior*, ed. C. M. Parkes & J. Stevenson-Hinde, pp. 171–84. New York: Basic Books.

Winefield, H. R. (1979). Social support and the social environment of depressed and normal women. *Australian and New Zealand Journal of Psychiatry*, **13**, 335–9.

Zeanah, C. H. & Barton, M. L. (1989). Introduction: internal representations and parent–infant relationships. *Infant Mental Health Journal*, **10**, 135–41.

11

Case management and network enhancement of the long-term mentally ill

GRAHAM THORNICROFT, WILLIAM R. BREAKEY AND
ANNELLE B. PRIMM

Introduction

Are people largely architects of their own social environments, as
Henderson has suggested (1992)? In this chapter we shall pursue this
issue by developing two arguments: first that a complex pattern of factors
influences the social networks of people with severely disabling mental
illnesses, and second that such networks may be enhanced through
careful case management approaches to treatment. If this is so, why
enhance such networks? Such enhancement may be important for three
reasons: to improve the availability of practical support from other
people, to improve patients' views of their own quality of life, and to
contribute towards alleviation of their affective symptoms. Where social
support resources are insufficient, staff may need to implement a
prosthetic network of professional and voluntary services (Harris &
Bergman, 1988).

In this chapter we shall outline the policy background for the care of
the seriously mentally ill in the United States, and examine the
definitions and practices of case management and its variants. Further,
we shall describe in detail a 2 year follow-up study of the social networks
of long-term psychiatric patients under the care of the COSTAR
programme in Baltimore, Maryland, a mobile treatment service for the
severely mentally ill; and we shall report the results of an evaluation of
patient outcome in relation to duration of contact with the programme,
and discuss the hypotheses generated by these results.

There has been considerable research interest in the quality of life,
problems of homelessness, organisation of services, use of case managers,
financial resource allocation, and governmental policy towards this
patient group. But there have been few attempts to evaluate the
effectiveness of mobile services for the seriously mentally ill in deprived
inner city areas, particularly in measuring their effects on social
networks (Avison & Speechley, 1987). This chapter begins to address
this deficit.

Defining case management

Case management can be defined as a strategy for distributing and coordinating services on behalf of patients (Modrcin *et al.*, 1985). It is a generic term that encompasses the following functions: the coordination, integration and allocation of individualised care within limited resources. Many more precise definitions have been put forward which emphasise aspects of this range of activities, and which reflect the various levels at which case management is intended to operate.

For individual patients, case management has been defined as the coordination of care for patients who require a multiplicity of services. At the project level, case management has been used to describe a method of organising the delivery of care for a defined patient group which clarifies and allocates the responsibilities of the staff team. At the programme level, case management has been characterised as an approach that provides services on the basis of need, which avoids duplication of effort between agencies, and which seeks to offer an adequate range of services to target groups of patients, such as those with diagnoses of both psychosis and substance abuse (Fariello & Scheidt, 1989).

There are three main definitional problems. First, the definitions of case management more often refer to treatment principles than to treatment practices (Modrcin *et al.*, 1985). Second, most accounts of case management are generalised elaborations of such principles and are not precisely defined (Bachrach, 1989). Third, descriptions of case management programmes for long-term mental illness refer to a very wide range of clinical practices (Robinson & Bergman, 1989). It is clear, therefore, that descriptions of 'case management' programmes should specifically set out their structure and working methods to allow useful comparison with other similar projects.

The principles of case management

The many variations in the practice of case management share a common set of underlying principles. Their starting point is that vulnerable patients with long-term psychiatric disorders need therapeutic interventions which optimise their social adjustment and minimise their functional disabilities. The caregiver is put in a facilitating relationship with a patient, where the common goal is assumed to be to maximise the patient's level of functioning (Intagliata, 1982; Bachrach, 1984; Kanter, 1989).

Practically speaking, case management for the long-term mentally ill has developed into a range of techniques which aim to ensure that patients with long-term psychiatric disorders receive consistent and continuing

Table 11.1. *Principles of case management*

Continuity of care
Accessible services
Staff–patient relationship
Titrating support to need
Facilitating independence
Patient advocacy
Advocacy for services

services for as long as they are required (Torrey, 1986), and that services do not focus inappropriately on patients with less severe conditions (Levine, 1981). The direct caregiver variants of case management, such as that used in the COSTAR mobile treatment programme, emphasise the *staff–patient relationship* as the key component through which effective care is channelled, in the tradition of social case work. *Brokerage models*, on the other hand, have placed less emphasis on personal contact with the patient and instead stress brokerage as the coordination of services delivered by other agencies. This model, however, has not developed a conceptual framework to link case work principles with a practice that de-emphasises personal contact (Modrcin *et al.*, 1985).

The principles most often described as being at the root of the case management concept are outlined in Table 11.1. Continuity refers both cross-sectionally to a comprehensive range of services for long-term mental illness, and longitudinally to emphasise the need for enduring and possibly indefinite care for a substantial proportion of this group (Anthony *et al.*, 1988; Challis, 1989).

The development of the case manager concept

Within the mental health services the case management coordination function was first formally recognised in the United States by the Community Mental Health Centers Act (1963), and its 1975 amendments explicitly required these centres to link with other agencies providing care for long-term patients. There has, however, been an increasing recognition in the United States over the last 25 years that community-based services for long-term mental illness have still too often been fragmented (Braun *et al.*, 1981; Kiesler, 1982; Robinson & Bergman, 1989). Methods of drawing together the health and social service care components were developed, especially in federally funded initiatives such as the Community Support Program (Tessler & Goldman, 1982). More recently in Britain it is striking that the practice of 'care management', which explicitly adopts a brokerage model of case

Table 11.2. *Core tasks of case management*

Identify patients (case finding)
Assess needs
Design care package
Coordinate service delivery
Monitor service delivery
Evaluate effectiveness of services
Modify care package
Repeat cycle unless services no longer needed

management within social services departments, has been adopted as government policy (Thornicroft *et al.*, 1993).

The core tasks of case management

There is considerable consensus about the range of tasks that case management can cover at the individual level, and which are summarised in Table 11.2 (Renshaw, 1987; Knapp *et al.*, 1990). Patient identification requires first the definition of the target group for the case management service. This may be clearly established from current contact with services, or may include, for example, forms of outreach to identify patients with no previous or current contact who nevertheless require psychiatric care.

The next step is to assess the social, clinical, vocational, physical health and residential needs of each patient (Brewin *et al.*, 1987). This may require interviews with several members of the care team to establish the extent of disability and appropriate past attempts at intervention in each domain. On the basis of this thorough assessment of need, the case manager decides, within the resources available, which services should be offered henceforth, how often, where and by whom. Where interventions are distributed between agencies, the details of each agreed service may be set out in joint care plans, or may be itemised in formal contract specifications (House of Commons, 1990). Whether the case manager acts as service broker or direct carer, the quality and effectiveness of care should be evaluated, formally or informally, after a suitable interval. It is often desirable, in addition, to use outcome measures of clinical and social function to establish the effectiveness of care (Hall, 1979).

Twelve axes to define case management

It may be said with some justification that there are as many ways to implement the principles of case management as there are case

Table 11.3. *Characteristics of the COSTAR service in relation to case management principles*

Case management axis	COSTAR programme implementation
Individual team case loads	Individual case loads with most patients well known to all staff
Direct/indirect care	Direct care predominates with a minor brokerage role
Intensity	Up to two contacts daily (average nine contacts per month)
Budgetary control	With director of programme
Health/social service balance	A part of Johns Hopkins Hospital Community Psychiatry Program
Status of case managers	Most are trained and experienced psychiatric nurse and social workers
Specialisation	Act as generic case managers except that nurses administer depot medication
Staff:patient ratio	Between 1:10 and 1:15
Patient participation	Patients actively collaborate in identifying treatment goals
Point of contact	Largely at patients' homes and other community sites
Level of intervention	Primarily individual and family with some system-level advocacy
Target population	Long-term psychiatric patients not treated by traditional hospital service

management programmes. Several authors have attempted to bring order to this disarray by developing contrasting models of case management (Lamb, 1980; Bachrach, 1980; Hargreaves *et al.*, 1984; Schwab *et al.*, 1988). For example, these studies commonly distinguish between direct personal care and indirect, or service broker, applications of case management, and the application of this typology to the COSTAR program is shown in Table 11.3. Indeed, it may be useful to consider each programme in terms of these twelve axes that, together, precisely define the characteristics of its practice.

Case management in practice: the COSTAR programme in Baltimore

Stein & Test (1980), with the Program for Assertive Community Treatment (PACT) in Madison, Wisconsin, demonstrated that *in vivo* community-based treatment approaches could be effective alternatives to traditional hospital and outpatient clinic-based psychiatric care. Since that time this model has been tested in Sydney and London (Hoult, 1986; Hoult *et al.*, 1983; Muijen *et al.*, 1992), and in Chicago (Witheridge & Dincin, 1985). Apparently these similar community-based programmes have been found to be effective in supporting severely mentally ill clients in a disadvantaged inner city environment. This success may in part be related to their effectiveness in assisting patients to develop supportive networks of social relationships, through case management and the adoption of a rehabilitation focus.

Community Support Treatment and Rehabilitation (COSTAR) is a community mobile treatment team, closely modelled on PACT, which combines case management and psychiatric treatment for a group of long-term mentally ill patients who are unable to utilise effectively the traditional outpatient mental health service system. The programme faces a dual challenge: it serves some of the most severely disabled patients in a community greatly stressed by urban problems (Breakey, 1989). Its catchment area is characterised by poverty, high unemployment, substandard housing, high crime rates, and significant substance abuse. COSTAR functions as a component part of The Johns Hopkins Community Psychiatry Program (CPP), a community mental health centre that emphasises teaching and research in addition to its service goal. CPP offers a constellation of services, including traditional outpatient clinic treatment, inpatient and partial hospitalisation in The Johns Hopkins Hospital, psychiatric emergency treatment 24 hours a day, school mental health services and mental health care to the homeless. Psychiatric rehabilitation services and supervised housing programmes are provided by a closely linked independent organisation. Within this network, COSTAR is able to respond to almost any need of a long-term mentally ill person.

Patients

At the end of its third year of operation, the COSTAR population included 47 men and 50 women, ranging in age from 20 to 80 years with an average of 43.8 years. Of these, 61% were diagnosed as suffering from schizophrenia, while most of the remainder had primary diagnoses of affective disorders. All COSTAR patients have demonstrated an inability to use traditional outpatient mental health services, judged by patterns of noncompliance, high re-hospitalisation rates, extensive use of emergency services, history of incarceration, poor coping skills, or ineffective social supports. The patient population includes people ranging from those who have maintained steady employment to those who are severely withdrawn, underactive, and whose lives have severely deteriorated. Some have serious medical illnesses or handicaps. Half of the patients live with a spouse or family members; a substantial proportion (40%) live alone in independent housing arrangements; and a minority (10%) live in special supervised housing arrangements. Most have grown up in the community where they now live, and have relatives and friends in the local area, although some have migrated from other parts of the city, or from more distant places.

Clinical methods

The treatment team includes nurses, social workers, other non-medical clinicians and psychiatrists. There are approximately 12 patients per clinical staff member. A team approach is employed, so that each case is familiar to each member of the team. Staff are active during normal business hours, but may also be contacted by patients or families at other times by a paging system. One of the greatest strengths of this flexible approach is the capacity of the team to tailor the treatment to the exact needs of each patient. Doses of medicines are matched to an individual's requirement for symptom relief; and with the prescription of PRN doses to be used at nurses' discretion, immediate modifications can be effected. Patients are treated in their own environment, staff–patient contacts often taking place in unconventional locations convenient for the patient. These *in vivo* settings provide an atmosphere in which staff can effectively assess mental status, provide therapeutic support, and model normal social behaviour.

Although COSTAR is a voluntary programme at treatment onset, many patients express some reluctance to engage with providers with a plan to follow them so closely. Often paranoid symptoms limit the capacity for early relationship engagement. COSTAR never forces its treatment. One method which has proved effective is to encourage the patient to indicate what needs are foremost. For some, improving housing may be a priority, while for others augmenting their monthly income with government benefits and entitlements for the disabled may be most compelling. Through the process of obtaining such resources, the patient establishes a trusting relationship with the therapist. Patients are then more likely to accept treatment in the form of medication and psychotherapy.

COSTAR clinical team members may also assist patients in carrying out activities of daily living. Feedback is given to the patient on their maintenance of personal hygiene. At times, COSTAR staff may directly assist the patient in doing so by supervising the purchase of toiletries as well as providing direct instruction on how to maintain a tidy appearance. Patients are also given rehabilitative assistance in gaining independence in the areas of meal planning and food shopping, housekeeping, laundry, negotiating public transport, and money management including budgeting, banking and bill-paying. Improvement in these areas greatly augments the social functioning of patients and their psychiatric stability.

Patients become socially more pleasant to be with, proud of a more attractive appearance, and pleased with the ability to manage their lives and families successfully.

The flexibility of care provided by COSTAR allows staff to increase or decrease the duration of each contact and frequency of visits according to what patient needs are. This is especially beneficial when patients begin to show early signs of relapse. Staff can work with the patient to avoid a full-blown crisis by seeing the patient more often and spending the time needed to employ crisis prevention techniques. If needed, psychiatric evaluation is available to assess the need for adjustment in medication or environmental circumstances to provide greater social support or monitoring during a period of instability. Once patients have been through such an episode, they learn to trust the capacity of the COSTAR service to address their needs when difficulty arises. This further galvanises the trusting bond.

The continuity of care provides functions not only cross-sectionally and longitudinally, but also across systems. In the event that a COSTAR patient requires admission to hospital, the COSTAR team can help facilitate as short a length of stay as possible by providing crucial information early on so that clinical interventions are swift, focused and goal-directed. Discharge is facilitated since COSTAR can ensure that patient treatment plans are instituted appropriately and patients will receive as close monitoring as can be provided after discharge.

COSTAR also serves as a small-scale psycho-rehabilitation programme in that many patients find it helpful to visit COSTAR daily to begin their day, take medication, and socialise with other members while enjoying a cup of coffee. Friendships are established which patients extend into outside visits to each other's homes, restaurants, and other settings. Group psychotherapy at COSTAR also helps to build support networks which provide further stabilisation and quality of life enhancement.

The most revealing assessments are often those done in the home. The functional capacity of a person living alone can be observed. Housing conditions that reinforce pathology may be found, such as poorly secured doors or windows that may add to the fear of a paranoid patient: understanding the position of the patient in a disorganised family system can help to explain current difficulties. In assessing a patient at entry to the programme, and throughout treatment, both psychiatric and medical symptoms are explored. Target symptoms are assessed and monitored constantly: changes result in an appropriate plan of action, which may entail further monitoring by a non-medical clinician or emergency assessment by a psychiatrist. The presence of experienced registered nurses on the COSTAR staff allows for early recognition of physical complaints and effective monitoring of chronic physical illnesses. Nurses can also provide effective health education on nutrition, substance abuse, personal hygiene, sexual relations, and specific physical and psychiatric illnesses. They enable the COSTAR programme to offer psychiatric treatment to patients whose physical handicaps render them housebound and/or bedridden.

One of the ways that COSTAR engages and provides continuing assistance to patients is through contact with and support for those who are closest to them, such as neighbours, care providers, landlords, friends or nearby shopkeepers, as well as family members of sexual partners. 'Nursing the carer' is a term COSTAR clinicians use to describe the concept of responding to the psychological needs of care providers and enabling them to continue coping with the difficulties of living with someone with a mental illness (Anderson *et al.*, 1986). COSTAR clinicians welcome the involvement of anyone interested in the patient and use a psycho-educational approach (Anderson *et al.*, 1986), including education about mental illness, medication and its effects, and ways of coping with problems. Family therapy and couples therapy are provided as need is identified.

Clinicians do not wait for crises to erupt but rather anticipate the care providers' need to ventilate their frustrations and to solve problems. COSTAR staff have on occasion referred family members for crisis counselling to other agencies. Nursing the care provider indirectly maximises the care of the patient. Staff members themselves become significant members of the patient's social network, supporting them through such highly stressful life events as births, deaths, weddings and family illnesses. COSTAR thus directly augments the patient's support network. However, COSTAR's involvement with patients is often directed towards an increase in the number of other people willing to assist them. As a patient achieves greater overall stability, family members and friends who have been alienated in the past are more likely to be supportive and to include the patient in regular social activities. Part of the COSTAR philosophy is that the greater the number of people in a patient's support network, the better the person's community adjustment will be (Cutler & Tatum, 1983).

Evaluation of COSTAR

Study aims

The aims of the study reported here are to establish the baseline socio-demographic, psychiatric and social network characteristics of the study population, to describe their social, cognitive and mental state, to relate these variables to duration of contact with the COSTAR programme, and to rate change in these characteristics at 2 year follow-up. The study design was to make a complete ascertainment of patients treated at the COSTAR programme in 1988, and to follow-up all available patients 2 years later, the large majority of whom were still then in contact with COSTAR. At follow-up most interviews were conducted using a laptop computer to enter data, a process which the majority of patients slightly preferred to paper data entry (O'Ryan *et al.*, 1992).

Method

Data were collected from interviews with the patients, key informants (either the clinician or a relative), and from case note review. Interviews were conducted at baseline and at 2 year follow-up by a research psychiatrist with no clinical responsibility for the patients. Most patients were interviewed at home, or at the COSTAR offices, but five were seen in hospital while in relapse, and one was assessed in Baltimore City Jail. The study population was all 97 patients within the COSTAR programme. They had entered the programme during the 30 months since its inception. The entry criteria to the programme are: (1) age 18–80 years, (2) primary diagnosis (DSM-III-R; American Psychiatric Association, 1987) of schizophrenia, schizo-affective disorder, affective disorder, or a psychosis not otherwise specified, (3) living within or close to the catchment area of the Johns Hopkins Community Psychiatry Program in East Baltimore, (4) no primary diagnosis of dementia or delirium, and (5) failure to comply with treatment in traditional outpatient settings, or a history of frequent relapses. In practice, the patients admitted to the programme are those who have failed to benefit from the usual outpatient services, or who have lost contact with services between admissions.

Of the 97 patients in the COSTAR programme, baseline interview information was not obtained from 17 (13 refused to be interviewed, two were not traceable, and in two cases the patients were in early relapse and an interview was not advised). Apart from the study group, in the first 30 months of COSTAR's operation, only nine patients had separated from the service (two died of cardio-vascular disease, six were transferred to long-term hospitals or nursing homes, and one was discharged at his own request).

The assessment instruments used in the study were: (1) sociodemographic data and psychiatric history at entry to the programme, (2) Brief Psychiatric Rating Scale (BPRS: Overall & Gorham, 1962), (3) Social Behaviour Schedule (SBS: Wykes & Sturt, 1986), (4) Mini Mental State Examination (MMSE: Folstein *et al.*, 1975), (5) the Social Network Schedule (SNS: TAPS, 1989), and (6) the Global Assessment Scale (GAS: Endicott *et al.*, 1976). For the comparisons between the short-contact (12 months or less) with COSTAR, $n = 45$) and long-contact (more than 12 months $n = 52$) groups, and between the baseline and follow-up data, Student's *t*-test was used for the continuous variables, and the chi-squared test for the categorical variables, using Statistical Analysis System (SAS) software.

Results

Service contacts

Most patients had been subjected to 'revolving door' treatment before joining COSTAR, and had had frequent and usually brief admissions (mean of six previous admissions). In terms of the patterns of service contact, there was a trend identified for the frequency of contact with COSTAR staff to decrease slightly over the 2 years of follow-up (i.e. from 10 to 9 contacts per month).

Symptoms and social behaviour

At least one quarter of patients retained severe problems in social behaviour, including, for example, underactivity, indifference to aims, poor personal hygiene and passive leisure interests, and the frequency of social behaviour problems changed little during the period of follow-up. There were no changes on several of the outcome indicators, including, for example, the BPRS and GAF scores (detailed tables available from author and editor).

Several patient-specific variables were able to distinguish patients with larger and smaller social networks at the baseline assessment. For example, the total number of social contacts in the last month were recorded, along with the number of people who would be missed if they were not seen again, and the total number of people seen in the preceding week. As a group, women had clearly larger and richer networks. Diagnosis also played a role: patients with affective disorders tended to describe larger networks than those with schizophrenia, among whom patients with paranoid delusions or bizarre thoughts were significantly socially impoverished (table available on request).

Abnormalities of social behaviour were also highly associated with fewer social contacts, and a reduced network size was found, for example, in patients who manifested underactivity, odd behaviour, hostility or poor hygiene (Table 11.4). Nevertheless, it was striking that over the course of the study marked and significant improvement in the quantity and quality of the social networks of many patients did occur (Table 11.5).

Discussion

While research on social network and social support is dominated by studies about non-psychotic disorders, this paper focuses on patients

Table 11.4. Social network in relation to social behaviour characteristics of patients at baseline assessment

Variable	*n*	Primary group size	Number of active contacts
Underactivity			
Present	31	10.6 (8.6–12.6)	3.8 (2.6–5.0)
Absent	47	14.4 (11.4–17.4)	5.5 (4.0–6.0)
Odd behaviour			
Present	8	7.9 (5.6–10.1)	2.9 (0.6–5.2)
Absent	67	13.7 (11.5–15.9)	5.0 (3.9–6.1)
Hostility			
Present	3	6.7 (2.7–8.7)	4.3 (1.4–7.2)
Absent	75	13.2 (11.2–15.2)	4.8 (3.7–5.9)
Poor personal appearance			
Present	30	9.5 (6.6–12.4)	3.1 (2.1–4.1)
Absent	45	15.5 (12.9–17.1)	6.0 (4.4–7.6)

Table 11.5. *Social networks and duration of contact with COSTAR*

	1988		1990	
Variable	Contact with COSTAR less than 1 year	Contact with COSTAR over 1 year	Contact with COSTAR over 2 years	*p*
Primary group size	10.7	15.0	23.4	<0.05
Weekly contacts	4.9	7.3	12.1	<0.05
Monthly contacts	2.3	1.4	5.0	<0.01
Friends	2.2	3.3	4.7	<0.05
Relatives	4.7	7.6	5.9	NS
Acquaintances	3.1	2.8	8.6	<0.05
Confidants	2.6	3.7	3.7	NS
People missed	8.1	10.8	12.6	<0.05

severely disabled by chronic psychotic conditions (Beels, 1981; Brugha, 1991). Such long-term patients require long-term clinical and research follow-up (Sokolove & Trimble, 1986). This study must be interpreted carefully, since it is uncontrolled and the follow-up period is still modest in the context of the psychiatric careers of most of the patients concerned (Thornicroft & Breakey, 1991). Even so, the results indicate that patients in longer-term contact with COSTAR did demonstrate some improved aspects of social functioning. From the SBS improved scores were recorded for slowness, destruction to property, mannerisms and restlessness at follow-up. These data are also consistent with the findings of Wykes & Sturt (1986), that SBS and mental state (Present State Examination) ratings did not correlate among a group of long-term mentally ill patients. It may be that there is a considerable delay between initial treatment and longer-term improvement in social function after contact.

The data substantially confirmed that with longer contact with COSTAR, patients did show markedly greater quality and quantity of their social networks. Indeed previous work has repeatedly found that social isolation is associated with poorer outcome for chronic schizophrenia (Henderson *et al.*, 1978; Brugha *et al.*, 1993). At the ecological level social isolation has been recognised by the aggregation of such patients in inner city areas. Second, the isolation of living alone has been associated with earlier psychotic relapse. Third, the isolation of single marital status is more common among those with chronic schizophrenia. Finally, contact with fewer friends has been correlated with poorer outcome for schizophrenic patients.

The converse association may hold: that intimate and supportive personal relationships can be associated with better outcome. This would have important implications for community-based psychiatric services. In planning both the discharge of long-term inpatients, and the transfer of such patients between wards and hospitals, existing support networks may need to be recognised and sustained. For patients whose condition has interrupted family and friendship ties, a primary function for the case manager may be the reconstitution of such social relationships (Intagliata, 1982). In particular, barriers to forming or maintaining intimate relationships may be an important focus for family interventions.

If COSTAR is effective in helping its patients to expand their networks of social relationships, with the presumed benefits to be derived from these relationships, it is worth considering how this benefit is obtained. COSTAR staff, in their role as clinicians as much as case managers, make a point of becoming known to family members, neighbours and others. This has several benefits for the service delivery: such persons are often in the front line if problems arise, and need access to assistance and advice. They may have become demoralised after months or years of trying to cope with an ill friend or family member. They may have been frightened by stigmatising and ill-informed notions of mental illness. The clinicians make a point of educating, informing and supporting friends, relatives and carers, and coopting them as collaborators in the process of treatment and rehabilitation. This may extend to those persons who have utilitarian relationships with the patient: shopkeepers, landlords, bank or social service workers. In addition, there are certain activities provided at COSTAR which foster the development of relationship skills. These include groups for the development of self-esteem, thought to be especially useful in an impoverished, racial minority population. There are also women's and men's groups which address issues of relationships, social skill building, etc. Some patients participate in a psychosocial rehabilitation programme where they have opportunities to participate in a variety of pre-vocational training activities which include the development of interpersonal skills necessary for employment. Activities such as these, whether or not they come under the rubric of case management, may have been instrumental in enabling patients to enhance their social networks.

That specific characteristics of patients appear to be associated with the nature of their social network raises intriguing research and clinical possibilities. Specifically, it seems that the social contacts of women may be less harmed by their mental illness than those of their male counterparts. The design of this study limits the weight which can be accorded to the results: we have no information on pre-morbid social circles, nor on the overall extent of symptomatic improvement from the first point of contact with COSTAR. Nevertheless, the data generate the hypothesis, testable in further studies, that women are buffered against the full impact of social network attrition experienced by men after the onset of serious mental illness. It is possible that mental illness in a women is less threatening to families and friends than mental illness in a man, perhaps because men are more likely to be violent. In the homelessness context, this may explain why homeless women often seem to be 'sicker' than homeless men: only the sickest women are actually expelled from the home. These data, showing that mentally ill women have larger networks than men, would support this idea.

The diagnostic data are less unexpected, but reinforce the frequent clinical impression that patients with paranoid and bizarre ideas are more often shunned by friends and family than patients with other types of delusion (Segal & Holshuh, 1991). The social behaviour attributes are also consistent with the account of family members who report that the most distressing features they encounter are intimidating behaviour and the frustration of patients' negative symptoms such as underactivity and poor personal hygiene.

Although causality in social network research is fraught with method-ological complexity (Henderson, 1980), the data presented here can be seen as hypothesis-generating. An aetiological cycle can therefore be postulated. Not only may inadequate social networks have an adverse effect upon the outcome of schizophrenia, but also certain characteristics of such schizophrenic patients may weaken their social networks and cause them to become more isolated. The success of the COSTAR mobile treatment model, with its emphasis upon direct care and contact with patients, and with patients' families in their homes (Table 11.3), may consist partly in encouraging social re-integration, so that the cycle is reversed, and this may offer a buffer against future relapses (Henderson & Brown, 1988).

Acknowledgements

We would like to acknowledge the support for this work of all the staff and patients of the COSTAR programme, and of Dr Paul R. McHugh, Director of the Department of Psychiatry and Behavioral Sciences at The Johns Hopkins Medical Institutions. The baseline study was carried out by G.T. while participating in an exchange programme between the Maudsley and Johns Hopkins Hospitals, and the follow-up completed while he was an MRC Training Fellow.

References

American Psychiatric Association. (1987). *Diagnostic and Statistical Manual of Mental Disorders*, 3rd edn., revised, Washington, DC: American Psychiatric Association.

Anderson, C. N., Reiss, D. J. & Hogarty, G. E. (1986). *Schizophrenia and the Family*. New York: Guilford.

Anthony, W., Cohen, M., Farkas, M., *et al.* (1988). The chronically mentally ill and case management: more than a response to a dysfunctional system. *Community Mental Health Journal*, **24**, 21–8.

Avison, W. & Speechley, K. (1987). The discharged psychiatric patients: a review of social, social-psychological, and psychiatric correlates of outcome. *American Journal of Psychiatry*, **144**, 10–18.

Bachrach, L. (1980). Overview: model programs for chronic patients. *American Journal of Psychiatry*, **137**, 1023–31.

Bachrach, L. (1984). Asylum and chronically ill patients. *American Journal of Psychiatry*, **141**, 975–8.

Bachrach, L. (1989). Case management: towards a shared definition. *Hospital and Community Psychiatry*, **40**, 883–4.

Beels, C. (1981). Social support and schizophrenia. *Schizophrenia Bulletin*, **7**, 59–71.

Braun, P., Kochansky, G., Shapiro, R., Greenberg, S., Gudeman, J., Johnson, S. & Shore, M. (1981). Overview: deinstitutionalisation of psychiatric patients, a critical review of outcome studies. *American Journal of Psychiatry*, **138**, 736–49.

Breakey, W. (1989). Integrating training and research with clinical services in a community setting. *Hospital and Community Psychiatry*, **40**, 1175–9

Brewin, C., Wing, J., Mangen, S., Brugha, T. & MacCarthy, B. (1987). Principles and practice of measuring needs in the long-term mentally ill:

the Medical Research Council Needs for Care assessment. *Psychological Medicine*, **17**, 971–98.

Brugha, T. (1991). Support and personal relationships. In *Community Psychiatry*, ed. D. Bennett & H. Freeman, pp. 115–61. Edinburgh: Churchill-Livingstone.

Brugha, T. S., Wing, J. K., Brewin, C. R., MacCarthy, B., LeSage, A. (1993). The relationship of social network deficits with deficits in social functioning in long-term psychiatric disorders. *Social Psychiatry and Psychiatric Epidemiology*, **28**, 218–24.

Challis, D. (1989). *Case Management: Problems and Possibilities*. Canterbury: PSSRU, University of Kent.

Cutler, D. L. & Tatum, E. (1983). Networks and the chronic patient. *New Directions for Mental Health Services*, **19**, 13–22.

Endicott, I., Spitzer, R., Fleiss, J. & Cohen, J. (1976). The global assessment scale. *Archives of General Psychiatry*, **33**, 766–71.

Fariello, D. & Scheidt, S. (1989). Clinical case management of the dually diagnosed patient. *Hospital and Community Psychiatry*, **40**, 1065–7.

Fischer, P. & Breakey, W. (1986). Homelessness and mental health: an overview. *International Journal of Mental Health*, **14**, 6–41.

Folstein, M., Folstein, S. & McHugh, P. (1975). Mini Mental State, a practical method for grading the cognitive state of patients for the clinician. *Journal of Psychiatric Research*, **12**, 189–98.

Hall, J. (1979). Assessment procedures used in studies on long-stay patients. *British Journal of Psychiatry*, **135**, 330–5.

Hargreaves, W., Shaw, R., Shadoan, R., Walker, E., Surber, R. & Gaynor, J. (1984). Measuring case management activity. *Journal of Nervous and Mental Disease*, **172**, 296–300.

Harris, M. & Bergman, H. (1988). Misconceptions about use of case management services by the chronic mentally ill. *Hospital and Community Psychiatry*, **39**, 1276–80.

Henderson, A. (1980). A development in social psychiatry: the systematic study of social bonds. *Journal of Nervous and Mental Disease*, **168**, 63–9.

Henderson, A. (1992). Social support: the concept and the evidence. *Epidemiologia e Psichiatria Sociale*, **1**, 161–3.

Henderson, A. & Brown, G. (1988). Social support: the hypothesis and the evidence. In *Handbook of Social Psychiatry*, ed. A. Henderson & D. Burrows. Amsterdam: Elsevier.

Henderson, S., Duncan-Jones, P., McAuley, H. & Kitchie, K. (1978). The patient's primary group. *British Journal of Psychiatry*, **132**, 74–86.

Hoult, J. (1986). Community care of the acutely mentally ill. *British Journal of Psychiatry*, **14**, 137–44.

Hoult, J., Reynolds, I., Chargouneau-Powis, M., *et al.* (1983). Psychiatric hospital versus community treatment: the results of a randomized trial. *Australian and New Zealand Journal of Psychiatry*, **17**, 160–7.

House of Commons (1990). The National Health Service and Community Care Act. London: HMSO.

Intagliata, J. (1982). Improving the quality of care for the chronic mentally disabled: the role of case management. *Schizophrenic Bulletin*, **8**, 655–74.

Kanter, J. (1989). Clinical case management: definition, principles, components. *Hospital and Community Psychiatry*, **40**, 361–8.

Kiesler, C. (1982). Mental hospitals and alternative care. *American Psychologist*, **4**, 354–60.

Knapp, M., Cambridge, P., Thomason, C., Beecham, J., Allen, C. & Darton, R. (1990). Care in the Community Newsletter No. 9. Canterbury: PSSRU, University of Kent.

Lamb, R. (1980). Therapist–case managers: more than brokers of services. *Hospital and Community Psychiatry*, **31**, 762–4.

Levine, M. (1981). *The History and Politics of Community Mental Health*. Oxford: Oxford University Press.

Modrcin, M., Rapp, C. & Chamberlain, R. (1985). Case management with psychiatrically disabled individuals: curriculum and training programme. Lawrence, Kansas: University of Kansas School of Social Work.

Muijen, M., Marks, I., Connolly, J. & Audini, B. (1992). Home based care and standard hospital care for patients with severe mental illness: a randomized controlled trial. *British Medical Journal*, **304**, 749–54.

O'Ryan, D., Baxter, L., Thornicroft, G. & Glover, G. (1992). The TAPS Project (14): computer-assisted evaluation of long-term psychiatric patients: acceptability to patients and staff. *International Journal of Methods in Psychiatric Research*, **2**, 145–9.

Overall, J. & Gorham, D. (1962). Brief psychiatric rating scale. *Psychological Reports*, **10**, 799–812.

Renshaw, J. (1987). Care planning and case management. *British Journal of Social Work*, **18**, 79–105.

Robinson, G. & Bergman, G. (1989). *Choice in Case Management*. Washington, D.C.: Policy Resources Incorporated.

Schwab, D., Drake, R. & Burghardt, E. (1988). Health care of the chronically mentally ill: the culture broker model. *Community Mental Health Journal*, **24**, 174–84.

Segal, S. & Holshuh, J. (1991). Effects of sheltered care environments and resident characteristics on the development of social networks. *Hospital and Community Psychiatry*, **42**, 1125–31.

Sokolove, R. & Trimble, D. (1986). Assessing support and stress in the social networks of chronic patients. *Hospital and Community Psychiatry*, **37**, 370–2.

Stein, L. & Test, M. (1980). Alternative to mental hospital treatment. I. Conceptual model, treatment program and clinical evaluation. *Archives of General Psychiatry*, **37**, 392–7.

TAPS (1989). *Fourth Annual Report of the Team for the Assessment of Psychiatric Services*. London: North East Thames Regional Health Authority.

Tessler, R. & Goldman, H. (1982). *The Chronic Mentally Ill: Assessing the Community Support Program*. Cambridge, Mass.: Ballinger.

Thornicroft, G. & Breakey, W. (1991). The COSTAR programme. I. Improving the social networks of the long-term mentally ill. *British Journal of Psychiatry*, **159**, 245–9.

Thornicroft, G., Ward, P. & James, S. (1993). Care management and mental health. *British Medical Journal*, **306**, 768–71.

Torrey, F. (1986). Continuous treatment teams in the care of the chronic mentally ill. *Hospital and Community Psychiatry*, **37**, 1243–7.

Witheridge, T. F. & Dincin, J. (1985). The Bridge: An assertive outreach
program in an urban setting. In *Training in Community Living Model: A
Decade of Experience*, ed. L. I. Stein & M. A. Test, pp. 65–76. San Francisco:
Jossey-Bass.
Wykes, T. & Sturt, E. (1986). The measurement of social behaviour in
psychiatric patients: an assessment of the reliability and validity of the SBS
schedule. *British Journal of Psychiatry*, **148**, 1–11.

12

Expressed Emotion: measurement, intervention and training issues

LIZ KUIPERS

I almost hoped he would get run over. That would be better than this person dying and yet reappearing with another personality. It's just hell.
(Mother talking about her son. Evidence of hostility as rejection)

It's brought us together ... As time goes on he's coming back, never 100%, but he's getting better and we'll wait and see.
(Mother talking about her son. Evidence of warmth)

She's a really nice person.
(Mother talking about daughter. Positive remark)

I will never get over the shock [of the illness].
(Mother talking about son. Evidence of emotional overinvolvement)

He became violent on a couple of occasions, smashed winders, smashed doors, nice antique chairs I had, several clocks, my radio. *Everything* my wife bought me he seemed to *smash*.
(Father talking about son. Critical comment)

He's verbally very critical, *accusing*, or just *blatantly* disregards what you are saying, just refuses to listen.
(Staff member talking about key patient. Critical comment)

Introduction

The topic of social support is a broad one, and many authors have referred to the literature on Expressed Emotion (EE) as one of its aspects. It is appropriate, therefore, that while discussing the research literature on social support in psychiatric disorder, and its implications for intervention, an overview on EE should be included. In this chapter I will focus on the measurement of EE and the range of social interventions it has generated, and discuss a model of training in these interventions which has been developed.

The examples above are all comments that contribute to a rating of EE. It is a measure which uses not only verbal but vocal aspects of speech:

the speed, pitch and tone of voice as well as the content of what is said. It seems likely that this reliance on affective qualities as well as on meaning has been one of the reasons EE has been useful, both in predicting relapse in schizophrenia (Kavanagh, 1992) and in a variety of cultures and languages (Kuipers, 1992).

EE was first 'retroduced' by G. Brown and colleagues, a process he describes in a later article (Brown, 1985). At the time the researchers were convinced that if social factors were to play a role in schizophrenia then it would have to be possible to measure such factors in 'ordinary' family interactions. This idea has now been vindicated in that EE has been found not only in families with schizophrenia, but also in a wide variety of both physical and psychiatric conditions, ranging from weight loss (Flanagan & Wagner, 1991) and diabetes (Sensky et al., 1991) to manic depression (Priebe et al., 1992).

How EE is measured

EE is rated from an audiotape of an interview with a carer. This interview (Vaughn & Leff, 1976), now shortened, called the Camberwell Family Interview (CFI), has a semi-structured questionnaire format which allows a flexible use of standard questions and probes and encourages an interviewer to listen to information as it emerges, and not to interrupt if areas of interest have been discussed spontaneously. The interviewer covers the start of problems, focuses on the previous 3 months, and asks about possible difficulties in the relationship such as irritability and tension. Symptoms and coping responses are discussed and recent examples are probed for if a carer is reticent or vague. How time is spent in a recent typical week is the basis of what is called the time budget, which allows assessment of time awake spent in the same room together for the patient and carer.

From the CFI, five scales can be rated as shown in the examples. These are critical comments (CC), positive remarks (PR) (both frequency ratings), and global ratings of hostility (H), warmth (W) and emotional overinvolvement (EOI). Of these CC, H and EOI have been the most predictive, and many studies now do not discuss W and PR. CC rely particularly on tone, and are defined as an unfavourable remark about a person's behaviour or personality. CC are usually the most prevalent rating. H can exist independently of CC, but is often associated with criticism; it is defined either as a generalisation of criticism or as a rejecting remark, and relies on content which is usually unequivocal. EOI is the most complex of the scales, combining aspects of overprotection, self-sacrifice and past exaggerated emotional responses as well as behaviour during the interview (such as crying) and dramatisation (such as extravagant praise, the tone and tempo of speech). Traditionally, the scales have been used as categories; high EE is defined as a cutoff of six or more CC, or a moderate amount of EOI (3 or more out of 5) or any hostility (maximum score 3). Some carers will exhibit a mixture of these high ratings. They define a family as high EE even if only one member is so rated.

EE and outcome

At the time of writing there have been over 30 studies of EE and its relationship to outcome in schizophrenia 9 months or a year after patients return to live with families. The studies have been done in both developed and developing countries. Kavanagh (1992) points out that 'the median relapse rate is 21% for low EE or less than half of the 48% rate in the high EE group' (p. 601). Although not all studies are confirmatory, most replications, particularly the most recent ones (Kuipers, 1992), are in the predicted direction. In a meta-analysis of 24 of the worldwide studies ($n = 1346$) Bebbington and Kuipers (1994) was able to confirm that EE is strongly predictive of relapse in schizophrenia; is equally predictive of relapse in men and women; and that the association with relapse is stronger when high EE relatives are in close contact with patients, whereas in low EE families contact seems to be protective. Finally the effect of medication in reducing relapse is evident only in high EE families. These findings add weight to some of the original observations in the early studies (Brown *et al.*, 1972; Vaughn & Leff, 1976). Overall, the outcome studies suggest that EE remains a robust predictor of relapse in schizophrenia, and is able to identify 'stressful' environments in a variety of different cultures.

What does EE mean?

When EE first appeared in the early 1960s it did not map on to other social or family measures. It has taken some time for EE's usefulness as a predictor of relapse in schizophrenia to be matched by an understanding of what it is. Jenkins & Karno (1992) point out that an explanation of EE 'requires a theoretical bridge from behaviour to meaning' (p. 12) and speculate that 'In our view, the unknown and theoretically overarching something or somethings indexed by the global construct of EE are culturally constituted features of kin response to an ill relative' (p. 16). As Jenkins (1991) has discussed, one of the features of the rating of criticism is its use of the vocal channel and lack of dependence on specific content of speech. This may account for its success in transcending cultural barriers, allowing different cultures to criticise a variety of attributes in ill relatives. However, while cultural aspects are obviously important and underestimated, it does not seem likely that they will supply an adequate explanation of EE. Studies that have helped elucidate meaning so far have concentrated on the relationship of EE to other measures, particularly during interaction tasks.

There is now quite a long list of studies showing that high levels of EE in carers are related to a variety of other aspects of family functioning, such as direct criticism of the patient by the relative (Rutter & Brown, 1966; Brown & Rutter, 1966); negative affective style in relatives (Strachan et al., 1986; Miklowitz et al., 1989); an unpredictable home environment (MacCarthy et al., 1986); negative escalation patterns (Hooley & Hahlweg, 1986); conflict-prone structure, negative emotional climate and rigid interaction patterns (Hubschmid & Zemp, 1989); poor listening skills in relatives (Kuipers et al., 1983); fears and anxieties in relatives, particularly when they do not attribute patients' behaviour to illness (Greenley, 1986); a characteristic attributional style (Brewin et al., 1991); and less effective coping (Bledin et al., 1990).

For patients, a high EE rating in carers is related to higher criticality and fewer autonomous statements (Strachan et al., 1989), and poorer social functioning (Barrowclough & Tarrier, 1990).

It is also apparent that, in contrast, low EE carers are not just neutral but can be seen to make more *supportive* and positive statements (Hubschmid & Zemp, 1989) and have an ability to defuse rather than escalate arguments (Hooley & Hahlweg, 1986). Low EE, in other words, is normally not just an absence of negative aspects but has the potential to have positive and beneficial effects on patients.

EE in staff

A recent interesting extension of the EE research has been to consider EE in other carers, notably staff. The staff involved have shared some of the characteristics of other carers, because they have been the key worker for patients in long-term settings, and have thus not only spent time with patients but also had a working relationship with the client of at least 3 months. In research into burden, it has been found that staff and relatives share the impact of many of the behaviour problems and disturbance of clients but, unlike relatives, staff have time off and holidays, i.e. respite, which relatives often ask for but rarely receive (MacCarthy et al., 1989).

A series of studies have shown that such staff display a range of EE attitudes, and that over 40% ($n = 35$) had a high rating (more than six critical comments was the high EE cutoff) about at least one key patient

(Moore *et al.*, 1992*a*). This replicates an unpublished finding by Watts (1988) and also a study by Herzog (1988) who found the majority of staff to be high EE. Beltz *et al.* (1991) also showed that there was no consistent relationship between staff and family levels of EE. In other words, patients did not reliably predict a high EE response in carers, although staff and family members sometimes shared high EE attitudes.

In a content analysis of 61 interviews elicited from 35 staff members (Moore *et al.*, 1992*b*), criticism in both high and low EE interviews was most frequently focused on socially embarrassing or difficult behaviour, and the clinical poverty syndrome (e.g. apathy, slowness, poor self-care) (Wykes, 1982). The category which attracted the most criticism was the repetition of inappropriate behaviour and attention seeking. This mirrors a result found in a study of EE in dementia: that the behaviour most often criticised by carers was repetitious speech and behaviour (Bledin *et al.*, 1990). In staff, high levels of criticism were significantly related to regarding the patients' difficulties as under their own control, and having negative rather than positive expectations of a patient's ability to manage independently. A prospective naturalistic study of differential outcome in two hostels, one characterised by a majority of high EE staff and the other by low EE staff, suggested that patients in the former hostel had a poorer outcome in the subsequent 9 months (Ball *et al.*, 1992).

Finally, an interaction study of staff and their key patients (Moore & Kuipers, 1992) found high EE staff more likely to make negative statements and less likely to make supportive ones. Low EE staff did not focus on their own negative feelings (if any) or on those expressed by the patient. These studies suggest that EE is a useful indicator of potential problems for staff and carers. They provide evidence that even the most difficult or disabled patients can be worked with constructively if staff are able to focus on some positive or likeable aspect of their behaviour or personality, rather than on the almost inevitable negatives.

Intervention studies

One of the most notable achievements of the EE measure has been its use in both structuring and evaluating the impact of social treatments in interventions with families. The intervention studies completed so far have been extensively reviewed (e.g. Kuipers & Bebbington, 1988; Lam, 1991; Kavanagh, 1992).

There have now been five well-documented controlled trials of family intervention with 2 year follow-up which have been successful (Leff *et al.*, 1982, 1985, 1989, 1990; Falloon *et al.*, 1982, 1985; Hogarty *et al.*, 1986, 1987; Tarrier *et al.*, 1988, 1989) and three without follow-up which have not been successful (Köttgen *et al.*, 1984; McCreadie *et al.*, 1991; Vaughan *et al.*, 1992).

In the successful studies, relapse rates in the intervention groups became no greater than that expected in patients from low EE families. Success was largely but not totally related to an improved family atmosphere, in that when it was measured, social performance was improved in patients (Doane *et al.*, 1985; Hogarty *et al.*, 1986) and subjective burden was reduced (Falloon & Pederson, 1985).

It is not entirely clear why unsuccessful studies did not improve patient or family functioning significantly. The Hamburg study of Köttgen and her colleagues (1984) involved a psychodynamic approach to treatment, and this may have been experienced by the rather younger patient group as intrusive and upsetting (Strachan, 1986). The other two studies claimed to have used techniques very similar to the successful studies; failure may have been the result of a lack of experience in the therapist or of particular attributes of the patient group. This raises questions of therapist training that will be discussed later. In the Sydney study (Vaughan *et al.*, 1992) patients in both intervention and control groups were not very compliant with medication. The intervention in the Nithsdale study (McCreadie *et al.*, 1991), which had limited success in engaging families, was also unsuccessful in lowering EE, although even here the total number of relapses was reduced somewhat for patients whose families accepted the intervention.

Successful interventions were sometimes associated with a reduction in EE or negative affective style (Leff *et al.*, 1982, 1990; Falloon *et al.*, 1982), sometimes not (Hogarty *et al.*, 1986). However, less successful interventions (Köttgen *et al.*, 1984; McCreadie *et al.*, 1991) did not reduce EE levels in relatives and too few reassessments were carried out in Sydney for valid analysis. This does suggest that a reduction in EE may be a sufficient but not necessary component of change.

The successful studies, although not offering the same programme of intervention and usually using different labels for their therapeutic endeavours, have nevertheless seemed to offer a similar range of inputs. These include:

1 A positive attitude to carers and patients: not blaming or indicting families for the problems.
2 Education: offering information in various formats, as a precondition for later therapeutic input.
3 Problem solving: a focus on current problems in the family and improving communication skills in order to begin to solve them.
4 Emotional processing: sometimes called cognitive behavioural strategies, or dealing with stress (Barrowclough & Tarrier, 1992), or referred to as part of problem solving (Falloon, 1985), this usually

tackles some aspects of the upset, distress and burden carried by families.
5 Medication: all studies help patients to remain on optimum medication levels while receiving social treatments.

All the above studies have published manuals which discuss their interventions in more detail (Anderson *et al.*, 1986; Falloon, 1985; Kuipers *et al.*, 1992; Barrowclough & Tarrier, 1992).

The initial hope that education would change outcomes by itself has not been fulfilled. The evidence is now fairly clear that giving carers information is often the starting point for later intervention and has high face validity for carers, but does not change long-term outcome (Smith & Birchwood, 1987; Cozolino *et al.*, 1988; Tarrier *et al.*, 1988; Lam, 1991).

What seems to be emerging is that successful family intervention is a complex process that requires skilled (and therefore trained) therapists, who have specific objectives and offer both problem solving and emotion-focused coping skills. Changes in one aspect can be useful, but the most improved outcome happens where both patients' and relatives' behaviour is modified interactively. Studies that improve only one aspect, such as social functioning and negative symptoms, do not necessarily improve family atmosphere (Tomaros *et al.*, 1988), and vice versa (Orhagen *et al.*, 1992). It seems likely that to effect changes that are both clinically useful and maintained over time certain minimum requirements have to be met, i.e. that staff are trained effectively in skills training, goal setting, problem solving and managing emotional issues, and that intervention includes the patient where possible (Vaughan *et al.*, 1992). Relatives' groups have been effective in reducing EE and improving patient role performance (MacCarthy *et al.*, 1989; Kuipers *et al.*, 1989), but are likely to suffer from poor engagement and 'miss' up to half of the families who might benefit (Leff *et al.*, 1989). Thus while cost-effective and socially supportive, such groups remain as one intervention option. There will always be those who need home visits and individual family work.

Further requirements of successful family work include, as stated above, the provision of education, problem solving, and cognitive restructuring of expectations and progress in order to recognise improvement when it occurs.

How to offer family intervention in schizophrenia

It can be argued that all families would benefit from assessment of need and intervention. However, clinical services are often faced with prioritising such needs. If it is not possible to offer help to all those with

Table 12.1. *Indicators of families with greatest need*

Relatives living with patients who relapse more often than once a year despite being compliant with maintenance neuroleptics
Relatives who frequently contact staff for reassurance and help
Families in which there are repeated arguments leading to verbal or physical violence; and any family that calls in the police
A single relative, normally a mother, looking after a patient with schizophrenia on her own

From Kuipers *et al.* (1992).

carers then some clinical indications of family settings where need is likely to be highest are set out in Table 12.1.

In our training manual for therapists (Kuipers *et al.*, 1992) we have separated practical issues (dealt with first) from emotional ones. In practice the issues are often intertwined. No more than an outline of the interventions suggested can be given here.

Engaging families

One of the key aspects of work with these families is the necessity of spending time at the beginning ensuring the family accepts some help. However skilled an intervention is, it cannot be effective unless a family is willing to take it up. Many families have a history of what they perceive as unhelpful or inadequate professional help in the past and may have very low expectations of things being different this time. Other families are unwilling to risk the uncertainty of new help, in case things become worse. Seeing families initially at a crisis point, such as admission to hospital, can be a useful starting point, as things have obviously not been going well. Families at this stage may be more willing to begin to discuss coping and prevention that at a time when things are 'as normal'. Potential therapists have to be flexible and persistent. Early refusal, or difficulties keeping to an initial appointment, can often be coped with by continuing to offer alternatives. It is certainly not helpful to be rigid about the timing or place of an early meeting with relatives. We have found that pleasant but persistent offers of help at this stage are more likely to lead to long-term engagement in later intervention.

Education

One of the most useful ways to engage a family is to offer education, and most studies have endorsed this. Education by itself does not impart much information or lead to long-term behaviour change (Smith &

Birchwood, 1987; Tarrier *et al.*, 1988), but it does help families feel more optimistic about the future (Berkowitz *et al.*, 1984) and helps relatives' feelings of mastery and self-esteem (Lam, 1991). Offering information also has high face validity and overtly satisfies relatives' consumer demands. The way in which information is provided seems less important. Various studies have offered workshops (Hogarty *et al.*, 1986), relative groups (Smith & Birchwood, 1987) or individual home visits (Leff *et al.*, 1982, 1989).

Various leaflets are now available to back up spoken information. The crucial part of an information session appears to be when some sort of active learning takes place, i.e. when relatives ask questions and receive specific information as a result. Education needs to be given flexibly and not according to some rigid format. This allows disagreements to be aired and dealt with. For instance, patients and families may not accept the diagnosis but may well accept there is a problem, and will be encouraged to know that they are not alone in having to deal with it. The use of patients as the 'expert' in these situations is worth fostering. It can be suggested that relatives ask patients to describe some of their psychotic experiences and patients can then tell relatives how they might help.

Relatives' groups are also very useful in encouraging relatives to discuss common themes, ask each other questions and exchange information, so that feelings of isolation and fear of the unknown can diminish (Kuipers *et al.*, 1989, 1992; Kuipers & Westall, 1992).

Specific interventions

Specific interventions will differ depending on the type of family, the range of members (e.g. spouse or a parental family; one, two or three generations), and the stage of the illness (first onset, or many years afterwards). However, there are some overall strategies that will need to be used. Even families who have lived with problems for many years may not have begun to sort them out and may resemble a new-onset family in terms of having unsuccessful coping skills and unrealistic expectations of progress.

Communication skills

The first task in any family meeting is to help participants to improve their communication skills. This may take many sessions and have to be reiterated. Family members may have to practise listening to each other, without interrupting, and talking directly to each other, not about each other. This helps to defuse negative statements in itself, and encourages everyone's participation in a session. For example, 'He is very difficult' has to be rephrased and is usually toned down if said directly to the person as '*You* are difficult at home sometimes'.

In some families communication patterns may be very disrupted or dysfunctional. Talking to each other may always lead to an argument and so may be avoided. Therapists may have to make and enforce 'ground rules', such as turn taking and listening, and be prepared to intervene and prevent arguments or negative comments. Having a co-therapist in the session can be particularly useful as they are an ally and can help defuse negative patterns, and model more constructive dialogue.

Task setting

One of the key vehicles of behaviour change in these interventions, and one that each research group has stressed, is some sort of family consensus followed by action taken around a particular task, normally called problem solving. Family members are encouraged to take turns in offering a list of current problems. These are then prioritised by the family and some specific alternative solutions are arrived at. These are then negotiated, agreed to and (it is hoped) practised as homework before the next session. This emphasis on the 'here and now' allows families to feel that current problems are being dealt with and encourages engagement and participation. It is also the case that however menial or prosaic the problem decided upon, the very fact that it has not yet been resolved points up other problems of family functioning which can be dealt with in due course. The fact that patients are (for example) not allowed to cross the road by themselves, to buy the cat food or to be left alone, or are not trusted to spend money sensibly or take medication, can then begin to be dealt with. This allows more constructive approaches to be practised and helps family members begin to experience success and then optimism, rather than failure and resignation.

Emotional issues

Living with schizophrenia can give rise to a wide variety of emotional responses, ranging from grief, guilt, anger, rejection, hopelessness and resignation, to unrealistic denial that there are any problems. Therapists need to know how to deal with these if intervention is to progress. While problem solving may be part of this process, in some families the feelings are so intense or long lasting that emotional issues have to be dealt with before any other work can be done.

Therapists can start the process by *normalising* even extreme emotional upset. Virtually all families will feel some aspects from the possible emotional range; it would be surprising if they did not, given the difficulties that many have to cope with. Finding out from therapists that such reactions are commonplace rather than unusual can be very reassuring and allays fears such as 'I thought I was going to go mad too'. Relatives' groups and other opportunities for relatives to talk to each other can also help this, as it becomes obvious that such feelings are universal and that it is possible to cope with and survive them.

A strategy that we have found useful for emotional issues is called *positive reframing*. This is where the meaning underlying even hurtful or extreme emotional statements is made clear by the therapists. Thus even comments such as 'I hate you' or 'I can't stand living with you' can be reframed to demonstrate that it is only because the person cares at all that such extreme sentiments are uttered. Often the way the illness has disabled or changed an individual might be the cause of the feeling, and this too can be discussed. For example, 'I can't stand living with you' might refer to how upsetting it is to watch a loved one suffer or behave differently, and might actually reflect grief over the loss the illness may have caused for both patient and relative. In most family sessions the fact that relatives and patients are trying to sort out the problems can be drawn upon, together with the fact that family members would not be attending if they were totally indifferent to the problem.

This is not to deny that in some family situations it may be impossible for care to continue. In some settings (particularly with a spouse) it may be true that a partner does want to leave and to reject the caring role. If these factors are prominent then even they can be reframed as a clear indication of strong feelings. An attempt can then be made, perhaps in the session, perhaps separately, to discuss how the caring role might be modified or, if necessary, how alternative care might be offered.

In terms of the EE rating, criticism and overinvolvement are particularly likely to have to be dealt with.

With *critical relatives*, the negative emotions are usually due to anger, frustration and (typically) a misunderstanding of negative symptoms. Education and continuing discussion, particularly of the cause of negative symptoms, together with help in restructuring expectations and in noticing progress even if it is slow, will begin to help change many of the feelings that fuel critical comments.

Overinvolvement is a more complex set of emotional responses, often surrounding guilt and unresolved grief. Parents are the most likely to exhibit it in an attempt to care for the patient, and offer help with perceived disabilities. Overinvolvement can be seen as a protective parental response similar to that made when the patient was a child and needed high levels of care. While this is a helpful reaction to acute illness, in the long term it locks a patient into the 'sick' role, removes adult responsibilities and roles, and can impede social recovery. At its most damaging it can place a patient in a permanently childlike role. If the carer is also unable to set limits on unacceptable behaviour, this can at times lead to overtly demanding or even violent behaviour on the patient's part. At other times it may just mean that a patient is shielded from normal adult decisions and roles. This is not only unrealistic for the patient, preventing the normal practice of these roles, but also places unrealistic burdens on a carer.

A useful strategy with an overinvolved carer is for therapists to examine 'the worst outcome'. What would happen, for example, if the patient were left alone for half an hour? Sometimes the worst outcome has actually happened and this is why the carer is so worried; but even then, the likelihood of it being repeated may be small, and safeguards might be possible. Often, however, the fear is not well founded and carers are worried about 'what if?' Some testing of this in a very careful and graded way as part of task setting, and in consultation with the patient, may not only begin to help a patient take responsibility and be more independent but may also demonstrate that the 'catastrophe' is not inevitable.

Therapists may also give relatives 'permission' to take some time off from the caring role, and take up old friends and interests. This can allow a patient to function in a more adult way. Again, practising these ideas and finding out that both carer and patient may feel or manage better as a result is the most effective way of beginning to help family functioning to change.

Training intervention skills

In order to make the above strategies more generally available, it is necessary to offer training to staff. Unlike pharmacological treatments, where quality control can be applied at the manufacturing stage, social treatments are likely to need extra skills and quality control has to rely on checking the therapeutic input. This is a much more complicated process. As can be seen from the research studies, unless staff are adequately trained to deliver treatments, there is the possibility that therapy will be less effective or ineffective (McCreadie et al., 1991; Vaughn et al., 1992). Thus the questions to be answered include, in order of priority:

1 What needs to be taught (how should training be structured) and what are the skills that need to be transmitted?
2 Can the skills be learnt by a 'second generation' of staff who are primarily practioners rather than researchers?
3 If the skills can be taught and learnt, are they practised? In other words how can the therapy process be monitored reliably to find out how effectively skills are being demonstrated during a family session?
4 Does it work? Can second and third generation therapists provide social treatments that are as effective, possibly more effective, than the original, successful, research trials? The alternative is to have successful social treatments that cannot be promulgated or are not widely available.

There is already some evidence that such an endeavour is possible.

Brooker *et al.* (1992), in a pilot study, used community psychiatric nurses and trained them to deliver social treatment to clients with schizophrenia living with families. The training consisted of family assessment, health education and family stress management techniques. Families living with a patient with schizophrenia were recruited in a quasi-experimental design (not randomised) to either an experimental or control treatment lasting 12 months. In the experimental group, target symptoms, personal functioning and social adjustment were reported to be improved. The relatives were more satisfied with services, saying they had better advice, emotional support and service coordination, and their own psychiatric morbidity was reported to have improved as well.

In our own group, we have been piloting a training scheme for psychiatric nurses, and are aiming to use the trained staff to offer social treatment compared with a control group, in a randomised design. This should enable us to evaluate the effectiveness of this service delivery. Families in both groups will be assessed for levels of EE and social functioning, both before and after treatment. The treatment will be offered in a local district psychiatric service, not a research setting, in order to test how effective such treatments might be during 'normal' service delivery.

In order to do this, myself and colleagues Julian Leff and Dominic Lam decided to use a model similar to that used with families. In other words we aimed at a partnership model with the trainees (nursing staff) – a collaborative and facilitative approach, not just a didactic one. We wanted to offer them the specific aims and focused skill training for dealing with families in order to 'add' to their existing skills and experience. All trainees were of at least staff nurse level in terms of their professional training. We aimed to involve participants in the training, encouraged mutual feedback, and evaluated each session in order that we could learn from and improve the training as we went along.

The method of training was a mixture of didactic and experiential material. The latter we have found particularly valuable, as a way both of active learning and also of accessing some of the reality of emotional states such as grief, anger or hopelessness. Thus most of the training included the use of a role play during sessions. The training was developed, as in the intervention studies, to offer information (education) first (ten sessions) and then to follow up with group supervision meetings. These carried on weekly, and the complete course lasted 9 months. During this time each staff member began to work in a co-therapy pair and each pair took on two or three families who were worked with and evaluated during the training course. Trainees were evaluated in terms of their attitudes and beliefs before and after the initial teaching and after the supervision sessions. During this time a further two teaching sessions were offered on how to run a relatives' group.

In the supervision sessions the emphasis was on constructive and positive change, not on criticisms, and on learning from each other. The facilitators participated in each session in order to encourage this. Facilitators were flexible, they asked for, and tried to respond to, feedback, and they dealt with any problems as they arose. Towards the end of the course, participants were encouraged to run sessions themselves and the former facilitators became part of the group.

The content of the course is itemised in a training manual (Kuipers *et al.*, 1993) and supplemented by the treatment manual discussed earlier (Kuipers *et al.*, 1992). Issues during the didactic teaching included engaging families, offering education, tackling problems, criticism, overinvolvement and defining emotional problems, as well as co-therapy issues and running a relatives' group. During supervision the following themes were covered: co-therapy, how to be a therapist not a guest, controlling a session, task setting, homework, negotiating skills, guilt, anger, dealing with conflict, bereavement, independence and leaving. Other issues were discussed as they arose.

To date two training courses have been run ($n = 20$) and a third has been completed by a nurse therapist from the original course. Two members of this latter course (second generation) have trained the next generation of therapists who are offering intervention to families in the controlled trial (third generation).

In order to evaluate this training, several research instruments have been developed. The first is a schizophrenia family work scale. This comprises an *adherence* scale of technical skills (such as tasks assignments) and a *competence* scale which includes aspects such as interpersonal effectiveness, negotiating style and handling of emotions. At this stage we have established acceptable inter-rater reliability on the ratings of these therapeutic processes. Consumer satisfaction is assessed using a Helpful Aspects of Therapy (HAT) scale. After each family meeting each participant is asked to specify helpful and unhelpful interventions. It has been possible to do a content analysis and assign comments reliably using this scale. To tap into the trainees' attitudes and beliefs, a 40 item multiple choice questionnaire (MCQ) has also been devised which assesses factual knowledge about schizophrenia and family work. Attitudes and beliefs are assessed before and after didactic teaching and after supervision.

In both pilot courses, trainees made a significant gain in knowledge as measured by the MCQ and also significant gains in the desirable direction in the attitudes and beliefs questionnaire, both at the end of the didactic course and at the end of the supervision. This improvement in knowledge and attitudes made during the teaching block was maintained throughout the 9 month course (Lam *et al.*, 1993).

Changes in therapeutic process, in consumer satisfaction and in family functioning will be assessed during the main trial, now that it has been shown that we can rate them reliably. Outcome results for the new trial will not be available for several years, because of the length of time required to train staff, offer therapy and obtain adequate follow-up data.

Training for direct care staff

The finding that EE in staff is comparable to that found in relatives offering direct care to patients also has implications for training. The research suggests it might be possible to help staff deal with long-term, even very difficult patients, in a constructive and positive way.

Higson & Kavanagh (1988) describe a brief programme which showed some marginally significant effects on residents in two hostels who participated in a brief (seven sessions) psycho-educational approach, and where residents' critical comments during subsequent interviews were slightly reduced.

It seems likely that adapting the model of work from the family intervention to long-term staff could produce similar effects. Evidence from staff showing high EE attitudes to patients suggests that negative symptoms and embarrassing behaviour were more likely to be criticised (Moore *et al.*, 1992*b*). Potentially these might be reappraised and understood better through education and the development of more realistic expectations. Helping staff manage difficult behaviour by problem solving and stress management, while also ensuring that they focus on positives, has yet to be attempted in any formal way, but might well improve both patient functioning and staff satisfaction in long-term care.

Conclusion

The measure of EE has proved a reliable and valid way of assessing stressful environments, and also of helping both to structure and to evaluate attempts to change them. Ironically, while EE has also attracted criticism for being too narrow a research tool (Smith *et al.*, 1993) and for itself stigmatising relatives (Hatfield *et al.*, 1987), it is impossible to deny its valuable role in fuelling new and successful interventions.

The training of staff to deliver social interventions to families and possibly to modify their own behaviour in working with the long-term mentally ill is just developing, and the results remain to be quantified. Both these areas raise issues about evaluating therapeutic processes, although doing so systematically is still in its infancy. It may be that

gaining experience in the evaluation of clinical process, and in EE-related
intervention, will be of benefit to those wishing to develop interventions
based on other aspects of social support. Meanwhile, EE continues to be
a measure which is useful and which stimulates research effort in a
demanding and needy clinical area. While this is the case EE is unlikely
to be superseded.

References

Anderson, C. M., Reiss, D. J. & Hogarty, G. E. (1986). *Schizophrenia in the
Family: A Practical Guide to Psycho-education and Management.* New York:
Guilford Press.
Ball, R. A., Moore, E. & Kuipers, L. (1992). EE in community care facilities:
a comparison of patient outcome in a 9 month follow-up of two residential
hostels. *Social Psychiatry and Psychiatric Epidemiology,* 27, 35–9.
Barrowclough, C. & Tarrier, N. (1990). Social functioning in schizophrenic
patients. I. The effects of EE and family intervention. *Social Psychiatry and
Psychiatric Epidemiology,* 25, 125–9.
Barrowclough, C. & Tarrier, N. (1992). *Families of Schizophrenia Patients:
Cognitive Behaviourial Intervention.* London: Chapman & Hall.
Bebbington, P. E., & Kuipers, L. (1994). The predictive utility of Expressed
Emotion in Schizophrenia: an aggregated analysis. *Psychological Medicine,* 24,
707–18.
Beltz, J., Bertrando, P., Clerici, M., Albertini, E., Merati, O. & Cazullo, C.
L. (1991). Emotiva Espresso e schizoprenia: dai familiari agli operatori
psichiatrici. Paper presented at Symposium on Expressed Emotion in Latin
based languages, Barcelona, Spain.
Berkowitz, R., Eberleien-Fries, R., Kuipers, L. & Leff, J. (1984). Educating
relatives about schizophrenia. *Schizophrenia Bulletin,* 10, 418–29.
Bledin, K., MacCarthy, B., Kuipers, L. & Woods, R. (1990). Daughters of
people with dementia: EE, strain and coping. *British Journal of Psychiatry,*
157, 221–7.
Brewin, C. R., MacCarthy, B., Duda, R. & Vaughn, C. E. (1991).
Attribution and Expressed Emotion in the relatives of patients with
schizophrenia. *Journal of Abnormal Psychology,* 100, 546–54.
Brooker, C., Tarrier, N., Barrowclough, C., Butterworth, A. & Goldberg, D.
(1992). Training community nurses for psychosocial intervention: a pilot
study. *British Journal of Psychiatry,* 160, 836–44.
Brown, G. (1985). The discovery of EE: induction or deduction? In *Expressed
Emotion in Families,* ed. J. Leff & C. Vaughn, pp. 7–25. New York: Guilford
Press.
Brown, G. W. & Rutter, M. L. (1966). The measurement of family activities
and relationships. *Human Relations,* 19, 241–63.
Brown, G. W., Birley, J. L. & Wing, J. K. (1972). Influence of family life on
the course of schizophrenic illness: a replication. *British Journal of Psychiatry,*
121, 241–58.
Cozolino, L. J., Goldstein, M. J., Neuchterlein, K. S., *et al.* (1988). The

impact of education on relatives varying in levels of EE. *Schizophrenia Bulletin*, **14**, 675–86.

Doane, J. A., Falloon, I. R. H., Goldstein, M. J. & Mintz, J. (1985). Parental affective style and the treatment of schizophrenia: predicting course of illness and social functioning. *Archives of General Psychiatry*, **42**, 34–42.

Falloon, I. R. H. (1985). *Family Management of Schizophrenia*. Baltimore: Johns Hopkins Press.

Falloon, I. R. H. & Pederson, J. (1985). Family management in the prevention of morbidity of schizophrenia: adjustment of the family unit. *British Journal of Psychiatry*, **147**, 156–63.

Falloon, I. R. H., Boyd, J. L., McGill, C. W., Razani, J., Moss, H. B. & Gildersman, A. M. (1982). Family management in the prevention of exacerbations of schizophrenia: a controlled study. *New England Journal of Medicine*, **306**, 1437–40.

Falloon, I. R. H., Boyd, J. L., McGill, C. W., Williamson, M., Razani, J., Moss, H. B., Gilderman, A. M. & Simpson, G. M. (1985). Family management in the prevention of morbidity of schizophrenia: clinical outcome of a two year longitudinal study. *Archives of General Psychiatry*, **42**, 887–96.

Flanagan, D. A. J. & Wagner, H. L. (1991). Expressed Emotion and panic-fear in the prediction of diet treatment compliance. *British Journal of Clinical Psychology*, **30**, 231–40.

Greenley, J. R. (1986). Social control and EE. *Journal of Nervous and Mental Disease*, **174**, 24–30.

Hatfield, A., Spaniol, L. & Zipple, A. M. (1987). Expressed emotion: a family perspective. *Schizophrenia Bulletin*, **13**, 221–6.

Herzog, T. (1988). Nurses, patients and relatives: a study of family patterns on psychiatric wards. In *Family Intervention in Schizophrenia: Experiences and Orientations in Europe*, ed. C. L. Cazzullo & G. Invernizzi. Milan: ARS.

Higson, M. & Kavanagh, D. J. (1988). A hostel based psychoeducational intervention for schizophrenia: programme development and preliminary finds. *Behaviourial Change*, **5**, 85–9.

Hogarty, G. E., Anderson, C. M., Reiss, D. J., Kornblith, S. J., Greenwald, D. P., Javna, C. D. & Madonia, M. J. (1986). Family psycho-education, social skills training and maintenance chemotherapy in the aftercare treatment of schizophrenia. I. One year effects of a controlled study on relapse and Expressed Emotion. *Archives of General Psychiatry*, **43**, 633–42.

Hogarty, G. E., Anderson, C. M. & Reiss, D. J. (1987). Family psycho-education, social skills training, and medication in schizophrenia: the long and the short of it. *Psychopharmacology Bulletin*, **23**, 12–13.

Hooley, J. M. & Hahlweg, K. (1986). The marriages and interaction patterns of depressed patients and their spouses: comparison of high and low EE dyads. In *Treatment of Schizophrenia: Family Assessment and Intervention*, ed. M. J. Goldstein, I. Hand & K. Hahlweg, pp. 85–95. Berlin: Springer.

Hubschmid, T. & Zemp, M. (1989). Interaction in high and low Expressed Emotion families. *Social Psychiatry and Psychiatric Epidemiology*, **24**, 113–19.

Jenkins, J. H. (1991). Anthropology: Expressed Emotion and schizophrenia. *Ethos*, **19**, 387–431.

Jenkins, J. H. & Karno, M. (1992). The meaning of Expressed Emotion:

theoretical issues raised by cross cultural research. *American Journal of Psychology*, **149**, 9–21.

Kavanagh, D. J. (1992). Recent developments in Expressed Emotion and schizophrenia. *British Journal of Psychiatry*, **160**, 601–20.

Köttgen, C., Sonnichsen, I., Mollenhauer, K. & Jurth, R. (1984). Group therapy with the families of schizophrenic patients: results of the Hamburg Camberwell Family Interview Study III. *International Journal of Family Psychiatry*, **5**, 84–94.

Kuipers, L. (1992). Expressed Emotion in Europe. *British Journal of Clinical Psychology*, **31**, 429–43.

Kuipers, L. & Bebbington, P. E. (1988). Expressed Emotion research in schizophrenia: theoretical and clinical implications. *Psychological Medicine*, **18**, 893–910.

Kuipers, L. & Westall, J. (1992). The role of facilitated relative groups and voluntary self help groups. In *Principles of Social Psychiatry*, ed. D. Bhugra & J. Leff, pp. 562–72. London: Blackwell.

Kuipers, L., Sturgeon, D., Berkowitz, R. & Leff, J. P. (1983). Characteristics of Expressed Emotion: its relationship to speech and looking in schizophrenic patients and their relatives. *British Journal of Clinical Psychology*, **22**, 257–64.

Kuipers, L., MacCarthy, B., Hurry, J. & Harper, R. (1989). Counselling the relatives of the long term mentally ill. II. A low-cost supportive model. *British Journal of Psychiatry*, **154**, 775–82.

Kuipers, L., Leff, J. & Lam, D. (1992). *Family Work for Schizophrenia: A Practical Guide*. London: Gaskell.

Kuipers, L., Leff, J. & Lam, D. (1993). Training manual for family intervention in schizophrenia. MRC Unit of Community and Social Psychology, London. Unpublished manuscript.

Lam, D. H. (1991). Psychosocial family intervention in schizophrenia: a review of empirical studies. *Psychological Medicine*, **21**, 423–41.

Lam, D., Kuipers, L. & Leff, J. (1993). Family work with patients with schizophrenia. *Journal of Advanced Nursing*, **18**, 233–7.

Leff, J. P., Kuipers, L., Berkowitz, R., Eberlein-Fries, R. & Sturgeon, D. (1982). A controlled trial of social intervention in schizophrenic families. *British Journal of Psychiatry*, **141**, 121–34.

Leff, J. P., Kuipers, L., Berkowitz, R. & Sturgeon, D. (1985). A controlled trial of social intervention in the families of schizophrenic patients: two year follow up. *British Journal of Psychiatry*, **146**, 594–600.

Leff, J., Berkowitz, R., Shavit, N., Strachan, A., Glass, I. & Vaughn, C. (1989). A trial of family therapy versus a relatives' group of schizophrenia. *British Journal of Psychiatry*, **154**, 58–66.

Leff, J., Berkowitz, R., Shavit, N., Strachan, A., Glass, I. & Vaughn, C. (1990). A trial of family therapy versus a relatives' group of schizophrenia: a two year follow-up. *British Journal of Psychiatry*, **157**, 571–7.

MacCarthy, B., Hemsley, D., Schrank-Fernandez, C., Kuipers, L. & Katz, R. (1986). Unpredictability as a correlate of Expressed Emotion in the relatives of schizophrenics. *British Journal of Psychiatry*, **148**, 727–30.

MacCarthy, B., Kuipers, L., Hurry, J., Harper, R. & Lesage, A. (1989). Evaluation of counselling for relatives of the long term adult mentally ill. *British Journal of Psychiatry*, **154**, 768–75.

McCreadie, R. G., Phillips, K., Harvey, J. A., Waldron, G., Stewart, M. &

Baird, D. (1991). The Nithsdale Schizophrenia Surveys. VIII. Do relatives want family intervention and does it help? *British Journal of Psychiatry*, **158**, 110–13.

Miklowitz, D. J., Goldstein, M. J., Doane, J. A., Nuechterlein, K. H., Strachan, A. M., Snyder, K. S. & Magana-Amato, A. (1989). Is Expressed Emotion an index of a transactional process? I. Parent's affective style. *Family Process*, **28**, 153–67.

Moore, E. & Kuipers, L. (1992). Behaviourial correlates of EE in staff–patient interaction. *Social Psychiatry and Psychiatric Epidemiology*, **27**, 298–303.

Moore, E., Ball, R. A. & Kuipers, L. (1992a). Expressed Emotion in staff working with the long-term adult mentally ill. *British Journal of Psychiatry*, **161**, 802–8.

Moore, E., Kuipers, L. & Ball, R. (1992b). Staff–patient relationships in the case of the long-term mentally ill: a content analysis of EE interviews. *Social Psychiatry and Psychiatric Epidemiology*, **27**, 28–34.

Orhagen, T., d'Elia, G. & Gustasfson, P. (1992). Psycho-education and EE. Personal communication.

Priebe, S., Wildgrube, C. & Muller-Oerlinghausen, B. (1992). Expressed Emotion and lithium prophylaxis: a follow-up study. Personal communication.

Rutter, M. L. & Brown, G. W. (1966). The reliability and validity of measures of family life and relationships in families containing a psychiatric patient. *Social Psychiatry*, **1**, 38–53.

Sensky, T., Stevenson, K., Magrill, L. & Petty, R. (1991). Family Expressed Emotion in non-psychiatric illness: adaptation of the Camberwell Family Interview to the families of adolescents with diabetes. *International Journal of Methods in Psychiatric Research*, **1**, 39–51.

Smith, J. & Birchwood, M. J. (1987). Specific and non-specific effects of educational intervention with families living with a schizophrenic relative. *British Journal of Psychiatry*, **150**, 645–52.

Smith, J., Birchwood, M., Cochrane, R. & George, S. (1993). The needs of high and low Expressed Emotion families: a normative approach. *Social Psychiatry and Psychiatric Epidemiology*, **28**, 11–16.

Strachan, A. M. (1986). Family intervention for the rehabilitation of schizophrenia. *Schizophrenia Bulletin*, **12**, 678–98.

Strachan, A. M., Leff, J. P., Goldstein, M. J., Doane, A. & Burrt, C. (1986). Emotional attitudes and direct communication in the families of schizophrenics: a cross-national replication. *British Journal of Psychiatry*, **149**, 279–87.

Strachan, A. M., Feingold, F., Goldstein, M. J., Miklowitz, D. J. & Neuchterlein, K. H. (1989). Is Expressed Emotion an index of a transactional process? II. Patient's coping style. *Family Process*, **28**, 169–81.

Tarrier, N., Barrowclough, C., Vaughn, C., Bamrah, J. S., Porceddu, K., Watts, S. & Freeman, H. (1988). The community management of schizophrenia: a controlled trial of a behaviourial intervention with families to reduce relapse. *British Journal of Psychiatry*, **153**, 532–42.

Tarrier, N., Barrowclough, C., Vaughn, C., Bamrah, J. S., Porceddu, K., Watts, S. & Freeman, H. (1989). Community management of schizophrenia in a two year follow-up of a behaviourial intervention with families. *British Journal of Psychiatry*, **154**, 625–8.

Tomaros, V., Vlachonikolis, I. G., Stefanis, C. N. & Madianos, M. (1988). The effect of individual psychosocial treatment on the family atmosphere of schizophrenic patients. *Social Psychiatry*, **23**, 256–61.

Vaughan, K., Doyle, M., McConathy, N., Blaszczynski, A., Fox, A. & Tarrier, N. (1992). The relationship between relatives' EE and schizophrenic relapse: an Australian replication. *Social Psychiatry and Psychiatric Epidemiology*, **27**, 10–15.

Vaughn, C. & Leff, J. (1976). The measurement of EE in the families of psychiatric patients. *British Journal of Social and Clinical Psychology*, **15**, 157–65.

Watts, S. (1988). A descriptive investigation of the incidence of high EE in staff working with schizophrenic patients in a hospital setting. Unpublished dissertation for Diploma in Clinical Psychology. British Psychological Society.

Wykes, T. (1982). A hostel ward for new long-stay patients. In *Long-term Community Care*, ed. J. K. Wing. *Psychological Medicine Monograph Supplement*, **2**, 59–97.

PART IV

INTERVENTION PRINCIPLES AND RECOMMENDATIONS

13

Social support processes and cognitive therapy

GLENYS PARRY

Therapeutic neglect of social resources and social support processes

It is asking a great deal of individual psychotherapists that they should be attuned to the potential resources in their patient's social network and alert to the implications of research on social support. To become skilful at working with one person intensively, using specific techniques within a specialised formal helping relationship, a therapist must spend many supervised hours with individuals, learning techniques of assessment and intervention. Therapists focus on the individual's development, learning, behaviour, emotional responses, perceptions and thoughts. They see people in the social vacuum of the consulting room, plucked from their usual social environment, building a picture of the patient's interpersonal processes and social world from self-report. This is not the perspective of the epidemiologist, the sociologist or even the community psychologist. Indeed, the patient's kith and kin are often seen by clinicians as part of the problem rather than a social resource (Heller, 1979).

Yet, perhaps increasingly, psychotherapeutic methods are being incorporated into community mental health services and care programmes (see Thornicroft *et al.*, this volume), where there is a requirement both to deliver effective forms of specialist therapies and to ensure that these are ecologically valid, working synergistically with social and community approaches, increasing the willingness or ability of patients to access support from others. To use Pearson's (1990) comparison, this complements approaches which intervene directly within community networks to increase the willingness or ability of actual or potential supporters to offer social support to patients (Attneave, 1969; Gatti & Coleman, 1976; Rueveni, 1979; Jeger & Slotnick, 1982; Lewis & Lewis, 1983).

The focus in this chapter is primarily on cognitive behaviour therapy techniques rather than on psychodynamic approaches, although links are made to cognitive analytic therapy (Ryle, 1990).

A promising feature of cognitive therapies for depression is in reducing the rate of relapse compared with drug treatments (Blackburn *et al.*, 1986; Jacobson, *et al.*, 1993). There is no doubt that depression can be responsive to psychological treatment, but we continue to search for improvements in long-term outcome and further reduction in relapse rates. It is likely that patients who lack social support at the end of therapy will remain vulnerable to further episodes, and less able to maintain their clinical improvement. For example, following cognitive therapy for depressed married women, subsequent depressive symptoms and relapse have been found to be predicted by poorer quality of the marital relationship at the end of therapy and less improvement in the relationship during the course of therapy (Rounsaville *et al.*, 1979; Hooley & Teasdale, 1989). Jacobson and his colleagues (1993) found that where husbands were highly facilitative at the end of therapy, their wives were less likely to have a recurrence of their depression. There is also some evidence that following interpersonal therapy, lower rates of relapse may be related to the therapist having used cognitive instructions and interpersonal tasks (Frank *et al.*, 1991).

This chapter will explore ways in which cognitive therapists are able to help their patients improve the amount and quality of social support available to them by tackling problematic sequences of situational appraisal, schema-activation, cognition, emotion and behaviour which result in potential support being unmobilised, rejected, devalued or abused. Some of the clinical examples are drawn from Parry (1989).

First, it is particularly important for the clinician to take a differentiated *process view* of social support rather than a static, global one (Jung, 1987). Second, whilst recognising the supportive functions of therapy itself, its importance in giving patients new tools in self-understanding and behaviour change and helping them develop new skills in accessing support is emphasised. Third, relating closely to the theoretical issues, techniques of assessing and formulating patient difficulties in mobilising and using social support will be described. These techniques also serve a therapeutic purpose in giving an unusual opportunity to the patient of seeing clearly the size and structure of their social network and the availability within it of different forms of support. Finally, I shall outline ways in which cognitive behavioural approaches can be used to improve social support processes within the individual's network, building on the information gained during assessment, and based on the formulation.

In common with other psychotherapists wishing to link social support theory and research with their therapeutic work, I draw as much on clinical experience as on empirical evidence. I believe it is necessary to do so when developing these links 'to avoid the polar errors of uncritical acceptance and immobilising tentativeness' (Pearson, 1990). However, it should be clear within this account when I am referring to research evidence and when the suggestions are derived from clinical work.

Social support processes and mental health difficulties

We can see that the attractive simplicity of the concept of social support is illusory, referring to a complex array of psychosocial processes reviewed elsewhere in this volume. For example, there are certainly profound differences between the perception of being supported and supportive acts objectively received from friends and family during a crisis (Lakey & Heller, 1988). Feeling supported is a psychological phenomenon, based on an internal representation of self in relation to others (Lakey & Cassady, 1990). Where the self is perceived as unloved or unvalued, there may be a tendency to discount or devalue support. Here we can remember Cobb's early (1976) definition of support in cognitive terms as 'information leading individuals to believe that they are cared for and loved'. People who perceive themselves as lacking social support have been found to be less socially competent than 'high support' individuals, to be more introverted, to have higher trait anxiety, to be intolerant of psychological problems in others, to report unhappier experiences of their childhood relationships with parents, to have more pessimistic views about the benefits of social relationships, to have a passive, uninvolved stance towards life events, to see these as a burden to be endured and to have external locus of control (Sandler & Lakey, 1982; Duckitt, 1984; Ganellen & Blaney, 1984; Sarason *et al.*, 1985, 1986, 1990).

Even for mentally well individuals, the experience of social networks and social support may not be entirely positive. There are at least three potential difficulties which are important for the clinician to understand. First, seeking and receiving help can have self-esteem costs (see also Gilbert, this volume); second, the availability of support can be reduced just when one needs it most; and third, social networks can be a source of stress and personal demand as much as a resource (e.g. see Veiel this volume).

There is evidence that help seeking and using in social psychology laboratory studies is more frequent than in naturalistic studies (Wills, 1992). It seems that people can often persist on their own with failed problem-solving attempts rather than effectively enlist support. The degree to which individuals will be able to mobilise needed help in adversity depends on a number of factors: social network structure (see Brugha, Chapter 1, this volume), the willingness or ability of potential supporters to offer help; and, the focus of this chapter, *individual* barriers to seeking help where beliefs, attitudes and behaviours prevent optimum mobilisation of support. Pearson (1990), giving examples of the latter, lists low self-esteem, fear and suspicion of others, self-centredness, fear of dependency, selfishness, insensitivity, poor personal hygiene, manipulativeness and making unreciprocated demands.

Not seeking help may be a sign of self-reliance but may also be for negative reasons: for fear of rejection, criticism, shame or of being controlled by others (Brown, 1978). Help-seeking, particularly in the absence of major external crisis (such as an illness, bereavement, job loss, divorce), is often seen as a sign of weakness by others (Fisher et al., 1988). However, a crisis legitimises help-seeking. People can reject aid because of negative donor motives, the inability to reciprocate, because of threats to autonomy or because the help is not offered spontaneously, all of which constitute threats to self-esteem (Fisher et al., 1983). All help has the potential for negative messages about the self.

Self-esteem regulation is interwoven with life stress and social support processes (Brown et al., 1986; and Lloyd, this volume). Mental health is not simply having high self-esteem but the ability to regulate self-esteem in the face of negative feedback from others (Mollon & Parry, 1984). Self-definition is a fundamental human motivator and a ubiquitous influence on the cognitive processing of social information. It continues at all times (usually unattended) in relation to feedback from the social world. Social relationships serve self-definition goals. These self-definitions are developmentally derived (see Champion, this volume) and often extremely resistant to change. Severe disruption in self-evaluation can activate negative self-schemata which can lead to ineffective or dysfunctional attempts to cope and negative attitudes to support.

Social exchange and social comparison processes are important here (Buunk & Hoorens, 1992; and Gilbert, this volume), and indeed many of the formulations of equity and social comparison theory can be understood in terms of self-esteem regulation (Fisher et al., 1983). Social support is part of an exchange relationship, where equity theory suggests that if a benefit is given, an equivalent benefit is normally expected in exchange (Walster et al., 1978). This is more true of work relationships and friendships than of kinship, where there are circumstances in which temporary imbalance is tolerable without negative consequences. Mentally well individuals tend to seek a global reciprocity in the amount of support given and received, preferring to believe, if anything, that they give more than they get. But those with a history of mental ill health are often in the position of having asymmetrical helping relationships, seeking and receiving support from others without reciprocation (Gottlieb, 1985). Psychiatric patients have sometimes, by the time they are referred to formal professional help, alienated members of their informal support system (Froland et al., 1979). Self-esteem is not maintained or enhanced by believing that one is getting more support than one is giving, or that one has less support available than other people.

We could also hypothesise that individuals with vulnerable self-esteem are less likely to mobilise help effectively. When offers of support trigger negative self-referent cognitions, affects such as shame, humiliation and embarrassment are aroused. Exposure to these aversive states can be avoided by rejecting (or even sabotaging) offers of support. The evidence on whether low self-esteem individuals do fail to mobilise help is equivocal. Fisher and colleagues (1988) argue that low self-esteem individuals are less threatened by seeking help and approach others for help faster, more frequently and with larger requests. However, it is possible to engage in a high level of inappropriate help-seeking and still to be ineffective at eliciting or using support. Other evidence suggests high self-esteem individuals are better able to mobilise support (Buunk & Hoorens, 1992).

There is also the difficulty of finding one's social support resources diminished, particularly at times of stress. The event itself often directly causes depletion of potential support, as in a bereavement or divorce. Buunk & Hoorens (1992) describe a tendency for people to find those who express negative affect less attractive and to seek affiliation with others who are perceived as either happier or more competent than themselves. Lane & Hobfoll (1992) provide a good example of a negative effect of stress on support in a sample of patients with a severe chronic illness. Both symptoms and resource loss were related to greater anger that alienated supporters. To the extent that support can be reduced just when it is needed most, it is even more important to mobilise and use help which is available as effectively and as appropriately as possible.

These issues point up the subtlety of the cost–benefit analysis which underlies decisions about when to seek help, of what type, from whom and when. A clinician needs to understand the different aspects of support outlined above (and discussed in depth elsewhere in this volume) well enough to be able to help a patient to remedy consistent and repetitive deficiencies in social support which are causing problems, by altering beliefs, thoughts and behaviours that are preventing access to potential social support. In the final part of this chapter problem-solving approaches to increase the amount of support available, without paying an unacceptable price in loss of self-esteem, will be described.

Principles of clinical practice: the empowering intervention

By incorporating ways of improving an individual's ability and willingness to access support, cognitive therapy can take more account of the role of natural kinship and friendship systems in maintaining mental health. This approach is not 'blaming the victim' for deficiencies in social care available to them. By giving people new knowledge and skills in asking for help appropriately, using it well and rewarding others for giving support, it is an empowering intervention, fostering self-efficacy and reducing dependency on professional helpers.

There is no doubt that being in therapy or counselling can in itself be a powerful non-specific experience of emotional and instrumental social support, irrespective of what specific techniques are used, what skills are taught or what new learning takes place. Simply to have the consistent and regular availability of high-quality listening and empathy, with the safe opportunity to confide and to be offered new perspectives, would be a socially supportive experience. It may well be through this generic mechanism that so-called non-specific effects of all therapies are achieved, and specifically the effects of counselling interventions. A discussion of the evidence can be found in the final chapter of this volume by Brugha. However, the cognitive therapist is aiming to use specific techniques to encourage the development of a more effective natural support system, rather than to fill a vacuum in the personal support system of the patient. Accordingly, in the individual support intervention discussed in this chapter, it remains the responsibility of the patient, and not the therapist, to mobilise support from the network.

An important principle underlying this form of intervention is that behavioural assignments should take account of the social norms of the network. Although there is nothing intrinsically difficult about this form of work, it is an area where it is easy to make poorly focused interventions because of the therapist's ignorance about the social ecology the patient inhabits. Support cannot always be artificially 'grafted on' to an existing network; if it is inappropriate it may be rejected (possible examples can be found in the chapters by Dalgard *et al.*, and Barnett & Parker, this volume). Any cognitive behavioural intervention must be planned carefully, on the basis of a social network and support analysis, to lead to a logical extension of natural support or mobilisation of existing potential support. For example, a therapist may be aware that the patient's network is small and restricted in friendship and sources of problem-solving information. A therapy goal about 'joining a club' or 'going to an evening class' may be entirely alien to the values of the patient's network. This does not mean such methods of extending a network are always inappropriate, but that it is always important to formulate clearly what the therapist/patient collaboration is trying to achieve in terms of the existing resources. In this example, it is often better to examine the network for potential 'bridging ties' to other networks. These are weak ties which offer potential access to new friends, activities and sources of information (Granovetter, 1973; Walker *et al.*, 1977).

Factors such as gender, ethnicity, sexual orientation and age should also be taken into account when planning behavioural social support

Table 13.1. *Assessment of social support and networks: examples of measures*

Henderson *et al.* (1980)	Interview Schedule for Social Interaction (ISSI)
Jenkins *et al.* (1981)	Social Stress and Support Interview (SSSI)
Barrera & Ainlay (1983)	Inventory of Socially Supportive Behaviours (ISSB)
Orritt *et al.* (1985)	Perceived Social Network Inventory (PSNI)
Landerman *et al.* (1989)	Duke Social Support Index (DSSI)
Pearson (1990)	Personal Support System Survey (PSSS)

assignments, as they will affect the appropriateness of the intervention. For example, women relative to men tend to engage in more intimate self-disclosure, hold more positive attitudes to seeking and receiving help, seek more and receive more help. Men are more likely to seek companionship support (Burda *et al.*, 1984; Butler *et al.*, 1985).

Assessing social networks and social support

Assessment prior to support-enhancing cognitive therapy is essential. It provides an accurate picture of the patient's social relationships and social support deficits and the relative contribution of the patient's difficulties and the network's failings in creating and maintaining these. Just as important, a good assessment begins a collaborative process of involving the patient in standing back from and examining his or her social world in a way which builds a shared formulation of why there are repeated problems in getting support.

The assessment includes mapping the patient's network and its structural features (such as size, density, proportion of kin), assessing the frequency and types of helping behaviours that the patient has experienced from others in the network, identifying areas of relative strength and deficiency, and pointing up discrepancies between the support available and the patient's perceived social support. To upgrade one's technique in this field requires a knowledge of appropriate measures which facilitate problem formulation during assessment and in monitoring change. More than this, though, the patient learning to use these tools is a central part of the intervention. There are many published scales, questionnaires and interviews which measure different conceptualisations of social support, most of which were designed for research rather than clinical use (see Table 13.1). In practice, the therapist need use only three: a social network analysis, a measure of perceived support and a measure of helping behaviours. These allow patient and therapist to triangulate the social support process for a given individual.

Alternatively, Pearson's (1990) clinically oriented measure (PSSS) covers much of the same ground.

Methods for mapping and analysing a social network are given elsewhere (Maguire, 1983; Parry, 1990; and Brugha, Chapter 14, this volume). Typically, a list of primary network members is elicited by recording the names of all the people the patient meets to talk to regularly. Relatives, friends, neighbours, colleagues and professionals are included, but not those with whom there is only superficial contact. People who are significant but rarely seen can be included – for example, relatives and friends who are geographically separated and those with whom the patient has lost touch as a result of the psychiatric episode. The map of the network is then drawn by establishing for each possible pair of people in the list, whether or not they have a personal relationship, independent of the patient. The frequency of contact with each network member and the network's geographical dispersion are also ascertained.

Next the assessment moves from the structure of the network to the functional nature of the relationships, and the extent of support mobilisation within the network. This aspect is made more precise by using a measure of support of various types received (as distinct from perceived support; for example Barrera & Ainley, 1983) in a prospective diary format, where the patient records each occasion on which a particular type of help is offered or elicited. Examples include 'Provided you with transport' (tangible assistance); 'Taught you how to do something' (directive guidance); 'Comforted you by showing you some physical affection' (non-directive support); 'Did some activity to help you take your mind off things' (positive social interaction).

The social network map is then examined in conjunction with the helping behaviour tally to analyse how much of the network has been mobilised and in which areas, and to pinpoint specific support deficits. Common dysfunctional patterns include (1) very small networks, (2) total lack of one or more type of support, (3) uneven mobilisation, sometimes to the extent that all support is being received from one or two people. The network measure is then used to identify potential sources of help with the patient's current problems and is the basis for planning future behavioural assignments in support elicitation (described in Maguire, 1983). The method of using unexploited resources within a network to help the client solve problems can best be conceptualised as coping assistance (Thoits, 1986) and is the individual therapy equivalent to the community networking interventions I describe elsewhere (Parry, 1988).

In addition to the two assessment tools already described, a measure of perceived support is also of great value, and there are many available. The Orritt et al. (1985) measure is a useful example, partly because it focuses on coping assistance, and also because efforts have been made to establish its psychometric properties. This measure requires the individual to identify those people to whom he or she could turn when under stress or in need of help, then goes on to establish the type of support available from each person, how often given, whether reciprocal and whether the relationship is characterised by negative feelings.

This type of questionnaire is useful primarily as a baseline measure of support perception. The cognitive behavioural intervention is aimed not just at altering the amount of support elicited from the network but at altering the patient's perception of that support. Hence an outcome measure is needed which taps this variable, ideally at the time of referral, as therapy starts, at the end of therapy and at follow-up. In addition, a comparison of the perceptual measure with the objective or behavioural measure (Cohen & Syme, 1985) can be the starting point for identifying dysfunctional cognitive processes about support. For example, the perceptual measure may reveal that the patient perceives a particular network member as relatively unsupportive, when the log of helping behaviours shows that this person has been providing high levels of support which is cognitively devalued by the patient.

At this stage, it is usually possible to incorporate hypotheses about problems in the patient's support system into the initial formulation, which will also include a cognitive formulation of the presenting psychological difficulty. In Cognitive Analytic Therapy (CAT: Ryle, 1990) this formulation is written down in the form of a letter to the patient which is intended to foster a collaborative therapeutic alliance. Whether or not the formulation is shared with the patient, it is vital to establish a rationale for examining and changing thoughts and behaviours in social support transactions which the patient finds credible. The other feature of CAT which is highly congruent with cognitive behaviour therapy is its detailed attention to monitoring and revising circular sequences of cognitive appraisal, schema activation, emotional response, secondary appraisal, formation of intentions, plans and goals (usually unattended), behaviour, consequences of behaviour, which in turn become antecedents for situational reappraisal. The form of assessment process recommended here will often yield very specific examples of repetitive forms of support-destroying sequences where the appraisal of potential support is very negative, where although the goal may be to receive support the expectations may be unrealistic, and where potential supporters are unaccessed, rebuffed, treated badly or unrewarded.

One would not wish to claim that the individual approach is the treatment of choice in all situations where there are manifest difficulties with social support processes. Table 13.2, showing social support difficulties relating to mental health problems and the appropriate intervention for remedial work, makes the point that cognitive therapy geared to social support improvement is only one of a number of strategies.

Table 13.2. *Assessed social support difficulties and possible interventions*

Assessed difficulty	Possible interventions
Network deficiences: small, fragmented, low density	Retribalisation; self-help groups: voluntary befriending agencies; community support
Routine 'everday' support is rejected/devalued/unperceived	Monitoring and challenging self/other cognitions
Failure to mobilise support following crisis; inability to signal needs; inappropriate choice of supporter; rejection of offered support	Analysis of support needs and potential supply in network; functional analysis of problematic cognition/action sequences from self-monitoring; support skills enhancement

Helping individuals to improve their social support processes

Therapy continues with a systematic examination of the individual's perception of being unsupported and identifies repetitive social interactions in which support is being devalued, rejected, abused or unmobilised. Fundamental to both aspects of the work is precision in identifying the specific ways, for this particular individual, that supportive acts are being interpreted as threatening self-esteem.

From the diary-keeping format of the helping behaviour inventory, the therapist is usually able to show the patient that there are members of the network who are not providing support, or that all the supporting rests on one or two individuals. Gaps in the pattern of support (e.g. no companionship support) have also been identified. This leads easily to a self-monitoring assignment where the frequency of specific problems is recorded. No behavioural change is asked for at this stage, but an accurate description of the behaviour is aimed for. Examples of this are given in Table 13.3.

The patient will need guidance on how to record all instances of potential help, even if he or she perceived the 'offer' as unhelpful, insincere, inadequate, etc. It also takes practice to write a clear description of one's own behaviour in these circumstances. Therapists are advised to complete the ISSB or a similar measure, as a diary, followed by this self-monitoring exercise in their own lives, as this makes it easier to help patients learn to self-monitor.

The self-monitoring exercise will reveal a pattern of dysfunctional behaviours in response to potential support. These will be tackled by behavioural skills training but, in addition, dysfunctional beliefs about the social support process should be examined. It is logical for this work

Table 13.3. *Examples of potential help and dysfunctional responses*

Potential for help	My response
My son J. did the washing up but he didn't do it properly	I was very angry with him and I had to do it all again myself
Mum asked if I needed anything from the shops whilst she was down there	I said not to bother because it would make too much for her to carry
Went to see M. (ex-colleague) and spoke about my problems since I lost my job. He said 'It takes time you know'	I stopped talking about how I felt because he didn't understand

to be done prior to graded behavioural assignments, although in practice the two phases often overlap and proceed in parallel.

Statements such as those below (taken from clinical sessions) will probably be familiar to most therapists:

> If he loved me, I wouldn't have to ask him to help me.
> I can't tell my [adult] children about my operation because it would worry them.
> Well, she did offer to babysit but I know she didn't really mean it.
> It's embarrassing to admit I can't cope.
> He only said he would take me out because he feels sorry for me.
> I feel bad going round to her house yet again because I can't give anything to her.
> You are only helping me because it's your job.

Here we see processes of attribution (see also Brewin, this volume) and equity beliefs which can be challenged successfully and the consequences of an alternative belief tested out. Each remark arises from a personal belief held by the patient about interpersonal relationships (see Ryle, 1990, for an account of these). All these beliefs lead to support being devalued or rejected, not out of wilful self-defeating wrongheadedness, but as a *self-protective* strategy. In my experience, the therapeutic alliance is strengthened if this is understood and acknowledged by the therapist. The messages about the self implied by admitting one cannot cope, accepting that someone feels sorry for one, or having to ask for help are identified, challenged, and alternatives tested. These alternatives may involve, for example, discovering the intrinsic value of the support regardless of the motives of the donor, accepting that less than perfect care is a normal aspect of reality, learning to tolerate self-consciousness and embarrassment, or the legitimate use of gratitude as payment in social transactions. Over a period of weeks, patients can learn from their own experience the value of reciprocating support or of rewarding others for giving support. It is very common for patients to feel that they have no way of reciprocating or of rewarding their supporters, but this is rarely the case in fact, since patients tend to underestimate how rewarding it is

Table 13.4. *Example of monitoring intermediate thoughts between potential help and response*

Potential help	Automatic thoughts	My response
Went to see M. and spoke about my problems since I lost my job. He said 'It takes time you know'	What the hell does he know about it? He just wants to get rid of me. He thinks I'm a wimp	I stopped talking about how I felt because he didn't understand

for supporters to have a positive response to appropriate help. Some patients who have early maladaptive schemata about personal relationships, which lead them to expect either abusive neglect or caring rescue from their supporters, will need specific help to value everyday supportive acts rather than rejecting and punishing others for not offering total rescue.

The use of the self-monitoring exercise allows detailed examination of particular instances of dysfunctional support behaviour and the attendant cognitions. When the behavioural recording is established, the patient can be asked to record the automatic thoughts which precede the behaviour, as in Beck's method (Beck *et al.*, 1979). One of the examples above is used as an illustration of this in Table 13.4. Alternatives to these thoughts are then examined with the patient, using conventional techniques of cognitive therapy.

Cognitive treatment for the present problem, for example depression, should precede the social support intervention, so that the patient is already familiar with the general technique. In practice, during cognitive therapy for depression, anxiety, personality difficulty or obsessional symptoms, examples of dysfunctional support sequences are volunteered and monitored by the patient, so that it becomes easier to pay them more systematic attention having become aware of the issues in clinical application of social support research findings.

As work on the individual's personal beliefs and automatic thoughts proceeds, new behaviours can be tested within the network. An excellent discussion of this issue by Winefield (1984) is recommended, as she describes ways in which new skills in eliciting support can be taught using behavioural assignments. She notes that traditional social skills teaching is unlikely to be helpful, and that behavioural interventions should focus on teaching patients (1) the social norms for intimacy and its reciprocation, (2) how much and when to complain, (3) how to attend to and display interest in the other person and (4) how to reward the other for helping by responding positively. It would be possible to do this in a group teaching format.

In individual therapy, the behavioural assignments are undertaken after behavioural self-monitoring and examination of the cognitive basis of interpersonal behaviour. I have found it best to introduce the points made by Winefield in the context of the examples brought by the patient during self-monitoring. Alternative responses can take place in the session, first by the patient (with prompts) thinking of an alternative, then acting it out in a role play with the therapist. Role reversal is useful here, with the therapist playing the patient's part and the patient acting as the would-be helper. Another of the examples given above all serve as an illustration:

Offers of help
Mum asked if I needed anything from the shops whilst she was down there.

My thoughts
She doesn't really want to help me. She thinks I'm lazy. If she really means it she will insist that it isn't any trouble.

My response
I said not to bother because it would to too much for her to carry.

Alternative thoughts
She's offering some help which I need. I would do the same for her.

Alternative response
Oh thanks Mum, that's great. I need some bread.

This is a simple example and in practice most are more complex, but the same principles apply. It is better to start with simple examples so that the patient can practice support elicitation responses, before giving more difficult assignments. Examples of these include when it is not appropriate to ask for support. This is an example of a support elicitation attempt which failed:

My sister said I was being very selfish not going to see Dad as I lived much nearer to him than she did and I was putting her in an impossible position. I said she didn't understand how upset he made me and I wish she would see my point of view.

A simple acknowledgement of the sister's feelings would have been more useful as there is a request for expressive support in her statement. Instead the patient responds with a counter-request, which violates the social norm of reciprocation and leads to a deterioration in the quality of support available to her in future from this sister. It becomes possible for the patient to give a different response only when she sees that she is repetitively acting in a way which always leads to a negative outcome for her, rather than meeting her goal of being understood by her sister.

Summary

In delivering conventional cognitive therapy for depression or anxiety, it is possible to use social network and support assessment tools to foster the client's awareness of ways in which he or she fails to perceive or mobilise support within social relationships. Dysfunctional sequences of appraisal, schema activation, cognition and behaviour can be identified, monitored and, with practice, revised.

References

Attneave, C. N. (1969). Therapy in tribal settings and urban network intervention. *Family Process*, **8**, 192–210.

Barrera, M. & Ainley, S. L. (1983). The structure of social support: a conceptual and empirical analysis. *Journal of Community Psychology*, **11**, 133–43.

Beck, A. T., Rush, A. T., Shaw, B. F. & Emery, G. (1979). *Cognitive Therapy for Depression*. New York: Guilford Press.

Blackburn, I. M., Eunson, K. M. & Bishop, S. (1986). A two year naturalistic follow up of depressed patients treated with cognitive therapy, pharmacotherapy and a combination of both. *Journal of Affective Disorders*, **10**, 67–75.

Brown, B. (1978). Social and psychological correlates of help-seeking behaviour among urban adults. *American Journal of Community Psychology*, **6**, 425–39.

Brown, G. W., Andrews, B., Harris, T., Adler, Z. & Bridge, L. (1986). Social support, self-esteem and depression. *Psychological Medicine*, **16**, 813–31.

Burda, P. C. Jr, Vaux, A. & Schill T. (1984). Social support resources: variation across sex and sex role. *Personality and Social Psychology Bulletin*, **10**, 119–26.

Butler, T. Giordano, S. & Neren, S. (1985). Gender & sex role attributes as predictors of utilization of natural support systems during personal stress events. *Sex Roles*, **8**, 721–32.

Buunk, B. P. & Hoorens, V. (1992). Social support and stress: the role of social comparison and social exchange processes. *British Journal of Clinical Psychology*, **31**, 445–57.

Cobb, S. (1976). Social support as a moderator of life stress. *Psychosomatic Medicine*, **38**, 300–14.

Cohen, S. & Syme, S. L. (1985). Issues in the study and application of social support. In *Social Support and Health*, ed. S. Cohen & S. L. Syme. Orlando, Fl: Academic Press.

Duckitt, J. (1984). Social support, personality and the prediction of psychological distress: an interactionist approach. *Journal of Clinical Psychology*, **40**, 1199–205.

Fisher, J. D., Nadler, A. & De Paulo, B. M. (eds.) (1983). *New Directions in Helping*, vol. 1, *Recipient Reactions to Aid*. New York: Academic Press.

Fisher, J. D., Goff, B. A., Nadler, A. & Chinsky, J. M. (1988). Social psychological influences on help seeking and support from peers. In *Marshaling Social Support: Formats, Processes and Effects* ed. B. H. Gottlieb, pp. 267–304. Newbury Park, CA: Sage.

Frank, E., Kupfer, D. J., Wagner, E. F., McEachran, A. B. & Cornes, C. (1991). Efficacy of interpersonal psychotherapy as a maintenance treatment of recurrent depression. *Archives of General Psychiatry*, **48**, 1053–9.

Froland, C., Brodsky, G., Olson, M. & Stewart, L. (1979). Social support and social adjustment: implications for mental health professionals. *Community Mental Health Journal*, **15**, 82–93.

Ganellen, R. J. & Blaney, P. H. (1984). Hardiness and social support as moderators of the effects of life stress. *Journal of Personality and Social Psychology*, **47**, 156–63.

Gatti, F. & Coleman, C. (1976). Community network therapy: an approach to aiding families with troubled children. *American Journal of Orthopsychiatry*, **46**, 608–17.

Gottlieb, B. (1985). Theory into practice: issues that surface in planning interventions which mobilize support. In *Social Support: Theory, Research and Applications*, ed. I. G. Sarason & B. R. Sarason. Boston: Martinus Nijhoff.

Granovetter, M. S. (1973). The strength of weak ties. *American Journal of Sociology*, **78**, 1360–72.

Heller, K. (1979). The effects of social support: prevention and treatment implications. In *Maximising Treatment gains: Transfer Enhancement in Psychotherapy*, ed. A. P. Goldstein & F. H. Kanfer. New York: Academic Press.

Henderson, S., Duncan-Jones, P., Byrne, D. G. & Scott, R. (1980). Measuring social relationships: the Interview Schedule for Social Interaction. *Psychological Medicine*, **10**, 723–34.

Hooley, J. M. & Teasdale, J. D. (1989). Predictors of relapse in unipolar depressives: expressed emotion, marital distress and perceived criticism. *Journal of Abnormal Psychology*, **98**, 229–35.

Jacobson, N. S., Fruzzetti, A. E., Dobson, K. Whisman, M. & Hops, H. (1993). Couple therapy as a treatment for depression. II. The effects of relationship quality and therapy on depressive relapse. *Journal of Consulting and Clinical Psychology*, **61**, 516–19.

Jeger, A. M. & Slotnick, R. S. (eds.) (1982). *Community Mental Health and Behavioral Ecology: A Handbook of Theory, Research, and Practice*. New York: Plenum Press.

Jenkins, R., Mann, A. & Belsey, E. (1981). The background description and use of a short interview to assess stress and social support. *Social Science and Medicine, Part E*, **10**, 404–15.

Jung, J. (1987). Towards a social psychology of social support. *Basic and Applied Social Psychology*, **8**(1/2), 57–83.

Lakey, B. & Cassady, P. B. (1990). Cognitive processes in perceived social support. *Journal of Personality and Social Psychology*, **59**, 337–43.

Lakey, B. & Heller, K. (1988). Social support from a friend, perceived support, and social problem solving. *American Journal of Community Psychology*, **16**, 811–24.

Landerman, R., George, L. K. & Campbell, R. T. (1989). Alternative models of the stress buffering hypothesis. *American Journal of Community Psychology*, **17**, 625–42.

Lane, C. & Hobfoll, S. E. (1992). How loss affects anger and alienates potential supporters. *Journal of Consulting and Clinical Psychology*, **60**, 935–42.

Lewis, J. A. & Lewis, M. (1983). *Community Counselling: A Human Services Approach*. New York: Wiley.

Maguire, L. (1983). Networking with individuals. In *Understanding Social Networks*. Beverley Hills, CA: Sage.

Mollon, P. & Parry, G. (1984). The fragile self: narcissistic disturbance and the protective function of depression. *British Journal of Medical Psychology*, **57**, 137–45.

Orritt, E. J., Paul, S. C. & Behrman, J. A. (1985). The Perceived Support Network Inventory. *American Journal of Community Psychology*, **13**, 565–82.

Parry, G. (1988). Mobilizing social support. In *New Developments in Clinical Psychology*, vol. 2, ed. F. N. Watts, pp. 83–104. Chichester: BPS Books/Wiley.

Parry, G. (1989). Cognitive behaviour therapy in the social context. In *Annual Series of European Research in Behaviour Therapy*, vol 3, ed. P. Emmelkamp. Amsterdam: Swets.

Parry, G. (1990). *Coping with Crises*. Leicester: BPS Books.

Pearson, R. E. (1990). *Counselling and Social Support: Perspectives and Practice*. Newbury Park, CA: Sage.

Rounsaville, B. J., Weissman, M. M., Prusoff, B. A. & Herceg-Baron, R. L. (1979). Marital disputes and treatment outcome in depressed women. *Comprehensive Psychiatry*, **20**, 483–90.

Rueveni, U. (1979). *Networking Families in Crisis: Intervention Strategies with Families and Social Networks*. New York: Human Services.

Ryle, A. (1990). *Cognitive Analytic Therapy: Active Participation in Change. A New Integration in Brief Psychotherapy*. Chichester: Wiley.

Sandler, I. N. & Lakey, B. (1982). Locus of control as a stress moderator: the role of control perceptions and social support. *American Journal of Community Psychology*, **10**, 65–80.

Sarason, B. R., Sarason, I. G., Hacker, T. A. & Basham, R. B. (1985). Concomitants of social support: social skills, physical attractiveness and gender. *Journal of Personality and Social Psychology*, **49**, 469–80.

Sarason, I. G., Sarason, B. R. & Shearin, E. N. (1986). Social support as an individual difference variable. *Journal of Personality and Social Psychology*, **50**, 845–55.

Sarason, I. G., Sarason, B. R. & Pierce, C. R. (1990). Social support: the search for theory. *Journal of Social and Clinical Psychology*, **1**, 133–47.

Thoits, P. A. (1986). Social support as coping assistance. *Journal of Consulting and Clinical Psychology*, **54**, 416–23.

Walker, K., MacBride, A. & Vachon, M. (1977). Social support networks and the crisis of bereavement. *Social Science and Medicine*, **11**, 35–41.

Walster, E. G., Walster, W. & Berscheid, E. (1978). *Equity: Theory and Research*. Boston: Allyn & Bacon.

Wills, T. A. (1992). The helping process in the context of personal relationships. In *Helping and Being Helped: Naturalistic Studies*, ed. S. Spacapan & S. Oskamp, chap. 2. The Claremont Symposium on Applied Social Psychology. Newbury Park, CA: Sage.

Winefield, H. R. (1984). The nature and elicitation of social support: some implications for the helping professions. *Behavioural Psychotherapy*, **12**, 318–30.

14

Social support and psychiatric disorder: recommendations for clinical practice and research

Traolach S. Brugha

In this, the concluding chapter of this volume, intervention, both its practice and its evaluation, will be discussed further. Evidence that *social support* influences psychiatric disorder and thus *outcome*, which was discussed in the first and intervening chapters, will be reconsidered throughout this final chapter in relation to the present and future scope for the evaluation and practice of intervention work. Second, building on the previous chapter, the general field of *psychotherapy research* will be considered, including studies that evaluate psychosocial interventions, in order to consider the relevance this body of work may have to the topic of social support interventions, and because most evidence for clinically proven effectiveness, and thus treatment recommendation, comes from this field. Third, the *lessons* available at present for current clinical practice and for future directions in clinical evaluation research, directly addressing the social support hypothesis, will be considered. This section will cover the extensive variety of *psychosocial interventions*, many of them not yet formally evaluated, ranging from community interventions to individual (traditional) psychotherapeutic interventions, which may exert benefits through positive alterations in the provision and the use made of social support to individual client/patients. Some principles that can currently be tentatively set down for *clinical practice* and *intervention* planning and evaluation will be discussed in the final section.

In the first chapter of this volume I summarised evidence concerning the relationship between social support and psychiatric disorder. The topics covered included: individual, environmental and heritable influences on social support; positive and negative aspects of support; reciprocal social support processes. The importance of individual factors and particularly that of self-esteem and of environmental factors such as the rank and status of actual or potential supporters has consistently emerged in the intervening chapters. Particular emphasis was given to the much more extensively research topic of *depression* and also to studies on psychiatric patients employing clinical measures. Recent new evidence, mainly from prospective cohort studies, was covered more comprehensively, because of the greater power of these studies to refute causal hypotheses. Previous more detailed reviews by this author were also referred to (Brugha 1988 to 1922). The present chapter is also based partly on earlier discussions of the topic of intervention (Brugha, 1991a, 1993).

The first chapter deferred discussion of the topic of psychotherapy, a subject given relatively little attention in the social support literature. There are two reasons for devoting some time to this topic. The first is that psychotherapy may indeed make use of concepts and mechanisms that are central to the social support model. This point has been discussed specifically by surprisingly few writers. Second, given the paucity of social support intervention studies among patients and the now extensive and rapidly growing psychotherapy evaluation literature, much of it demonstrating real clinical advantages that have been experimentally confirmed, it is possible that we may *already* have in these treatments effective ways of reducing social support deficits, albeit by working with and through the patient him- or herself, as discussed in Parry (this volume). This section is also offered in the hope that it will stimulate researchers to devise ways to test this suggestion more formally in future evaluation projects and, where it exists, to publish existing data that have not yet appeared in the scientific literature.

Psychotherapy evaluation research

There is a somewhat surprising gulf between workers who have contributed to our empirical knowledge about the association between social factors and psychiatric disorder and those who concern themselves with psychosocial treatments. Some notable exceptions to this will be mentioned in this section. The literature in this area is devoted principally to non-psychotic disorders. In a recent volume summarising evidence on psychological aspects of depression, Gotlib & Hammen (1992) have devoted a chapter to behavioural and interpersonal approaches to the treatment of depression. Of course clinical practice and epidemiologically based scientific research are both highly absorbing and demanding areas of activity; it is hardly surprising that so few people are able to find the time to master the problems that need to be understood and worked on in each of the two areas.

Some contributors to the empirical psychotherapy and social treatment evaluation literature have discussed this gulf also. For example, Beckham (1990), in summarising his own views about the psychotherapy of depression evaluation literature, critically tackled the so-called primary premise of therapy, namely the assertion that a treatment achieves symptomatic remission by alteration of a targeted aetiological variable (cognition, interpersonal functioning, etc.). In his view the primary premises for psychotherapies of depression have not been proven. Shepherd (1993) has recently returned to the closely related and fundamental question of treatment *specificity*, urging further work to be conducted on the nature of the *placebo* effect in treatment trials. The failure to demonstrate specific differences in treatment effectiveness in comparative studies has been debated in the psychotherapy evaluation literature (Stiles *et al.*, 1986). The present author would argue that, just as in very specific forms of anxiety disorder highly effective, specific and efficient behavioural interventions have developed (Hawton *et al.*, 1990), which are at least, to some degree, related to 'targeted aetiological variables', one might expect similar *specific* effects to emerge from similarly devised interventions in depression.

Although behavioural, cognitive behavioural and interpersonal psychotherapies all have stated rationales, one does not sense, in reading the literature, that there is a constant cycle of activity designed to feed back to clinicians and therapists (and treatment manual designers) the more recent and consistent empirical and epidemiological findings of possible causal processes in these areas. However, there are some exceptions. Methods of social intervention (Kuipers *et al.*, 1992; Falloon, 1988) and psychotherapies based upon interpersonal (Klerman *et al.*, 1984; Gotlib & Hammen, 1992), dyadic (Hahlweg *et al.*, 1988) and family aspects of interaction can be particularly recommended to readers interested in a more detailed discussion than will be covered below.

Social support and the nature of interpersonal therapies

A number of authors have suggested that a fundamental component of psychotherapy is the provision of social relationship or social support resources (Henderson, 1977; Cross *et al.*, 1982; Winefield, 1987). Holmes (1993) has discussed the importance of attachment theory, which may be said to provide a biological basis for psychotherapy. In his well-known volume *Persuasion and Healing*, also referred to by Beckham (1990), the American psychiatrist Jerome Frank argued that most therapies have in common a caring therapist–patient relationship (Frank & Frank, 1991). According to Frank, psychotherapy counteracts demoralisation by providing an emotionally charged confiding relationship with a helping person; a healing setting; a rational conceptual scheme or myth; and a ritual.

The present author would propose that in order to foster 'an emotionally charged confiding relationship with a helping person', which is a fundamental statement of the nature of a supportive dyad, the participants require a special motivation to overcome their resistance to doing so. For the therapist, apart from the material gain and enhanced status that therapy brings, a belief in the importance of his or her own specific skills must surely heighten the intensity of interest taken in the client – hence the importance of technique, a rational conceptual scheme and so on. The client must at least not be a 'non-believer', although it may be sufficient that there is an 'expert' or person of higher rank present taking this unique interest in him or her. For therapy to have an enduring effect, the client/patient's experience of this rewarding relationship must lead to behavioural change elsewhere in the family and peer network. There is no scope properly to develop this (possibly not very original) suggestion much further here, although some selective evidence that may be relevant will be discussed below.

In a small Randomised Controlled Trial (RCT) comparing insight-oriented therapy and behaviour therapy (Cross *et al.*, 1982), patients were asked questions about the process of therapy. Outcome was essentially the same in the two groups, as found in most other similar trials. Interest focused, also as it often does, therefore, on the *process measures*. Clients were asked, in hindsight (e.g. 4 months after completing treatment), what factors were important in contributing to improvement, focusing on aspects of technique and focusing on the therapist, or relational aspects. Relational aspects clearly stood out in the comments of patients who received insight-oriented therapy. Relational aspects were also apparent in the behaviour therapy group; clients did not rate technical aspects of treatment as important in either setting. Interestingly, clients did not place any value on the efforts by the therapists to influence other people (e.g. family, friends or employer). The authors concluded that their study gave partial support to the idea that relational factors are viewed as underlying improvements, regardless of the specific treatment method employed.

Links between psychotherapy and social support

Winefield (1987) has discussed parallels and differences in the helping process linking psychotherapy and social support specifically. Both provide esteem enhancement and both provide informational support. Both involve a helping and close relationship. Crucial differences include the relative expertise of therapist and 'natural helper', that therapy has to be paid for and that, from the standpoint of attachment theory, the professional role implies a greater emotional distance.

Given the possibility that social support and psychotherapy share these commonalities, we may ask a number of questions. What evidence is there that the clinical effectiveness of psychotherapies can be explained by the enhanced provision of 'social support' to the patient, either directly by the therapist or indirectly by others through the way therapy alters the interpersonal behaviours and/or cognitive behaviours of the patient? And, in addition, what specific skills of therapists are of therapeutic importance and what ingredients of training are essential? Answers to such questions might help us to judge whether existing effective therapies represent, in part at least, positive social support interventions, albeit by another name.

Marziali (1987) developed a social support measure for use with psychiatric patients entering and completing psychotherapy. A self-completion questionnaire was developed with scales covering the number of friends and close attachments available, and an estimate of satisfaction with these people. The structure and content were similar to that of the Interview Schedule for Social Intervention (ISSI: Henderson *et al.*, 1981), also briefly described earlier (Brugha and Barnett & Parker, this volume). Forty-two patients undergoing brief psychotherapy completed the scales, before and after treatment. All four major scales (satisfaction and availability of friends and of an intimate, respectively) were significantly altered, with three of four showing medium improvements in effect size. The authors concluded that this open study showed that psychotherapy leads to improvements in levels of social support. Clearly an open study such as this is capable of a number of interpretations, but the study did 'fail' to show that levels of social support are not altered by such a treatment.

To conclude this section, it is apparent that a small number of workers have begun to publish articles which address the notion that psycho-therapy and social support are interrelated and, more controversially, perhaps interdependent topics. A case has been made for taking greater account of the findings of epidemiological research and thus developing and evaluating more theory-driven interventions. In the next section specific individual and other forms of psychotherapy will be referred to in the light of these background comments, and their relevance to the topic of support interventions will be argued further.

Specific psychosocial interventions in the wider community

As this book begins with a social and environmental perspective and from there introduces the (perhaps) equally important individual perspective, we shall begin with a discussion of interventions at a wider community level and then gradually return to the topic of the last section, including the potentially promising field of psychotherapy research, as it relates to interpersonal functioning. The specificity and precision of interventions will be seen to increase as we move towards family, marital and individual approaches. A particularly important aspect of this has been the development of intervention and *treatment manuals*, essential for both evaluation of and training in these techniques.

Community-based and 'macrosocial' interventions

An attempt to appraise the effectiveness of case-level (client-centred) and community-level social care has been provided in a review of the (mainly British) social work literature by Goldberg (1987). Whilst it was possible to identify an example of a case-level evaluation that showed measurable improvements in later community survival (i.e. outcome) for identifiable individuals, it proved more difficult to find such evidence in community-oriented practice. The latter (structural intervention) may have the advantage of influencing earlier referral of individuals at risk (presumably an analogue of population screening), but a well-established principle in the quality of care literature states that reliable indications of benefit are more likely to come from process 'outcome' data on individuals (Brugha & Lindsay, 1994).

Rook (1984) has discussed ways in which the *community environment* and the *structure* of the working environment can be modified so as to enhance and facilitate more social interaction for the lonely. Similarly, 'unintentional network building' can follow from projects that give people who are isolated in the community, a task that can only be carried out by cooperation, sharing and thus meeting in the form of new social groups, as in groups with charitable and voluntary tasks (Rook, 1984).

The role of the 'community worker', acting in a specific neighbourhood (or a cluster of physically related residential units) is discussed by Parry (1988), who also contrasts such formal interventions with the potential contribution to community functioning of 'natural helpers' such as bartenders and hairdressers. Recently Milne & Mullin (1987) have reported on a successful, structured training programme in which hairdressers were trained in the provision of social support to their customers. The programme was evaluated experimentally and its success indicated by enhanced experimental group customers' ratings of the perceived helpfulness of their hairdressers. Mother-to-mother befriender schemes in Great Britain in Leicester (Homestart) and subsequently in South London (Newpin) have also been described by Van der Eyken and Pound et al. (in Newton & Craig, 1991) and by Cox et al. (1991). These studies, inevitably, do not incorporate refined methods for identifying those most likely to benefit from intervention. They rely on a considerable level of altruistic behaviour by others. Unfortunately, such altruism may be less likely to be found in communities that have been damaged by poverty, unemployment and violence, although they may have the greatest potential need for such interventions.

In a review article on social and *community intervention*, Heller (1990) makes the point that certain social contexts and community structures may enhance support; an example given is that of providing unemployed men with work, which may be viewed as far more 'supportive' than providing a 'support group'. This article is also important for arguing that enhancing individual skills and competencies may not be of value because, so often, strong adverse cultural norms or adverse social conditions serve to maintain undesirable behaviour. This particularly seems to apply to those who because of their gender, ethnic status, age or low socio-economic group status are prevented from using what would otherwise be more effective interpersonal strategies. This then leads to a call for research (and in due course interventions and new government-backed social policies) at the macro-community level rather than at the micro-personal level. The methodological problems, not to mention the implications, for true community-based interventions are considerable.

Self-help groups and voluntary organisations

Although self-help groups have emerged in order to assist both treatment-seeking and 'normal' or treatment-non-seeking persons in the general population, the topic will be considered here as part of the subject matter of community interventions. A number of descriptions of informal and *voluntary* support systems for the chronically mentally ill living in the community have been described by Mitchell & Birley (1983) and by Cutler & Beigel (1978). Readers interested in a more detailed overview of this topic should consult Kuipers & Westall (1993) in order to obtain the perspective of those involved in developing large, national self-help organisations, devoted to major diagnostic categories including schizophrenia, manic depressive illness and autism.

Self-help groups have been with us for many decades but without serious attempts to evaluate their effectiveness (Galanter, 1988). A small number of controlled studies incorporating the concept of self-help, or mutual help, have appeared in the literature (Galanter, 1988; Marmar *et al.*, 1988; Spiegel *et al.*, 1981), with the latter two studies employing randomisation procedures. Although each group included therapists, in the study by Spiegel and colleagues, members were encouraged to support one another both within and between meetings. Members were psychologically distressed women with advanced breast cancer; a major theme of the meetings was the topic of death. Social isolation, problems of communication with physicians and the impact on the marriage and family were also important themes. Countering isolation was one of the aims of the group. Psychological outcome, including improved mood, was significantly better in the intervention cases as compared with the controls (Spiegel *et al.*, 1981) (although mortality was initially slightly higher in the intervention group). A long-term follow-up analysis showed that the group members had significantly enhanced survival (Spiegel *et al.*, 1989). In another study, 61 of 76 women with prominent symptoms of anxiety or depression were randomised to either brief dynamic psychotherapy ($n = 31$) or to a mutual-help group treatment (Marmar et al., 1988). In terms of both symptomatic and social functioning, outcome was essentially the same in the two groups.

In the first chapter of this volume I described and discussed a series of experimental social support programme evaluations by *community psychologists* (Sullivan et al., 1992; Heller et al., 1991; Price et al., 1992). The target populations were, respectively, elderly isolated women, physically abused women and the recently unemployed. Two of the studies produced the expected experimental outcomes, with the last showing clear evidence for a treatment effect on depression prevention in the recently unemployed (Price et al., 1992). However, all of these studies raise questions about the extent to which social support effects can be studied specifically, in much the same way as has been discussed earlier in this chapter in relation to the psychotherapy evaluation literature. This evidence will be returned to shortly in a discussion of the sorts of supportive interventions that could or should be specific in future intervention work.

From primary detection/prevention to treatment for conspicuous attenders

In spite of some encouraging evidence for their benefits, it is hard to know whether such community-based interventions and policies could be demonstrated to be of value to those seen in psychiatric clinical practice. At attempt to evaluate their introduction, or their transfer to populations that include the group of primary concern in this volume, might at best provide indirect evidence for their effectiveness, by monitoring case register prevalence rates of psychiatric disorder or possibly other *outcome indicators* (Jenkins, 1990) during the period of intervention. By implication, it would be necessary to show that those community characteristics that appear to be damaging to mental health (for example stigma against the mentally ill, famine, war, or other physical and social environmental problems: Freeman, 1985) when ameliorated through specific community-level interventions, result in health-enhancing outcomes for community members.

In relation to physical health of the community, cigarette smoking is a good example (Lichtenstein et al., 1991) because of the importance of changing the values and beliefs of a society (and thus also of politicians) before such an epidemic can be eradicated. Nevertheless, improvements to the community and social environment are arguably worthwhile in themselves and should not have to await proof of their clinical value. The interest that politicians and administrators have taken in the work of community psychologists, and the potential value of community psychology methods in conducting social action initiatives, has been discussed elsewhere by Jason (1991).

'Community' support systems and community mental health

The further use here of the term 'community' may be misleading. The move from *institutional* to community care has developed more for historical, economic and governmental policy reasons than because of scientifically proven evidence for efficacy of care – a large topic which cannot be covered here. The intention and policy aims of such 'support systems' or, more correctly, *services* is to identify and solve medical, psychological and social problems, which are then managed at an *individual* or *family* level. The community is altered in the sense that individuals who formerly resided, and were kept occupied, in large isolated institutions (or separate communities) are expected to, but not always assisted to, function within the wider community, making use of the same housing, shopping, leisure and other amenities that are used by the wider society. This is in contrast to intervention with (non-consulting) needy or deprived communities at a macro-social level, as discussed briefly in the previous paragraphs.

The President's Commission on Mental Health (1978) in the United States promoted a policy to foster natural *support systems* in the wider community. The topic takes us into a much more general aspect of community and social psychiatry, discussed elsewhere (Bennett & Morris, 1983). The term 'system' is intended to denote the principle that provision for the physical, social and psychological needs of individuals who are ill or disabled, and therefore at risk of being unable to fend for themselves, is well organised, managed and coordinated. The systematic assessment of such needs and the principles involved in meeting them at an individual, couple or family level will be discussed further in the final section, in which we shall return to the topic of community mental health services. The coordination and delivery of such systems of care is also the subject of the chapter by Thornicroft *et al.* in this volume.

Day care and outreach services

Although the term 'day care' is a reference to a service setting and not a specific intervention, the flexibility and scope for social contact it provides deserve particular mention here (Lavender & Holloway, 1988). Elsewhere in this volume there is a discussion of case management and of services reaching out into the community, which are designed to help long-term patients improve their general level of functioning and their personal social networks (Thornicroft *et al.*, this volume). In a recent study on men and women with severe and persistent mental illness, in which improvements were noted in client involvement in their peer social milieu, factors within the individual were largely irrelevant in explaining the extent to which they became more socially involved (Levin & Brekke, 1993). However, increased involvement by clients was related to their perceptions of the support and of the clarity of the expectations and rules laid down by staff in the setting.

Social network interventions

Social network intervention has been discussed in the journal *Family Process* by several workers (Speck & Rueveni, 1969; Erickson, 1984) and in a more detailed volume by Rueveni (1979). Erickson's paper is a useful source of additional reference material, helpfully discussed. The paper by Speck & Rueveni is essentially a detailed description of the problems and the therapeutic sessions that took place with a 'schizophrenic family' [*sic*]. Apart from the family, extended kin, neighbours and friends of the family were invited to participate. The aim of therapy was to strengthen the wider network of social relationships and loosen the 'double binds in significant dyads or triads' within the existing (i.e. family) network. According to those who participated in the first six sessions, the 26-year-old 'schizophrenic' daughter changed for the better in a number of ways: she would talk more in front of people, she was encouraged to and succeeded in going out of the family home to a job, she enjoyed more being with people and discovered that she had many friends. Whether therapy sessions should incorporate others in this way is debatable, but until tested and evaluated need not be dismissed. The emphasis on 'doing something' rather than just on 'talking about' social isolation and withdrawal (or, for some, entrapment) may also be important and worth more deliberate consideration. A particularly positive aspect of this approach may lie in the more positive expectations and understanding of the network towards the disabled individual: a truly supportive community.

   Others have also discussed therapy beyond the dyad or family (Pattison *et al.*, 1975; Pattison, 1977; Rook, 1984; Heller, 1990). Pattison *et al.* (1975) argued that most American families were based on an extended psychosocial kinship system and that the separate nuclear family was something of a rarity. They argued that family therapy should extend beyond the nuclear family because the extended psychosocial kinship system was a normal source of help and support to families facing stress and challenge. Pattison (1977) has also provided a more elaborated formulation of social-system therapy taking into account the structure of the psychosocial kinship system, with different kinds of intervention depending on the level or type of the system at which intervention seemed to be needed. The aim of any therapy was to 'achieve communication and congruence of goals among all the people with whom the patient may have contact'. Thus the patient would be better able to utilise the resources available in the system. More recently, Halevy-Martini and colleagues (1984) have emphasised that an important final stage in network therapy is the shifting of the locus of control from the therapeutic team to the network itself.

Recently two North American programmes that were designed to enhance the social networks of patients with severe mental illness, including in particular schizophrenia, have been described in detail (Thornicroft *et al.*, this volume; Wasylenki *et al.*, 1992). Both include useful comments on the problems that can arise in clinical practice. A guide to the application of network techniques for use by British social workers has recently been produced by Seed (1990).

Specific psychosocial interventions in institutional or office settings

Recently Bond and colleagues (1991) have reminded us of a cultural divide between traditional therapies, which are based in office or institutional settings, and the more radical redeployments into the world outside, exemplified by *Assertive Community Treatment*. Much of what follows can be traced to the more widely understood institutional tradition, but is of great relevance to our topic, nevertheless.

Group psychotherapy

Group psychotherapy (Yalom, 1975) represents a bridge between personal and environmental approaches that is intriguing but, from the process point of view, difficult to evaluate. Closed groups, in which interaction outside therapy sessions is strongly disapproved of, belong more to the category of individual rather than environmental interventions, and yet are partly based on the premise that insight and learning come best through an open sharing with others and the support, understanding and listening that they provide in the group setting. On the other hand, in open groups, such as those described in Chapter 9 of this volume by Dalgard and colleagues and, more particularly, support groups for cancer patients (Spiegel *et al.*, 1981, 1989), there is little or no reason to discourage the development of social relationships that may have begun within the group, provided confidentiality is respected and individuals are protected from exploitation.

Support for supporters?

The needs of natural supporters (usually female members of the patient's family) are often neglected and ought properly to be provided for also (Fadden *et al.*, 1987; MacCarthy, 1988; MacCarthy *et al.*, 1989*a*). Often the unmet needs of relatives are material – for example for welfare assistance, for respite care (a break from a chronically ill or dependent patient) or for information and advice. However, contact with staff and emotional burden are also important targets of assistance (MacCarthy, 1988; MacCarthy *et al.*, 1989*b*). Many of the methods to be used have already been mentioned, including individual and group work. However, advice, education about the illness and practical assistance with material and welfare problems may also greatly relieve burden on a supporter and thus indirectly benefit the patient (MacCarthy *et al.*, 1989*b*).

The family work interventions that have been developed for the families of high Expressed Emotion patients with schizophrenia incorporate a number of these methods and have been shown to be of consistent benefit to the patients of these families in clinical trials (Kuipers & Bebbington, 1988; Kuipers, this volume). A recent review of facilitated relatives' groups can be strongly recommended (Kuipers & Westall, 1993). Details of the beneficial effects on relatives and patients have been reported (MacCarthy *et al.*, 1989*b*). The beneficial effects of supporting the supporters are discussed in relation to an open intervention study evaluating the effects of providing social support to relatives and friends caring for discharged patients with schizophrenia or schizoaffective disorder (Jed, 1989). A number of different forms of support were given to caregivers of the elderly in another study, in which a control group that received no additional support was available for comparison (Montgomery & Borgatta, 1989). Reduction in subjective burden was found in all the intervention groups but not in the control group. Smith & Birchwood (1990) have also described a service model for delivering support to relatives of individuals with schizophrenia.

Family therapy

In family therapy, issues of control and the freedom to engage in age-appropriate social relationships outside the family can also be key matters for discussion and for change within the maturing family. The principles of family therapy, ranging from radical to conservative approaches, have been discussed comprehensively by Crowe (1988). The topic of behavioural family therapy and its empirical evaluation has been extensively written about also (Falloon, 1988). One can argue that strategies that reduce levels of dysfunction within a family are likely to change it into being a more supportive environment, and an environment that its more mature members can be free to move in and out of in order to fulfil their external needs for support and personal development; unfortunately, recent attempts to search the published literature have failed to uncover any examples of empirical evidence from intervention studies focusing on this potentially important aspect of social support to a key individual. Similar arguments can be stated in relation to *sexual therapy* (Crowe, 1988), a much neglected topic in the field of social support research. It has been pointed out that *sexually abused* women expend considerable effort to prevent angering their spouses and that such effort often compromises potentially supportive relationships with other network members (Coyne & Downey, 1991).

Family work

Before mentioning the family work approach, it should be emphasised that family work interventions do often occur in the home and not in the professional's base or office. Elsewhere in this volume there is a discussion by Kuipers of this form of assessment and intervention. Specific indications for using this programme, which includes both educational components and meetings with the family, are included in the contribution to this volume by Kuipers, and need not be reiterated here.

Marital therapy

Most studies on social support focus particularly closely on sexual or marital relationships (Brown *et al.*, 1986), although some emphasise the wider range of family social relationships also. In *marital psychotherapy* a range of interpretive and prescriptive methods have been described and evaluated (Crowe, 1976; Hahlweg *et al.*, 1984; O'Leary & Smith, 1991). Marital therapy has recently been shown to be an effective treatment for depression in couples with marital discord where the wife is diagnosed as suffering from major depression (O'Leary & Beach, 1990). In a comparison with cognitive therapy there was significantly greater marital satisfaction following therapy and at a 1 year follow-up; symptomatic improvement was good under both conditions and did not significantly favour either treatment. An interesting, although anecdotal observation has been made by Follette & Jacobson (1988) in a discussion of behavioural marital therapy. They have observed many marriages between dominant husbands and powerless, oppressed wives, in relationships with a very low rate of reinforcement: 'Rather than emphasising social skills deficits or other defects in the depressed women, we are moving toward a model that increasingly emphasises the aversive family and social environmental context in which depression often occurs'.

Personal interventions: the individual psychotherapeutic approach

The potential importance to our topic of psychotherapeutic approaches, that is interventions directed at the patient rather than at supporters, has been discussed above and by Parry (this volume). Here, we expand on the nature of the processes involved, which can be of several kinds. A *cognitive* psychotherapeutic approach may be designed to alter key social cognitions, such as dysfunctional attitudes and beliefs about the value of close personal relationships with others. (Parry, this volume). A *social skills* training package (Corrigan *et al.*, 1991), or a *problem-solving* training package (Catalan *et al.*, 1991), may be designed to overcome skills deficits that may be restricting a patient from developing or making effective use of more supportive relationships. *Interpersonal* psychotherapy, by providing the patient with a social relationship that is safe to learn within, may also lead to enhanced skills in obtaining additional sources of support from others. These three kinds of strategies have also been discussed in relation to helping the lonely and socially isolated (Rook, 1984). Detailed treatment manuals are now available that describe a number of these treatment modalities.

For example, Interpersonal Psychotherapy of Depression (IPT: Klerman *et al.*, 1984) was developed by workers who had previously found that exit life events were associated with an increased risk of depression. IPT is conducted in a one-to-one, psychotherapeutic setting, with timetabled sessions, in which exploratory and interpretive rather than prescriptive (as in cognitive and behavioural therapies) techniques are employed. Thus it is closely based on traditional psychotherapy, which emphasises the importance of the client–therapist relationship, or *transference*. The initial assessment focuses on frequency and quality of *social interaction*, personal expectations of key *social relationships*, areas of *dissatisfaction*, and finally on what the patient wants from each social relationship. Many of these variables are covered in standard social network inventories also (Brugha *et al.*, 1987). Grief and *loss*, *disputes*, changes in roles, and deficits such as *loneliness* are also examined. Arguably, therefore, the subject matter of IPT is of particular relevance to this volume.

Formal training for IPT (Klerman *et al.*, 1984) has been available only in North America, and it would seem that the delayed publication of the treatment manual may have contributed to the regrettable and otherwise inexplicable lack of training in IPT treatment in Europe, However, training, a treatment manual and evidence for efficacy do exist for a form of exploratory psychotherapy that has close parallels to IPT, and which has been developed in Great Britain (Shapiro & Firth, 1987).

IPT has been evaluated in a series of clinical treatment and maintenance trials for depression. In many of these it has been shown to produce significant clinical improvement in depression (Gelder, 1990). The use of interpretive rather than prescriptive techniques in IPT has not in itself been systematically evaluated. The IPT process has been shown to overlap very little with *cognitive* psychotherapeutic methods (Elkin *et al.*, 1989); nevertheless there do not appear to be significant differences in their relative effects on outcome (Beckham, 1990). In a recent report on the efficacy of IPT as a maintenance treatment for recurrent depression, the *process* of therapy was studied also through ratings of audiotaped sessions with the guidance of a Therapy Rating Scale, which rated, for example, the therapist's exploration of the patient's social network with respect to a particular problem experienced by the patient (such as depression) (Frank, 1991). The study showed that when the patient and therapist were successful in maintaining a high level of interpersonal focus, monthly maintenance sessions of IPT (Frank, 1991) had substantial prophylactic benefit. Further work, which includes data on social support, is anticipated.

The content of Cognitive Behavioural Psychotherapy (CBT) for depression (Beck *et al.*, 1979) does focus frequently on cognitions about the self, in relation to other key persons; a number of examples can be found in Parry (this volume). Classic examples of such social faulty cognitions are rating oneself as less able than others in the absence of confirmatory evidence and, for example, thinking that 'they wouldn't be interested in me or they wouldn't like me anyway'. We cannot say to what extent the inclusion in cognitive therapy of efforts to alter such faulty 'social cognitions' contributes to its effectiveness in the treatment of depression, although there are good theoretical grounds for supposing that distortions of social cognitions, *per se*, are a key factor in maintaining some states of depression (see a more complete discussion of cognitive social processes and their importance to the topic of support by Brewin, this volume).

In an open, process study of 17 depressed and anxious patients undergoing CBT, that was designed to disaggregate the interpersonal and technical effects of cognitive therapy (countering negative cognitions), Persons & Burns (1985) found that both changes in automatic thoughts and in the patient's relationship with the therapist made significant contributions to mood changes. More recently Burns & Nolen-Hoeksema (1992) found that therapeutic empathy had a moderate-to-large causal effect on recovery from depression in a group of 185 patients treated with CBT. Patients of therapists who were the warmest and most empathic improved significantly more than the patients of therapists with the lowest empathy ratings, when controlling for initial depression severity, homework compliance, and other factors. Other

310   T. S. BRUGHA

psychotherapy treatment manuals also reveal a considerable emphasis
on interpersonal issues in the therapeutic process, as in the previously
mentioned interpretive psychotherapy evaluated by Shapiro & Firth
(1987).

An influential exposition of the possible use of CBT in addressing
problems in social support has been provided by Parry (1988), now
further developed by Parry in this volume. In addition to identifying and
challenging cognitions that may lead to support from others being
devalued, unused or abused, this form of cognitive therapy focuses
specifically on teaching clients new skills in eliciting and making use of
support from others.

Social skills and problem solving training

The use of social skills training and assertiveness skills training would
appear to be an important area for evaluation, as social skills are often
deficient during, for example, an episode of depression (Zeiss &
Lewinsohn, 1988). However, Zeiss & Lewinsohn found that observed
deficits in social skills returned to normal after recovery. Furthermore,
attempting to improve these skills during an episode did not achieve any
outcome-specific effect on depression (Zeiss et al., 1979). No example of a
study evaluating the effects on social support and the outcome of
psychiatric disorder of training in assertion skills could be located at the
time of writing. However, as pointed out in the first chapter of this
volume, the relationship between social support and assertiveness is
complex and it may be premature to attempt to specify a mode of
intervention at this stage. A recent meta-analysis of studies of the
effectiveness of social skills training failed to support the hypothesis that
this treatment significantly reduces later psychiatric symptom levels
(Corrigan, 1991).

Problem solving training by psychiatrists has been shown to be more
effective than routine care by a general practitioner in patients with
recent onset emotional disorder judged to have a poor prognosis
(Catalan et al., 1991). No studies on problem solving training for
psychiatric disorders have provided data on possible effects on social
support.

Formal evaluation: the challenges

Designing experimental interventions based on social support theory and epidemiological findings

The relative rarity of formal, experimental research, based explicitly on
the social support model, which could be 'theory driven' or empirically

derived from the findings of epidemiological studies, may make what is being set out here appear somewhat tentative and even controversial in nature. The somewhat unpredictable nature of attempts to help people by enhancing or in some way modifying their support systems must be acknowledged. As already pointed out, two formal trials have been conducted by psychiatric research groups (Parker & Barnett, 1987; Dalgard *et al.*, 1986 and Benum *et al.*, 1987), both discussed further in this volume by Barnett & Parker and Dalgard *et al.* A limited number of small laboratory experimental studies have also shown that support can be manipulated with a positive effect on psychological performance (Sarason & Sarason, 1986) and on affect (Bowers & Geston, 1986; Lakey & Heller, 1988) in non-psychiatric, normal and high-risk group subjects. To these can be added several more recent Randomised Controlled Trials (RCTs) in the community, conducted by community psychologists, that were referred to earlier and in the first chapter of this volume. These are revisited in the final section of this chapter in a discussion of techniques that may be effective in support interventions.

Methodological challenges

There are two methodological difficulties. First, outside of the strict and atypical confines of RCTs, one cannot be certain of the underlying reason for clinical improvement, for example in episodic psychiatric disorders. Second, even within experimental studies there remains uncertainty about *specific* treatment effects over and above 'placebo' effects, as discussed above. It is particularly important to be open to questioning what one is achieving and of course to support fully any formal attempts to evaluate more rigorously the efficacy as well as the specific nature of such interventions.

Thus, although a number of process studies, just mentioned, suggest that interpersonal aspects may be significantly related to beneficial effects in individual psychotherapy, more specific experimental verification is needed. Unfortunately this has, so far, appeared to be a technically difficult task; studies designed to disaggregate the specific therapeutic ingredients of psychotherapy have not been as fruitful as one would have hoped. For example, the multicentre major depression treatment trial reported by Elkin *et al.* (1989) contained, in addition to IPT, CBT and imipramine (antidepressive drug) treatments, a fourth treatment termed 'routine support', which consisted of regular, non-specific, supportive contacts with a psychiatrist. All four treatment groups showed substantial reductions in depressive symptoms, although the support group benefited slightly less than the others (particularly in more severe cases). The study was not designed to evaluate support, but in general does show that the more technically demanding psychotherapies of IPT and CBT do not result in *substantially* better outcomes. Thus a highly *specific* 'aetiologically focused' social intervention has yet to emerge for such disorders.

In the final section of this chapter, an intervention model will be outlined that aims to encapsulate the lessons that have been learnt to date and which might be of benefit to clinical practice with patients suffering from psychiatric disorders and to the management and evaluation of services. Throughout, at appropriate points, comments will be made that may also have relevance to the design of formal evaluative studies.

Clinical practice and intervention

General principles

Very few writers have attempted to discuss how support interventions might evolve in practice. Vaux (1988) has emphasised the importance of two principles in particular – persuasion and the use of tactics – in order to achieve real change.

Before considering the important issues of goal setting, assessment and treatment planning, some general principles need to be discussed. Clinical and psychosocial assessment and intervention can and should be conducted together in an *integrated* way. The recommendation that psychological and physical treatments should often be provided at the same time in relation to Family Work (Kuipers *et al.*, 1992) and IPT (Klerman *et al.*, 1984) is worth supporting as a general principle also. Apart from ameliorating symptoms and behaviours that may be socially isolating, medication may even have positive and direct social benefits as, for example, in the suggestion that antidepressives may improve assertiveness (Schubert, 1989).

Within clinical psychiatry, knowledge of the biological, developmental and psychosocial basis of *psychopathological* disorders makes it easier for us to adapt the style of social assessment to individuals who, for any of these underlying reasons, may respond in apparently counterproductive ways to enquiries about their social support systems. For example, symptoms such as pathological guilt, subjective retardation, irritability, simple ideas of self-reference and magical thinking, may significantly affect the quality and quantity of social interaction between a patient and his or her social network, as well as significantly distorting the record of these events that the patient can provide. Equally, this principle may also extend to other members of the network who are distressed or have problems in psychological functioning. Although such clinical problems may distort the quality of information obtainable concerning a patient's support system, this in no way reduces the importance of pursuing such information with care and attempting to act on it in a positive way.

A second important principle that must be considered is the extent to which a patient's *vulnerability to stress* or the nature of his or her psychopathology may *contraindicate* any significant attempts to increase social stimulation (with its inevitable demands) from others. Some examples of this might include patients suffering from acute exacerbations of symptoms with a persecutory content, or those with fundamental social handicaps that greatly limit their capacity to interact with others, as for example occurs in cases of Asperger syndrome (or schizoid personality disorder) (Wing, 1981).

A third important principle is that, wherever possible, use be made of RCT proven methods first, in which manuals and training are available, followed by other well-described methods that have been studied independently and reliably in relation to *process* and outcome. To the best knowledge of the present author, only one manual has been designed explicitly to cover a 'social support' intervention (Spiegel *et al.*, 1989): the supportive group work with women with advanced breast carcinoma, discussed above. Three interesting components are worth noting: participants are encouraged to meet outside the group and support one another; the group meetings offer a unique opportunity for women with a problem in common to share their experiences and feelings with others who clearly know what it feels like to be in this situation; the therapists also offer a separate support group for the nearest relatives. The principles underlying a generic self-help group for women in a deprived housing scheme are described by Dalgard *et al.* (this volume).

Apart from the work of Spiegel and colleagues in Stanford, no one has 'manualised' a so-called social support intervention. One cannot offer to do so here. However, a tentative basis for possible progress in that direction can be gleaned also from this and from other contributions, particularly in the final part of this volume (Kuipers, this volume; Parry, this volume). An attempt to produce a single unimodal manual based on the 'social support' model may be both naive and the wrong strategy at this stage. If the social support literature is pointing to a variety of interventions not covered by existing 'manualised' treatments, then perhaps interested workers should begin developing 'theory driven' and 'empirically driven' interventions, possibly for specific target populations.

Some empirical examples might usefully be touched on here. Given what appear to be the different support needs of men and women, young and old, ill and recovered (or at-risk but not yet ill), and given that individuals may not know what they need or may not be able to get permission/flexibility within their existing relationships to fulfil these needs, there might be a case for a 'manualised' intervention that assesses the needs of an individual at a particular point in time. Such a mode of intervention could then assist that person to meet those needs through a

314   T. S. BRUGHA

process that could include also direct involvement with other network members. For example, Coyne (1988) discusses ways of covertly helping individuals who appear to be trapped in a damaging relationship to find their needs elsewhere because they are unable to find them in the marriage. Thus, the housewife whose husband or children or parents cannot meet her support needs (Veiel, this volume) could be helped to obtain positive support through a peer group network (Dalgard *et al.*, this volume). Similarly, a man who is, or perceives himself to be, 'tied down' when he returns home (or feels that he cannot go out again in the evening because of his partner's apparent resentment) might need help to negotiate with his partner ways of getting out to mix more with his peers or 'buddies', by giving something else back to his family in return (equity), by giving more attention to their needs. Single or separated men (Brugha *et al.*, 1990) could be helped to achieve stable partnerships by means of a cognitive social intervention with the aim of helping them to contribute more equitably to such a relationship, as well as to appraise more realistically what can be expected of a partner. For both, the apparently contradictory values of home life and the peer group outside may also need addressing.

It follows, therefore – and this is a fourth principle – that one should be able to make it possible for the client/patient (and indeed the service provider) to *exercise choice* over the intervention methods available: this should range from personal or individual approaches to environmental manipulations that, by implication, involve relevant others in the social network, such as the spouse or partner. For example, this author would argue that an exclusive focus on the psychological functioning of the patient implies that it is his or her sole responsibility to correct deficits in social relationships, even when any harm or deficiencies that they produce is verbally acknowledged by the therapist. Community interventions should not be ruled out when adverse social circumstances are clearly having a deleterious effect on the health of others, for example in a community that is being harassed racially. The topic of patient choice will also be taken up later again in relation to the implementation of clinical interventions.

Also following from the preceding discussion about choice in achieving potentially effective interventions, a fifth point should be made concerning the underlying principles of intervention. It can be argued that one of the problems with the interpretation of existing RCT data, particularly in relation to the very important, large, multicentre psychotherapy trials, is that a single treatment modality is given to all available patients fulfilling a particular set of clinical criteria, such as Major Depression or Schizophrenia, without regard to particular exacerbating or pathoplastic factors in each individual case. The purpose of such studies is to test *efficacy*. In clinical practice it is perfectly reasonable, and indeed desirable, to *tailor the intervention* to the particular case (and to some extent psychotherapy treatment manuals lay down *a priori* rules for doing this, within the treatment setting). For a more complete discussion that also emphasises the topic of client choice, see Brewin & Bradley (1989).

The social support intervention literature raises similar difficulties. For example, in the study quoted in the first chapter of this volume, which failed to show a significant treatment interaction in elderly women randomised to receive peer support by telephone (Heller *et al.*, 1991), the authors concluded, using their own observational data from this population, that they may have used the wrong intervention. Apparently the most important social support deficit in these women's lives was inadequacy of contact with close family members, typically their own daughters. According to Wills (1991), commenting on the same study, the peer group support offered had been devised on the basis of research on the buffering effects of social support against adversity in adults – of far less relevance to an elderly population, for whom such coping advice would be less important. Thus, in the absence of clearer data on effective interventions, it is the practice of the present author to try to identify the most salient interpersonal difficulties and deficits that face patients and to use whatever psychological and social strategies appear best suited to reducing these: hence the considerable importance of assessment that covers clinical, psychological (individual) and social (environmental) aspects. The resulting intervention process can sometimes be slow and prolonged. Clearly this must be perceived by the patient or client as both *rewarding*, and *relevant* to their perceived problems.

A final important principle is that the *location* at which care is provided should also be determined, where practicable, by the ability and capacity for independence of the patient. In essence, help should only be brought *to* patients who for good reason are unable to make their own way to a service at which it could be provided at less cost and more efficiently. Thus the provision of day and outreach services should be based on the promotion and maintenance of *independence* (and the discouragement of *dependence*) in service users, with the additional advantage that attendance at the service can bring the user into contact with a wider range of potential companionship and mutual support. According to Holloway (in Wainwright *et al.*, 1988) users of day care services mentioned social contact as the most important and valued aspect of such services for them. However, access to services should also be flexible and from a client's point of view enabling and empowering, particularly in relation to unexpected crises and initial contacts.

The aim of social support intervention

A set of aims both for the patient's social functioning and for those in the wider social network should be recorded. Common to all such plans is the

316 T. S. BRUGHA

Table 14.1. *The assessment of the possible causes of current deficits in social support*

1. Severe depressive, anxiety or psychotic symptoms
2. Faulty, untested social attributions (cognitions)
3. Interpersonal behavioural response styles
4. Social skills deficits/problem solving skills deficits
5. Dysfunctional dyadic interactions
6. Damage/neglect by others (i.e. childhood, adolescence, contemporaneous)
7. Deficits or problems, if any, in relationship resources
8. Social isolation (not due to self/skills deficits)
9. Poverty/racism/homelessness/imprisonment/unemployment/isolated parent
10. Review and consider other causes: family, peers, employment, etc.
11. Summarise what appear at present to be the significant contributory factors

aim of bringing about an improvement in the patient's own perception of the quality and rewarding nature of transactions with others (i.e. perceived support), particularly with those with whom it is appropriate to share information about feelings, worries and hopes. In addition, not only does the quality of confiding social relationships appear to matter, but a carefully judged extension of the range of different kinds of social relationships and their functions (sometimes referred to as multiplex relationships) should be aimed for, as these also appear to be indicative of a better level of functioning. Thus aims can be both individual and environmental. Aims should be realistic, and thus the time that it may take to achieve them should be carefully considered. In the case of more severe or long-term disorders it may be better at first to discuss limited, short-term aims only. They should be recorded and the patient or client should retain a record. Recording of aims also allows them to be monitored reliably.

Once it is clear what one wants to achieve in principle, it is easier to decide what information is required in the individual clinical case, before deciding on the precise goals and objectives of intervention and on how to achieve them *in practice*.

Assessment

As was discussed in earlier chapters, there are potentially many causes for deficits in social support. They range from those in the individual, perhaps due to faulty or distorted cognitions or causal attributions, or deficits in social problem solving skills, to those in the environment, such as an overbearing, abusive or neglectful spouse (see Table 14.1). Wills (1991) has also argued for taking account of individual factors, such as locus of control, together with environmental aspects of support provision in community-based support interventions. Whilst it is probably true that there are many perfectly healthy members of the general population who suffer from deficits in levels of social support, it is very unusual to fail to find significant deficits of this kind amongst psychiatric patients seeking treatment. Particularly important, however, are those who have proven unresponsive to treatment. A social perspective may be a particularly powerful route to unlocking 'treatment resistance': thus Hobfoll & Jackson (1991) discuss the central importance of *self-empowerment*, arguing that people are already sophisticated copers and tend to resist intervention. Intervention success will depend on a combination of the .extent of internal resources (from the patient or client) and external resources in the form of that intervention and its intensity. Goal and objective setting will need to take such a formulation into account, as will the choice of treatment strategy.

Table 14.1 sets out some of the points that should be considered in an extensive assessment of social and psychological aspects of a particular case. Clinical and diagnostic and individual issues will be discussed first, followed by the more environmental aspects, with particular emphasis on the systematic assessment of the social support system. Individual aspects are taken first because patients consulting services with conspicuous and acknowledged problems will often expect this.

In view of the key role of carers, it is worth considering suggesting on a routine basis that an appropriate relative, partner or peer group member is invited to attend also during an initial assessment, wherever that may occur. The client's consent should be obtained for this.

The importance of clinical symptoms and a summary clinical diagnosis has already been mentioned, as these may have come to have a direct influence on social functioning. A striking example, already noted earlier, will be that of a developmental impairment that is temporally stable in its effects. Sometimes confused clinically and diagnostically with schizophrenia are the rarer *neurodevelopmental* disorders of social development, probably a form of autism, which have come to be known by the term *Asperger syndrome* (Frith, 1991) after the Austrian paediatric physician, Hans Asperger. Apart from the importance of their correct recognition to appropriate treatment, these individuals are of particular interest because of the fundamental social impairments that they share with each other: abnormalities of reciprocal social interaction and non-verbal communication. Not surprisingly, because of these life-long impairments (which tend to become more conspicuous from early adolescence onwards, as social pressures and demands increase), affected individuals have hardly any close peer relationships. Relationships with the family often break down in early adult life and this may result in a fruitless referral to psychiatric services, where staff are often not trained or equipped to recognise and respond appropriately. Some patients have a peculiar fascination with social relationships but somehow lack a meaningful comprehension of their nature. These difficulties would have to be taken into account by any investigator interested in studying the social networks of such adults.

To the points made earlier about symptoms, could be added that amongst the episodic, functional psychiatric disorders, one should consider the consequences of a phobic, avoidant, anxiety state and particularly social phobia; the anergia, social withdrawal and irritability of depression; and the inappropriate and sometimes socially embarrassing behaviour shown by patients in the acute phase of a psychotic episode, whether affective, delusional or hallucinatory. The course of these symptoms and syndromes should also be taken into consideration, with regard to their onset, recovery (relapse prevention), specific precipitating factors and causes.

When interviewing the client or patient, links between symptoms, memories, events (including *stressful life events*), thoughts and experiences should be explored so that symptoms are viewed not just as signs or labels for a disorder – although this is not to dismiss their value for that purpose. The topic of *adjustment reaction* (or stress or situational reaction) should be considered at this point by enquiring, in relation to each key symptom or behavioural observation, the extent to which it can be judged to be 'out of keeping with circumstances'. As other writers have suggested, one can also use the interview to reframe a client's statements according to a particular model that is used in treatment; one can then monitor the client's reaction to help assess likely response to such interventions when active treatment is initiated. For example, Follette & Jacobson (1988) have described how they make use of 10 minute video recordings of couples talking about their day and solving a problem, which show examples of power and *dominance behaviours* (ignoring and not allowing interruption) and their ability to make use of conflict resolution skills.

Description of the social support network

Outlined here is a procedure for eliciting the psychosocial variables that indicate lack of social support during the clinical assessment of each patient. Similar suggestions, emphasising a number of important psychological principles also, are found in the chapter by Parry (this volume).

Description of the social support system can begin by adding to information already gathered about the family – focusing on the location of members, their frequency of contact, and the kinds of transactions that occur, and then moving on to a consideration of the strength of social relationships in terms of 'felt attachment', the ability and tendency to *confide*, and the degree to which these qualities appear to be *reciprocated*. Where the patient is married or has a close sexual relationship, particular attention is given to the social relationship with this partner under these headings. (It may also be worthwhile interviewing such a confidant and establishing whether the illness has had a negative impact on their own sources of support.)

The enquiry then moves out towards the wider social network of close friends, neighbours and work associates (particularly if they are also regarded as 'friends', 'acquaintances', 'mates', etc). Again, it seems useful to enquire about recent social interaction, its nature and context, and in particular whether there have been planned social events involving these others which are not a necessary part of work, or routine events in the community (e.g. club and church attendance). Where, as is often the case, a major significant life event has occurred recently, the transmission of information between other members of the network concerning such events can also be enquired about, in order to map the structural properties of the network.

There are two elements to the enquiry about social support: the first concerns itself with action taken by the patient (help- and support-eliciting, where this seems to be appropriate) and the second concerns the behaviour and action of others. With reference to material aid (*tangible support*), it can be particularly revealing to enquire about the degree to which transactions of this kind have actually occurred in both directions (termed 'equity' in a dyadic social relationship). In trying to achieve a judgement about the quality of *emotional support*, it is important to ask questions that reveal something of the capacity of those involved to identify sources of distress, to tolerate unpleasant news and the feelings that go with it, and to empathise with the person who is distressed. A variety of both open and closed questions should be employed, the latter being used to focus, on the one hand, on how easy or difficult it is for the patient to listen to someone else who has something distressing to discuss, and on the other hand on whether the patient felt that the other person was really listening and was interested in something important that he or she wished to discuss.

Examples of interaction should always be asked for. When the questions focus on what actually happened during a recent crisis, they may reveal a great deal about other potentially important elements such as coping style, self-esteem and the degree to which elements of an individual's psychopathology directly impinge on social interaction. The belief that one is not being listened to or that one's ideas and feelings are not being acknowledged may also be associated with conflict. It may be easier to identify *negative interaction* by approaching it with questions about the 'listening qualities' of others, in addition to questions about the extent to which others try to exert social control over the individual. Not surprisingly, low self-esteem, conflict and a tendency for competitiveness may go hand in hand. Efforts by the patient to appraise and tackle such problems should be recorded.

Recognising the social dimension from the point of view of individual service users is important but difficult. Preliminary data (unpublished) gathered by the present author and colleagues, in order to test the validity of a social network inventory in such a setting, revealed some interesting difficulties. As part of the Camberwell High Contact Survey (Brugha *et al.*, 1988, 1993), staff were asked to identify important social relationships between a named patient and other patients or staff. Patients were also routinely asked such questions about themselves, by means of questions derived from the Interview Measure of Social Relationships (IMSR: Brugha *et al.*, 1987). It became quite apparent that staff were frequently identifying social relationships that did not exist (in the view of the patient). Leff and his colleagues (1990) have reported similar findings. The principal lesson to be derived at present is that the patient's own perceptions and views should be sought. This is a particularly important but often overlooked issue where the transfer of one or a group of patients to a different service facility is being decided upon. Taking account of patients' views is a topic discussed further below in relation to patient choice, engagement and compliance.

Intervention planning and evaluation

In Table 14.2 a structure or model is outlined to help an exploration of the relationship between *aims* and *interventions* in each individual case. The development of a successful, realistic, treatment strategy may be fostered by the flexible use of this model, which can be regularly reviewed with the passage of time. Intervention can be intended and thus under the control of the professional: but *unintended interventions* or influences that can not be controlled must also be noted and taken into account.

Agreeing goals with patients and clarifying targets of intervention

On the basis of the general principles laid down earlier and with specific information about the patient's own current social network and supports, current clinical condition and other relevant influences on support suggested in Table 14.1, it should be possible to produce a 'social formulation' that summarises the patient's difficulties and possible routes for action. A clearly listed set of manageable objectives with a realistic time frame in which to review their outcome should be recorded at this stage, making use of Table 14.2 in the planning process. The implementation of such a planned intervention is discussed in the next section.

Choosing strategies and implementing a plan of intervention

Having decided on aims, completed an assessment and then identified specific treatment objectives, specific methods should be chosen that are designed to try to achieve these objectives (bearing in mind the need to

Table 14.2. *A model for the relationship between goals and 'intervention'*

Goals	Interventions
Enhanced social support	
Perceived social support	Matching client and case worker, therapist or carer in relation to: ethnicity, social class/social rank, gender, educational level, common life experiences (e.g. migration, unemployment, disease)
Network size	
Family/kith	Expressed emotion/conflict reduction; realistically dealing with problems with power, subservience, dependency and trust; getting out more
Other/kin	Buddies, play and recreation; work, neighbours, church, etc.
Support functions	
Specific aid	Care or case management: money, shelter, medicine, training
Guidance	Cognitive Behavioural Treatment: causal inferences, self-esteem, a good network
Listening, empathy, confiding	Choice of partner; choice of therapist/counsellor/priest/shaman

Table 14.3. *Specific strategies to be used in implementing supportive interventions*

1. Managing medication flexibily (consider patient choice and knowledge)
2. Who else (with consent) to see (for intervention and ongoing assessment)
3. Alliance formation and not blaming or colluding
4. Who sees them (together or separately?)
5. Education about the disorder and its prognosis
6. Learning to see problems more clearly
7. Communication: improved listening
8. Conflict resolution and problem solving activities
9. Tolerating pain/stress management
10. Techniques from individual (cognitive and interpersonal), couple and family work
11. Helping supporters (acknowledging their burdens)
12. Maintaining therapist/counsellors within their separate professional roles

consider both the short-term and long-term effects on the course of the psychiatric disturbance). Strategies to be considered are listed in Table 14.3. The IPT manual (Klerman *et al.*, 1984), the Family Work manual (Kuipers *et al.*, 1992) and Gilbert's views on the social outcomes of power and belonging (1992) have been particularly influential in the clinical work of this author.

The methods used will be familiar also to those working in the fields of *Psychiatric Rehabilitation, Assertive Community Treatment* and *Community Psychiatry*: training and skill enhancement, monitoring of goals and making use of feedback from others. For those more severely impaired who do not or can not respond to these learning strategies, sheltered social amenities and the use of visual and verbal reminders and cues by staff or relatives should be provided, possibly on a long-term basis (Brewin *et al.*, 1987).

Examples of the kind of action to be taken can range from a relatively brief set of guidelines to the patient on how to make better use of potential social resources in their existing network, to a more detailed series of counselling sessions incorporating both insight building and specific directions on social behaviour and social interaction with others. Readers should note, however, Brewin's comment (this volume) that urging closer contact with others may also have deleterious effects. Such a series of counselling sessions will also importantly provide both the opportunity for monitoring the results of directive advice and the possibility of modifying it, in order to increase the patient's effectiveness in transactions with others. There may, of course, be some parallels between this approach and that of social skills and problem-solving training. The important distinction between them lies in the way the approach is tailored specifically to the particular social relationships that the patient is developing with others in their network. Techniques based on cognitive therapy are covered by Parry (this volume).

On the basis of the research evidence cited earlier, it will sometimes be more beneficial (with the patient's consent) to intervene directly through others by working with a couple or a family. Involving key members of a community, or others at the place of work, could also be considered. An example of the latter is the way in which social isolation due to the stigma of being labelled a psychiatric patient can be overcome by making direct links with employers, key figures in personnel departments, or employee organisations. Where these strategies are effective, they may lead others in the social network to change their ideas (or perhaps more specifically their own expectations) about the patient's personality. The adoption of a more realistic and also a less negative set of attitudes may well be highly therapeutic, as in the experimentally verified Family Work of Leff and his colleagues (1982) on high *Expressed Emotion* (discussed by Kuipers, this volume). Working with the patient in a problem solving framework may also help to anticipate and reduce interpersonal conflict (Falloon & Fadden, 1993).

Patient choice over treatment

In some areas, and particularly in relation to the treatment of depression, there may be several different treatments of established effectiveness available. Service resources available locally may be a limiting factor, however. For example, some patients with clinically significant, or major, depression may choose not to take antidepressive medication or, rarely nowadays, may have medical contraindications to such treatment. Psychosocial interventions can be considered as a first-choice treatment in such cases (the alternative so often being that if the patient's views are not taken into account they may continue to struggle alone and ineffectively with their difficulties).

The value of medication should not be dismissed too easily, however. Patients sometimes have incorrect ideas about which treatments work, how they work, or indeed about whether formal treatment is appropriate (and sometimes they are right about this!) Engaging the patient or client successfully, if a treatment plan is worth pursuing, does demand particular attention, but is more likely to occur when his or her preferences are *listed* to and are not devalued.

Engagement and compliance

For the less compliant or more socially disabled client/patient a more effective starting point may be to ask what their goal in life is and then consider the steps needed to achieve it. To the patient who is reluctant to see their mood symptoms as out of keeping with circumstances, the following questioning strategy may be of assistance: 'Do you sometimes notice moods that go up and down? Do you always know exactly why they go up and down? Can you always predict when some event will make them go up and down?' Then, if applicable, 'Does it surprise you then that your mood problem may be partly physical and partly due to the circumstances of your life? Surely treatment should be on both lines, reflecting both kinds of reasons?' In much the same way, there can be patients, perhaps, who through being treated previously on strictly somatic and physical lines, do not appear aware of possible connections between problems, or losses, in their lives and their symptoms, particularly when somatic symptoms predominate. Standard inventories of stressful experiences and social support deficits, systematically used, may uncover these. Subsequent dialogue between the clinician and patient will be necessary to make such connections more immediate and accessible to relevant interventions.

Successfully engaging the patient or client in this way at an early stage seems to be an important factor in determining outcome and deserves more time and effort than might otherwise appear necessary.

Process monitoring and 'side effects'

Quality assurance and *quality of care* depends very much on close attention being given to the quality of assessment and treatment processes (Brugha & Lindsay, 1995). Things can go wrong, not just in

relation to physical treatments (i.e. drug side effects) but also in relation
to psychological and social interventions. The management of more
severe disorders, inevitably involving more than one member of a team of
staff, raises the spectre of institutionalised harmful effects. As will be
mentioned at the end of this chapter, good management of staff will
probably mean that their trust and support towards one another enables
them to be in a better position to be supportive to patients at a time when
the social network may no longer be able to cope. Poorly trained,
overworked and poorly supported staff may also get into difficulties with
clients who are re-enacting remembered interpersonal conflicts that have
occurred in earlier key relationships in their own lives. Inexperienced
staff may not feel able to share these with appropriate colleagues. This
deprofessionalisation of the 'treater–client relationship' may lead to
abuses of trust and harm to the client at a vulnerable time. Very careful
attention should be given to the supervision of trainee and inexperienced
staff, particularly when working with severely disturbed, long-term
patients who themselves may have been the *victims of abuse* by dominant
figures in their own lives (Palmer *et al.*, 1993). A particularly powerful
training and process monitoring medium involves the use of audio-visual
monitoring, which can later be reviewed by supervising staff. Such
records can even be helpful to clients, couples or larger intervention
groups to reinforce, between sessions, what has been learnt. They may
also be made use of in later 'maintenance' sessions, during subsequent
contacts with treatment staff.

Evaluating and maintaining intervention effectiveness

Information acquired initially about the social support system should be
rechecked regularly, possibly as often as each meeting with the therapist
(Parry, this volume). This provides important information about
achieving targets and also serves to remind the patient what they need to
be concentrating their own efforts on. Progress achieved will also be a
source of encouragement to the patient, although as was already pointed
out here and in the first chapter of this volume, change in the social
network may be a very slow process.

Obviously *clinical status* must also be assessed. Strictly speaking, the
term 'outcome' should only be used when there is empirical evidence of a
treatment effect (Brugha & Lindsay, 1995). It may be that any benefits
of support enhancement are long-term, and for this and other reasons it is
important to establish some system, perhaps through collaboration with
a primary health care practitioner, for monitoring long-term clinical
status, or outcome, over the subsequent months and years after treatment
has ended.

Outcome indicators in clinical practice have yet to be systematically
developed and evaluated but their use is bound to increase with the

growing emphasis in health care systems on the need for evidence of effectiveness and 'value for money' (Jenkins, 1990). It is very important to *follow up* clients, even those who drop out of treatment, if at all possible. Patients with psychiatric disorder should clearly understand that relapses are not uncommon and that they need to 'take care of themselves'. This does not imply failure. If a recurrence of symptoms or related problems occurs and does not clear up using what has been learnt previously, the client should be encouraged to return for further assessment and possibly further intervention. Good treatment records, including videotapes, may be very helpful here. The primary health physician and members of the family should also be aware of the value of further intervention on the same lines, as they would also be in relation to the benefits of further indicated medication if symptoms have recurred.

Developing, evaluating and managing services

Given the slow growth of research evidence, already discussed in this and earlier chapters, concerning the possible effectiveness of support enhancement on clinical course and outcome, those providing any service that aims to carry out such work must give serious attention to the evaluation of that service. Standardised measures of both symptoms and other aspects of psychopathology will need to be used in conjunction with social support inventories of known psychometric properties (Brugha, 1989). Ideally, the data gathered should be aggregated and analysed statistically. A great deal can also be learnt from a detailed longitudinal case study analysis of individual patients, not omitting those many patients who drop out of treatment at an early stage (Brugha *et al.*, 1992).

Experimental evaluations

Clinical trials must also be carried out, as there can be no substitute for what is learnt from Randomised Controlled Trials experiments (RCTs). This area is ripe for such work; there are no major ethical dilemmas, as the interventions involved are unlikely to be significantly harmful and it is genuinely not known what, if any, positive benefits the outcome of further trials will reveal. The design problems have already been discussed, focusing particularly on the difficulties involved in disaggregating evidence of specific treatment efficacy from general effects. Readers should also refer to the first chapter (Brugha, this volume).

Quality assurance and audit

Even when the scientific basis for the *efficacy* of an intervention has been established in a randomised study, evidence for *effectiveness* in routine practice must be (but rarely is) obtained (Brugha & Lindsay, 1995). The *processes* involved in intervention must be closely monitored in order to ensure that practice conforms to good models of care, through institutionally based criterion audit programmes. At an individual level, both patients and therapists can be asked to complete questionnaires and forms that provide accounts of the content of sessions and of what appear to be the effects of the intervention at the end of each session. Therapists working with this model should also discuss their work and share these data regularly. Audiotape or audio-visual recordings of sessions may also be a very helpful addition to the audit process. However, one should be careful to avoid becoming overwhelmed by the wealth of data collected in this way. Practitioners and staff should also devote regular time to keeping 'up to date' (Sackett *et al.*, 1992). Both the medical and the psychological literature should be regularly scanned. General guidance on how to keep up to date efficiently has been provided by Sackett and colleagues (1992) in a recent update of their primer on *Clinical Epidemiology*.

Systematic need assessment and service planning

In order that *Community Mental Health Services* or systems function effectively the specific medical, psychological, social and welfare (material) needs of patients and their carers in the community must be assessed in a coordinated way. *Systematic Needs Assessment* (Brewin *et al.*, 1987) fits into the traditional framework of clinical medicine, also used by paramedical professionals, including social workers, psychologists, occupational therapists and community-based nurses. The term 'care planning' is being used increasingly. In the presence of clinically significant mental illness that is interfering with the individual's capacity to function independently, problems in psychological and social functioning that could contribute to social isolation, such as an inability to initiate, form and maintain social interaction, lack of use of public and recreational amenities, and observed slowness and underactivity can be reliably identified (Brewin *et al.*, 1987, 1988; Brugha *et al.*, 1988; MacCarthy *et al.*, 1989*a*). The appropriateness of care and evidence for its effectiveness should be judged using later assessments of health status (i.e. outcome). Any needs that have been identified can then be taken into account in the planning and management of the service. Professionals who are responsible for monitoring the *public health*, in defined geographic areas, can also make use of aggregated data on needs assessment and care planning, from such services, in order to achieve a more rational distribution of funds and related resources through planning and the negotiation and drafting of purchaser/payer contracts or service agreements.

Staff support and managing the service

Services also need to be managed, and in the view of this author, good management begins at team level. Bad team functioning means wasted resources, deteriorating staff morale and inevitably deficiencies in outcomes and care processes. In a well-managed service staff and teams regularly and openly examine the way they work together. They also consider how they relate to the larger organisation and service, the implications of what they do for the resources available, including, obviously, financial considerations. But perhaps the last thing that should be said is that staff who do not work together with trust and respect for each other's efforts and skills can not be said to support one another. They are likely to have far more difficulty in being supportive to and in teaching support skills to their patients and their families and their social networks. The potential value of these principles in *Quality Assurance* is discussed elsewhere (Brugha & Lindsay, 1995). Smith & Birchwood (1990) have described a relatives' support service for individuals with schizophrenia which incorporates integration with other agencies, training and supervision of 'front-line' professionals and a quality assurance programme.

Conclusions and future prospects

The nature of support and the factors that appear to influence its development over the life course make up a complex system that involves environmental as well as personal components. A distinction has been made between the value of emotional support provided particularly by close personal social relationships and the practical and profession-provided support that long-term and socially disadvantaged psychiatric patients need from formal 'social support systems' that are nowadays typically community based but provided by experienced, responsible, professional staff.

The main aim of this final chapter was to discuss clinical and psychosocial management, a much neglected topic from the research point of view, although one that is implicit in the work and functioning of many clinical and social agencies of human care. It has provided some background to the work of such services. A series of principles and guidelines that emphasise a self-questioning and self-critical approach were set out. The need for evaluation of support-enhancing interventions has been emphasised throughout; some of the principles and difficulties involved in such work have also been considered. Perhaps, and rather controversially, it has been argued that the absence of evidence for *specific* effects in the evaluation of psychosocial interventions points both to the value of a larger theory of social influence, which is embodied in the topic of social support as well as acknowledging the difficult task of evaluating its particular effects.

The future use and development of the concept of social support will

328   T. S. BRUGHA

depend on a more equitable balance between observational studies and experimental research. Both types of research have their advantages as well as their limitations. But without a new effort devoted to the experimental evaluation of the social support hypothesis, the future development of this promising subject must be awaited in an atmosphere of uncertainty that will be slow to dispel.

References

American Journal of Community Psychology (1991). Support interventions (whole issue). *American Journal of Community Psychology*, **19**, 1–167.

Beck, A. T., Rush, A. J., Shaw, B. F. & Emery, G. (1979). *Cognitive Therapy of Depression*. Chichester: Wiley.

Beckham, E. D. (1990). Psychotherapy of depression research at a crossroads: directions for the 1990s. *Clinical Psychology Review*, **10**, 207–28.

Bennett, D. & Morris, I. (1983). Support and rehabilitation. In *Theory and Practice of Psychiatric Rehabilitation*, ed. F. N. Watts & D. Bennett, pp. 189–211. Chichester: Wiley.

Benum, K., Anstrop, T., Dalgard, O. S. & Sørensen, T. (1987). Social network stimulation: health promotion in a high risk group of middle-aged women. *Acta Psychiatrica Scandinavica, Supplement 337*, **76**, 33–41.

Bond, G. R., Witheridge, T. F., Dincin, J. & Wasmer, D. (1991). Assertive community treatment: correcting some misconceptions. *American Journal of Community Psychology*, **19**, 41–52.

Bowers, C. A. & Geston, E. L. (1986). Social support as a buffer of anxiety: an experimental analogue. *American Journal of Community Psychology*, **14**, 447–51.

Brewin, C. R. & Bradley, C. (1989). Patient preferences and randomised clinical trials. *British Medical Journal*, **229**, 313.

Brewin, C. R., Wing, J. K., Mangen, S. P., Brugha, T. S. & MacCarthy, B. (1987). Principles and practice of measuring needs in the long-term mentally ill: the MRC Needs for Care Assessment. *Psychological Medicine*, **17**, 971–81.

Brewin, C., Wing, J., Mangen, S., Brugha, T. S., MacCarthy, B. & Lesage, A. (1988). Needs for care among the long-term mentally ill: a report from the Camberwell High Contact Survey. *Psychological Medicine*, **18**, 457–68.

Brown, G. W., Andrews, B., Harris, T., Adler, Z. & Bridge, L. (1986). Social support, self-esteem and depression. *Psychological Medicine*, **16**, 813–31.

Brugha, T. (1988). Social support. *Current Opinion in Psychiatry*, **1**, 206–11.

Brugha, T. (1991a). Support and personal relationships. In *Community Psychiatry: The Principles*, eds. D. Bennett & H. Freeman, pp. 115–61. London: Churchill-Livingstone.

Brugha, T. S. (1991). Human ethology. *Current Opinion in Psychiatry*, **4**, 313–19.

Brugha, T. S. (1993). Social support networks. In *Principles of Social Psychiatry*, ed. J. P. Leff & D. Bhugra, pp. 502–16. London: Blackwell.

Brugha, T. S. & Britto, D. J. (1992). Social support, environment and conditional associations. *Current Opinion in Psychiatry*, **5**, 305–8.

Brugha, T. S. & Lindsay, F. (1995). Quality of psychiatric care (invited review). *Social Psychiatry and Psychiatric Epidemiology*, in press.

Brugha, T. S., Sturt, E., MacCarthy, B., Potter, J., Wykes, T. & Bebbington, P. E. (1987). The Interview Measure of Social Relationships: the description and evaluation of a survey instrument for assessing personal social resources. *Social Psychiatry*, **22**, 123–8.

Brugha, T. S., Wing, J. K., Brewin, C. R., MacCarthy, B., Mangen, S., LeSage, A. & Mumford, J. (1988). The problems of people in long-term psychiatric care: an introduction to the Camberwell High Contact Survey. *Psychological Medicine*, **18**, 443–56.

Brugha, T. S., Bebbington, P. E., MacCarthy, B., Sturt, E., Wykes, T. & Potter, J. (1990). Gender, social support and recovery from depressive disorders: a prospective clinical study. *Psychological Medicine*, **20**, 147–50.

Brugha, T. S., Bebbington, P. E., MacCarthy, B., Sturt, E. & Wykes, T. (1992). Antidepressants may not assist recovery in practice: a naturalistic prospective survey. *Acta Psychiatrica Scandinavica*, **86**, 5–11.

Brugha, T. S., Wing, J. K., Brewin, C. R., MacCarthy, B. & Lesage, A. (1993). The relationship of social network deficits with deficits in social functioning in long-term psychiatric disorders. *Social Psychiatry and Psychiatric Epidemiology*, **28**, 218–24.

Burns, D. & Nolen-Hoeksema, S. (1992). Therapeutic empathy and recovery from depression in cognitive behavioral therapy: a structural equation model. *Journal of Consulting and Clinical Psychology*, **60**, 441–9.

Catalan, J., Gath, D. H. & Anastasiades, P. (1991). Evaluation of brief psychological treatment for emotional disorders in primary health care. *Psychological Medicine*, **21**, 1013–18.

Clarkin, J. F., Haas, G. L. & Glick, I. D. (1988). Assessment of affective disorders and their interpersonal contexts. In *Affective Disorders and the Family: Assessment and Treatment 8*, ed. J. F. Clarkin, G. L. Haas & I. D. Glick, pp. 29–50. New York: Guilford Press.

Corrigan, P. W. (1991). Social skills training in adult psychiatric populations: a meta-analysis. *Journal of Behaviour Therapy and Experimental Psychiatry*, **22**, 203–10.

Cox, A. D., Pound, A., Mills, M., Puchering, C. & Owen, A. L. (1991). Evaluation of a home visiting and befriending scheme for young mothers: Newpin. *Journal of the Royal Society of Medicine*, **84**, 217–20.

Coyne, J. C. (1988). Strategic therapy. In *Affective Disorders and the Family: Assessment and Treatment*, ed. J. F. Clarkin, G. L. Haas & I. D. Glick, pp. 89–114. New York: Guilford Press.

Coyne, J. C. & Downey, G. (1991). Social factors and psychopathology: stress, social support, and coping processes. *Annual Review of Psychology*, **42**, 401–25.

Cross, D. G., Sheehan, P. W. & Khan, J. A. (1982). Short- and long-term follow-up of clients receiving insight-oriented therapy and behaviour therapy. *Journal of Consulting and Clinical Psychology*, **50**, 103–12.

Crowe, M. (1976). Behavioural treatments in psychiatry. In *Recent Advances in Clinical Psychiatry*, ed. K. Granville Grossman, pp. 169–99. London: Churchill-Livingstone.

Crowe, M. (1988). Indications for family, marital and psychosexual therapy. In *Handbook of Behavioural Family Therapy*, ed. I. R. H. Falloon, pp. 51–77. New York: Guilford Press.

330 T. S. BRUGHA

Cutler, D. I. & Beigel, A. (1978). A church based program of community activities for chronic patients. *Hospital and Community Psychiatry*, **29**, 497–501.

Dalgard, O. S., Anstoup, T., Benum, K., Sørensen, T. & Moum, T. (1986). Social psychiatric field studies in Oslo: some preliminary results. Paper read at Second International Kurt Lewin Conference, Philadelphia.

Elkin, I., Shea, T., Watkins, J. T., Imber, S. D., Sotsky, S. M., Collins, J. F., Glass, D. R., Pilkonis, P. A., Leber, W. R., Docherty, J. P., Fiester, J. S. & Parloff, M. B. (1989). National Institute of Mental Health Treatment of Depression Collaborative Research Program: general effectiveness of treatments. *Archives of General Psychiatry*, **46**, 971–82.

Erickson, G. (1984). A framework and themes for social network intervention. *Family Process*, **23**, 187–98.

Fadden, G., Bebbington, P. & Kuipers, L. (1987). Caring and its burdens: a study of the spouses of depressed patients. *British Journal of Psychiatry*, **151**, 660–7.

Falloon, I. R. H. (1988). Recent advances in therapy and prevention. In *Handbook of Behavioural Family Therapy*, ed. I. R. H. Falloon. New York: Guilford Press.

Falloon, I. R. H. & Fadden, G. (1993). *Integrated Mental Health Care*. Cambridge: Cambridge University Press.

Falloon, I. R. H., Hole, V., Mulroy, L., *et al.* (1988). Behavioural family therapy. In *Affective Disorders and the Family: Assessment and Treatment*, Ed. J. F. Clarkin, G. L. Haas & I. D. Glick, pp. 117–33. New York: Guilford Press.

Follette, W. C. & Jacobson, N. S. (1988). Behavioural marital therapy in the treatment of depressive disorders. In *Handbook of Behavioural Family Therapy*, ed. I. R. H. Falloon, pp. 257–84. New York: Guilford Press.

Frank, E. (1991). Interpersonal psychotherapy as a maintenance treatment for patients with recurrent depression. *Psychotherapy*, **28**, 259–66.

Frank, E., Kupfer, D. J., Perel, J. M., *et al.* (1990). Three year outcome for maintenance therapies in recurrent depression. *Archives of General Psychiatry*, **47**, 1093–9.

Frank, J. D. & Frank, J. B. (1991). *Persuasion and Healing: A Comparative Study of Psychotherapy*. Baltimore: Johns Hopkins University Press.

Freeman, H. L. (1985). *Mental Health and the Environment*. London: Churchill-Livingstone.

Frith, U. (1991). *Autism and Asperger Syndrome*. Cambridge: Cambridge University Press.

Galanter, M. (1988). Zealous self-help groups as adjuncts to psychiatric treatment: a study of recovery. *American Journal of Psychiatry*, **145**, 1248–53.

Gelder, M. (1990). Psychological treatment for depressive disorder. *British Medical Journal*, **300**, 1087–8.

Gilbert, P. (1992). *Depression: The Evolution of Powerlessness*, pp. 459–82. Hove: Lawrence Erlbaum.

Goldberg, E. M. (1987). The effectiveness of social care: a selective exploration. *British Journal of Social Work*, **17**, 595–614.

Gotlib, I. H. & Hammen, C. L. (eds.) (1992). *Psychological Aspects of Depression: Toward a Cognitive-Interpersonal Integration*. Chichester: Wiley.

Hahlweg, K., Revenstorf, D. & Schindler, L. (1984). The effects of behavioural marital therapy on couples' communication and problem solving skills. *Journal of Consulting and Clinical Psychology*, **52**, 553–66.

Hahlweg, K., Baucom, D. H. & Markman, H. (1988). Recent advances in therapy and prevention. In *Handbook of Behavioural Family Therapy*, ed. I. R. H. Falloon, pp. 413–48. New York: Guilford Press.

Halevy-Martini, J., Hemley-Van-Der-Velden, E. M., Ruhf, L. & Schoenfeld, P. (1984). Process and strategy in network therapy. *Family Process*, **23**, 521–33.

Hawton, K., Salkovskis, P. M., Kirk, J. & Clark, D. M. (1990). *Cognitive Behaviour Therapy for Psychiatric Problems; A Practical Guide.* Oxford: Oxford University Press.

Heller, K. (1990). Social and community intervention. *Annual Review of Psychology*, **41**, 141–68.

Heller, K., Thompson, M. G., Vlachosweber, I., Steffen, A. M. & Trueba, P. E. (1991). Support interventions for older adults: confidante relationships, perceived family support and meaningful role activity. *American Journal of Community Psychology*, **19**, 139–46.

Henderson, S. (1977). The social network, support and neurosis. *British Journal of Psychiatry*, **131**, 185–91.

Henderson, S., Byrne, D. G. & Duncan-Jones, P. (1981). *Neurosis and the Social Environment.* Sydney: Academic Press.

Hobfoll, S. E. & Jackson, A. P. (1991). Conservation of resources in community intervention. *American Journal of Community Psychology*, **19**, 123–32.

Hogg, J. R. & Heller, K. (1990). A measure of relational competence for community-dwelling elderly. *Psychology and Ageing*, **5**, 580–8.

Holmes, J. (1993). Attachment theory: a biological basis for psychotherapy? *British Journal of Psychiatry*, **163**, 430–8.

ason, L. A. (1991). Participating in social change: a fundamental value of our discipline. *American Journal of Community Psychology*, **19**, 1–16.

Jed, J. (1989). Social support for caretakers and psychiatric rehospitalization. *Hospital and Community Psychiatry*, **40**, 1297–9.

Jenkins, R. (1990). Towards a system of outcome indicators for mental health care. *British Journal of Psychiatry*, **157**, 500–14.

Klerman, G. L., Weissman, M. M., Rounsaville, B. J. & Chevron, E. S. (eds.) (1984). *Interpersonal Psychotherapy of Depression.* New York: Basic Books.

Kuipers, L. & Bebbington, P. (1988). Expressed emotion research in schizophrenia: theoretical and clinical implications. *Psychological Medicine*, **18**, 93–109.

Kuipers, L. & Westall, J. (1993). The role of facilitated relatives' groups and voluntary self-help groups. In *Principles of Social Psychiatry*, ed. D. Bhugra & J. Leff, pp. 562–71. Oxford: Blackwell Scientific.

Kuipers, L., Leff, J. & Lam, D. (1992). *Family Work for Schizophrenia. A Practical Guide.* London: Gaskell.

Lakey, B. & Heller, K. (1988). Social support from a friend, perceived support, and social problem solving. *American Journal of Community Psychology*, **16**, 811–24.

Lavender, A. & Holloway, F. (1988). *Community Care in Practice. Services for the Continuing Care Client.* Chichester: Wiley.

Leff, J., Kuipers, L., Berkowitz, R., Eberlein-Fries, R. & Sturgeon, D. (1982).

A controlled trial of social intervention in the families of schizophrenic patients. *British Journal of Psychiatry*, **141**, 121–34.

Leff, J., O'Driscoll, C. & Dayson, D. (1990). The TAPS project 5: the structure of social-network data obtained from long-stay patients. *Psychiatry*, **157**, 848–52.

Levin, S. & Brekke, J. S. (1993). Factors related to integrating persons with chronic mental illness into a peer social milieu. *Community Mental Health Journal*, **29**, 25–34.

Lichenstein, E., Nettekoven, L. & Ockene, J. K. (1991). Community intervention trial for smoking cessation (COMMIT): opportunities for community psychologists in chronic disease prevention. *American Journal of Community Psychology*, **19**, 17–40.

MacCarthy, B. (1988). The role of relatives. In *Community Care in Practice*, ed. A. Lavender & F. Holloway, pp. 207–30. Chichester: Wiley.

MacCarthy, B., Brewin, C. R., Lesage, A., Brugha, T. S., Mangen, S. & Wing, J. K. (1989*a*). Needs for care among the relatives of long-term users of day care: a report from the Camberwell High Contact Survey. *Psychological Medicine*, **19**, 725–36.

MacCarthy, B., Kuipers, L., Murry, J., Harper, R. & Lesage, A. (1989*b*). Counselling the relatives of the long-term adult mentally ill. *British Journal of Psychiatry*, **154**, 768–75.

Marmar, C. R., Horowitz, M. J., Weiss, D. S., Wilner, N. R. & Kaltreider, N. B. (1988). A controlled trial of brief psychotherapy and mutual-help group treatment of conjugal bereavement. *American Journal of Psychiatry*, **145**, 203–9.

Marziali, E. A. (1987). People in your life: development of a social support measure for predicting psychotherapy outcome. *Journal of Nervous and Mental Disease*, **175**, 327–38.

Milne, D. & Mullin, M. (1987). Is a problem shared a problem shaved? An evaluation of hairdressers and social support. *British Journal of Clinical Psychology*, **26**, 69–70.

Mitchell, J. F. & Birley, J. C. T. (1983). The use of ward support by psychiatric patients in the community. *British Journal of Psychiatry*, **142**, 9–15.

Montgomery, R. J. V. & Borgatta, E. F. (1989). The effects of alternative support strategies on family caregiving. *Gerontologist*, **29**, 457–64.

Newton, J. & Craig, T. K. J. (1991). Prevention. In *Community Psychiatry*, ed. D. H. Bennett & H. L. Freeman, pp. 488–516. Edinburgh: Churchill-Livingstone.

O'Leary, K. D. & Beach, S. R. H. (1990). Marital therapy: a viable treatment for depression and marital discord. *American Journal of Psychiatry*, **147**, 183–6.

O'Leary, K. D. & Smith, D. A. (1991). Marital interactions. *Annual Review of Psychology*, **42**, 191–212.

Palmer, R. L., Coleman, L., Chaloner, D., Oppenheimer, R. & Smith, J. (1993). Childhood sexual experiences with adults: a comparison of reports by women psychiatric patients and general practice attenders. *British Journal of Psychiatry*, **163**, 499–504.

Parker, G. & Barnett, B. (1987). A test of the social support hypothesis. *British Journal of Psychiatry*, **150**, 72–7.

Parry, G. (1988). Mobilizing social support networks. In *New Developments in Clinical Psychology*, vol. 2, (ed.) Fraser N. Watts, pp. 83–104. New York: Wiley.

Pattison, E. M. (1977). A theoretical-empirical base for social system therapy. In *Current Perspectives in Cultural Psychiatry*, ed. E. F. Feulks, R. M. Wintrob, J. Westenmayer & A. R. Favazza, pp. 217–53. New York: Spectrum.

Pattison, E. M., De Francisco, D., Wood, P., Frazer, H. & Crowden, J. (1975). A psychosocial kinship model for family therapy. *American Journal of Psychiatry*, **132**, 1246–51.

Persons, J. B. & Burns, D. D. (1985). Mechanisms of action of cognitive therapy: the relative contributions of technical and interpersonal interventions. *Cognitive Therapy and Research*, **9**, 539–51.

President's Commission on Mental Health (1978). Report of the Task Panel on Community Support Systems. In *Task Panel Reports*, submitted to the President's Commission on Mental Health. Washington, D.C.: US Government Printing Office.

Price, R. H., Vanryn, M. & Vinokur, A. D. (1992). Impact of a preventive job search intervention on the likelihood of depression among the unemployed. *Journal of Health and Social Behaviour*, **33**, 158–67.

Rakos, R. F. (1991). *Assertive Behaviour: Theory, Research and Training*. London: Routledge.

Rook, K. (1984). Promoting social bonding: strategies for helping the lonely and socially isolated. *American Psychologist*, **39**, 1389–407.

Rueveni, U. (1979), *Networking Families in Crisis*, New York: Human Sciences Press.

Sackett, D. L., Haynes, R. B., Guyatt, G. H. & Tugwell, P. (1992). *Clinical Epidemiology: A Basic Science for Clinical Medicine*, 2nd ed. Boston: Little, Brown.

Sarason, I. G. & Sarason, B. R. (1986). Experimentally provided social support. *Journal of Personal and Social Psychology*, **50**, 1222–5.

Schubert, D. S. P. (1989). Increase assertiveness by medication. *Integrative Psychiatry*, **6**, 223–8.

Seed, P. (1990). *Introducing Network Analysis in Social Work*. London: Jessica Kingsley.

Shapiro, D. A. & Firth, J. (1987). Prescriptive v. exploratory psychotherapy: outcomes of the Sheffield psychotherapy project. *British Journal of Psychiatry*, **151**, 790–9.

Shepherd, M. (1993). The placebo: from specificity to the non-specific and back. *Psychological Medicine*, **23**, 569–78.

Smith, J. & Birchwood, M. (1990). Relatives and patients as partners in the management of schizophrenia: the development of a service model. *British Journal of Psychiatry*, **156**, 654–60.

Speck, R. V. & Rueveni, U. (1969). Network therapy: a developing concept. *Family Process*, **8**, 182–91.

Spiegel, D., Bloom, J. R. & Yalom, I. (1981). Group support for patients with metastatic cancer. *Archives of General Psychiatry*, **38**, 527–33.

Spiegel, D., Bloom, J. R., Kraemer, H. & Gottheil, E. (1989). Effect of psychosocial treatment on survival of patients with metastatic breast cancer. *Lancet*, **II**, 889–91.

Stiles, W. B., Shapiro, D. A. & Elliott, R. (1986). Are all psychotherapies equivalent? *American Psychologist*, **41**, 165–80.

Sullivan, C. M., Tan, C., Basra, J., Rumptz, M. & Davidson, W. S. II
(1992). An advocacy intervention programme for women with abusive
partners: initial evaluation. *American Journal of Community Psychology*, **20**,
309–32.

Vaux, A. (1988). *Social Support: Theory, Research and Interventions*. New York:
Praeger.

Wainwright, T., Holloway, F. & Brugha, T. (1988). Day care in an inner
city. In *Community Care in Practice*, ed. A. Lavender & A. Holloway.
Chichester: Wiley.

Wasylenki, D., James, S., Clark, C., Lewis, J., Goering, P. & Gillies, L.
(1992). Clinical care update: clinical issues in social network therapy for
clients with schizophrenia. *Community Mental Health Journal*, **28**, 427–40.

Wills, T. A. (1991). Comments on Heller, Thompson, Trueba, Hogg and
Vlachos-Weber, 'Peer support telephone dyads for elderly women'. *American
Journal of Community Psychology*, **19**, 75–84.

Winefield, H. R. (1987). Psychotherapy and social support: parallels and
differences in the helping process. *Clinical Psychology Review*, **7**, 1631–44.

Wing, L. (1981). Asperger's syndrome: a clinical account. *Psychological
Medicine*, **11**, 115–29.

Yalom, I. D. (1975). *The Theory and Practice of Group Psychotherapy*. New York:
Basic Books.

Zeiss, A. M. & Lewinsohn, P. M. (1988). Enduring deficits after remission of
depression: a test of the scar hypothesis. *Behaviour Research and Therapy*, **26**,
151–8.

Zeiss, A. M., Lewinsohn, P. M. & Munez, R. F. (1979). Non-specific
improvement effects in depression using interpersonal skills training,
pleasant activities schedules, or cognitive training. *Journal of Consulting and
Clinical Psychology*, **47**, 427–39.

Index

Attachment (*cont.*)
  as biosocial goal, 121
  in childhood
    early: implications for later life,
      66; importance, 64–65
    effect of separation, 71
    five to ten year period, 65–66
    and later social functioning,
      64–72
    patterns affecting later social
      support networks, 66–69;
      effect of stress, 66–67
    peer group factors, 65
    peer relationships, 71–72; *see also*
      Peer relationships
    and poor marital quality, 71
    preschool period, 65
    and quality of social support in
      adult life, 70–72
    security of attachment, 64–66;
      classification, 65
    socialisation, 67
    socioeconomically disadvantaged
      and stable families,
      differences, 66–67
    temperament, 67
  early infancy, 97–98
    and later personality
      development, 97
    and later social cognition, 97–98
  impact of historical events, 82
  infant–mother, 221, 223–224
  intergenerational continuities,
    69–70
  parent–child, 215–217
  theory, intervention study, 215
Attribution therapy, 110
Automatic thoughts, 290
Autonomy, 50

Beck Depression Inventory, 220
Befriending psychiatric patients, 131
Behavioural genetics, 13
Behavioural theories, 8
Belonging, basis and attachment,
    affiliation and cooperation,

131–135
Beneficial effects of social support,
    156–157
Berkeley Guidance Study, 71
Biological factors and social support
    development, 15
Biosocial goals and strategies, 120,
    121–122
Boosting status, 130
Breast cancer, adjustment processes,
    model, 54–55
Brief Psychiatric Rating Scale, 248

Camberwell Family Interview, 9
Care, see Institutional care
Care/help eliciting and affiliation,
    132
Carers
  of the elderly, need for support, 28
  Expressed Emotion, 260
  involvement, initial assessment, 317
  need for support, 306
  training for direct care staff, 271
  see also Training
Caretakers other than parents, 68
  effect on security of attachment,
    68–69
Caring/giving behaviour and
    affiliation, 131–132
Case management
  case manager, development of
    concept, 241
  core tasks, 242
  COSTAR programme in
    Baltimore, 243–247
  see also COSTAR
  defining, 240
    twelve axes, 242–243
  principles, 240–241
Causal direction and life events,
    45–46
CFI, *see* Camberwell Family
    Interview
Charity work, 131–132
Childhood, 72–77
  effects of poor quality

Diagnostic and Statistical Manual,
    19
'Discreditable' people, 103, 104
Divorce, model applied to situation,
    55–56
Drug abuse and teenager's peer
    network structures, 174–194
    findings, 178–181
    see also Adolescence; Teenagers
DSM-III, *see* Diagnostic and
    Statistical Manual

EE, *see* Expressed Emotion
Effectiveness, intervention, evaluating
    and maintaining, 324–325
Effectiveness of service, 325
Efficacy of service, 325
Efficacy testing of intervention,
    314–315
Ego mechanisms of defence, 51–52
Emotional support
    definition, 42–43, 73
    and interpersonal relationships,
        3–4
    see also Expressed Emotion
Environmental influences, and social
    support determinants, 12,
    13–15
Epidemiological psychiatrists, studies
    by, 26–27
Evaluation of services, 325–327
    experimental, 325
    see also Intervention
Evolution of need for social support,
    117–141
    affiliation, attachment and
        cooperation: the basis of
        belonging, 131–135
    development, 117–118
    perspective, 118–124
        biosocial goals, strategies and
            algorithms, 121–123
        social and cultural
            considerations, 123–124
    rank, 124–131
Exchange theory, and social support,
    8

Experimental studies based on
    randomised designs, overview,
    26–28
Expressed Emotion, 257–276
    by relatives, and quality of
        support, 108–109
    in carers, 260
    family work interventions, 306
    intervention studies, 261–263
        results, 261–262
        successful studies and reduction
            in EE, 262–263
    meaning, 259–260
    measuring, 258–259
    in schizophrenia, 258
        see also Schizophrenia
    in staff, 260–261
    training for direct care staff, 271
Expressive support, definition, 43
Eysenck Personality Inventory, 220

Families and attachment, 66
    differences between disadvantaged
        and stable, 66–67
Family influences on support,
    empirical evidence for, 98–101
Family relationships
    adolescence and depressed mood,
        80
    see also Father; Mother; Parents
Family therapy, evaluation, 306–307
Family work approach, evaluation,
    307
Family work interventions, Expressed
    Emotion, 306
Father
    importance of same-sex
        relationship in adolescence, 82
    role in attachment, 68
Father's support, effect on boys and
    girls, 98–99
Friends in childhood, importance,
    72–73

General Health Questionnaire, 165
Genetic relatedness and care giving,
    133